Angiotensin-Converting Enzyme Inhibitors: Scientific Basis for Clinical Use

Second Edition

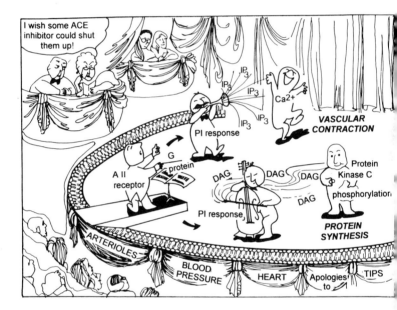

Angiotensin-Converting Enzyme Inhibitors: Scientific Basis for Clinical Use

Second Edition

by
Lionel H. Opie MD, PhD, FRCP
Professor of Medicine
University of Cape Town
Director
Hypertension Clinic
Groote Schuur Hospital;
Cape Town, South Africa;
Visiting Professor (1984–1994)
Stanford University Medical Center
Stanford, California

Introduction by Victor Dzau, MD
Foreword by Alberto Zanchetti, MD

WILEY-LISS

A JOHN WILEY & SONS, INC., PUBLICATION
New York • Chichester • Brisbane • Toronto • Singapore

Authors' Publishing House
New York

DISCLAIMER

Although every effort has been made to ensure that the indications and doses for the various drugs are correct, the ultimate legal responsibility for the correct use of drugs lies with the prescribing physician. Likewise, the institutions with which the author is or has been associated have no direct nor indirect responsibility for the contents of this book nor for the mode in which any drugs in this books are used.

The author's aim has been to achieve a totally unbiased text. Readers are requested to communicate any inadvertent bias directly to the author.

ISBN: 1-881063-004-6 (APH)
       0-471-11195-3 (WILEY-LISS)

Printed in the United States of America

Distributed worldwide by Wiley-Liss

CONTENTS

GENERIC AND TRADE NAMES OF ACE INHIBITORS

Generic name	Trade names
Alacepril	Cetapril
Altiopril	Lowpres
Benazepril	Cibace, Cibacen, Cibacene, Lotensin*
Captopril	Capoten*, Lopril, Lopirin, Captopril
Ceranapril	—
Cilazepril	Inhibace, Inibace, Vascace
Delapril	Adecut
Enalapril	Innovace, Pres, Renitec, Renivace, Vasotec*, Xanef
Fosinopril	Monopril*, Staril
Lisinopril	Longes, Prinivil*, Zestril*
Perindopril	Acertil, Coversum, Coversyl, Prestarium, Prexum, Procaptan
Quinapril	Accupril*, Accuprin, Accupro, Acuitel
Ramipril	Altace*, Delix, Ramace, Triatec, Tritace
Spirapril	Renpress, Sandopril
Trandolapril	Odrik, Gopten
Zofenopril	—

* = in USA

"I hope the author is not tempted to put his pen down because a second edition will soon be required to keep pace with the new developments in this rapidly evolving topic."

Review of the First Edition, British Medical Journal, 1992

"Voici mon secret. Il est tres simple: on ne voit bien qu'avec le coeur. L'essentiel est invisible pour les yeux."

Le petit prince, Antoine de Saint-Exupery

"This is my secret. It is very simple; one only sees clearly through the heart. The essentials are invisible to the eyes."

INTRODUCTION

One of the major discoveries of this century in cardiovascular pharmacology was the isolation of the nonapeptide angiotensin-converting enzyme (ACE) inhibitor from the snake venom of Bothrops jararaca. This discovery translated into the development of synthetic orally active drugs that inhibit the renin-angiotensin system in humans. In the early 1980s, the first ACE inhibitor, captopril, was introduced. This was followed by enalapril, lisinopril, and by now there are more than fifteen ACE inhibitors with different pharmacological properties. This class of drugs has emerged as one of the most important to modern cardiovascular medicine. Its efficacy in the treatment of hypertension, congestive heart failure, ventricular dysfunction, postmyocardial infarct, and diabetic nephropathy has been established. In addition, it has demonstrated potential in the treatment of coronary ischemia, resenosis, atherosclerosis, and cardiac hypertrophy.

Modern biology has revolutionized our understanding of physiology and pathophysiology. The powerful tools of molecular and cell biology applied in concert with traditional physiology and pharmacology have led to new insight into cardiovascular diseases. One important outcome of this research is an improved understanding of the biology and pharmacology of the renin-angiotensin system (Dzau and Pratt, 1991). Molecular and cell biological studies show that angiotensin is not only a contractile agonist but also a growth promoter of heart and blood vessel. Angiotensin-II growth action is mediated by the expression of protooncogenes and autocrine growth factors such as platelet-derived growth factor, basic fibroblast growth factor, and transforming growth factor beta 1. Angiotensin-II also modulates extracellular matrix composition. These trophic effects regulate long-term cardiovascular function and structure and may account for the slow pressor effect of Angiotensin-II. Recent research demonstrates that Angiotensin-II is also produced at local tissue sites. The tissue angiotensin concept has provided new understanding of the renin-angiotensin system and the action of ACE inhibitors. Specifically, it is now appreciated that a major determinant of ACE inhibitor effect is the inhibition of tissue ACE. Accordingly, blockade of local Angiotensin-II production may influence cardiac and vascular function and remodeling. Furthermore, recent data show that tissue ACE inhibition not only suppresses Ang II synthesis but may also activate the bradykinin-nitric oxide system, which can exert additional cardiovascular protection.

Given the rapid development of this area of research and clinical discipline, there is a great need for a comprehensive and up-to-date book that reviews the "scientific basis for clinical use" of ACE inhibitors. Professor Opie has masterfully accomplished this difficult task in the Second Edition of this book. The practical use of ACE inhibitors is discussed in the context of pathophysiology. The contents of this book illustrate the important link between fundamental research and clinical application in this area. The development of ACE inhibitors has indeed revolutionized cardiovascular therapeutics and enhanced fundamental research in cardiovascular pathophysiology. Molecular and cell biology research has identified new and rational targets for ACE inhibition. Pharmacological research of ACE inhibitors has generated new hypotheses in cardiovascular medicine. Indeed, the efficacy of ACE inhibition in the prevention of cardiac failure after myocardial infarction is a powerful illustration of the basic science-clinical medicine synergism. The clinical trials (SAVE, AIRE, ISIS-IV, SOLVD) are the direct result of basic animal studies. The recent observation from SAVE and SOLVD that recurrent myocardial infarction is significantly reduced in patients treated with ACE inhibitors has stimulated additional fundamental molecular and cellular investigations of the role of angiotensin in atherogenesis, coronary ischemia, and vascular complications. This area of research has successfully brought together cardiologists, nephrologists, physiologists, and geneticists.

Experimental and clinical studies have demonstrated the broad involvement of angiotensin in cardiovascular pathophysiology ranging from hypertension to coronary ischemia to congestive heart failure. Previously, Dr. Eugene Bruanwald and I (1991) proposed that organic heart disease is the consequence of a continuous chain of pathiphysiological events that is usally initiated by risk factors leading to atherosclerosis, coronary artery disease, myocardial ischemia, and infarction. The ventricular dysfunction and remodeling that develop as a consequence of myocardial infarction may result in ventricular dilatation and, eventually, symptomatic heart failure. Indeed, angiotensin plays an important role in may of these cardiovascular responses and contributes to the pathophysiology of disease expression and progression. Accordingly, it is logical to expect that inhibitors of the renin-angiotensin system may interrupt this chain of pathophysiological events and prevent the progression to significant ischemic heart disease, congestive heart failure, and end-stage cardiac disease. Indeed, the contents of this book address the effects of ACE inhibition on many of these pathophysiological processes.

ACE inhibitors have made an important impact in cardiovascular medicine. Its clinical use has reduced morbidity and mortality and improved the quality of life of patients with cardiovascular disorders. In my opinion, this class of drugs has earned the labeling of "cardioprotective drug of the 1990s." With the rapid and impressive progress in this field, as witnessed by the extensive updates between the first two editions of this book, it is certain that we can anticipate the publication of the next edition with excitement and enthusiasm.

1. Dzau VJ, Pratt RE. Renin angiotensin. In: Fozzard HA, Haber E, Jennings RB, Katz AM (eds.), *The Heart and Cardiovascular System*. New York: Raven Press, 1991; 1817-1850.
2. Dzau VJ, Braunwald E. Resolved and unresolved issues in the prevention and treatment of coronary heart disease: a workshop consensus statement. *Am Heart J* 1991; 121:1244-1263.

Victor J. Dzau

"When the gloss is taken away from the advertisements, what is really left?" is the question posed in the Preface to the First Edition. The answer is simple—there is more and more solid evidence for the therapeutic and prophylactic use of ACE inhibitors. The exciting new aspect that has caught the eye of cardiologists is that these agents can actually prevent overt heart failure from developing, and improve postinfarct prognosis, as shown in the SOLVD, SAVE, and AIRE studies. Use in the acute stage of infarction is the subject of the ISIS-IV and GISSI-3 megatrials, reported at the American Heart Associate meeting in November, 1993. And increasingly there is evidence that insulin-requiring diabetes with nephropathy can be protected from ultimate end-points, including death. Probably ACE inhibitors are exerting their protection at least in part by hitherto unexpected mechanisms, possibly at the site of the vascular endothelium or the interaction between the endothelium and platelets. Increasing molecular evidence points to the role of ACE activity in myocardial and vascular growth. This combined basic and clinical progress has led to the need for this Second Edition.

PREFACE TO THE FIRST EDITION

Angiotensin-converting enzyme (ACE) inhibitors are now established therapy in two of the most common cardiologic conditions, namely hypertension and congestive heart failure. In hypertension, these agents are rapidly increasing their share of the market, and in congestive heart failure, they have proven benefits on mortality besides being relatively simple to use. Although they are considerably more expensive than diuretics for hypertension or digoxin for congestive heart failure, they seem to be progressively displacing these less expensive agents. Despite the evident importance of ACE inhibitors, there appears to be no objective and comprehensive guide to their use.

The present book was written with the conviction that clinicians need more objective and detailed information about ACE inhibitors. Physicians are bombarded with apparently conflicting claims, and it is difficult to find data comparing the efficacy of different agents. What clinicians need to know to make rational choices are the simple facts. This book utilizes the style and format already proven successful in *Drugs for the Heart* (W.B. Saunders) now in its Third Edition, and *The Clinical Use of Calcium Channel Antagonists* (Kluwer Academic Publishers), Third Edition now in preparation. The experience in preparing these books has shown that pharmaceutical companies also benefit from objective and comparative evaluation of the data.

Thus, the major aim of this book is to present the clinician with the information needed for the practical use of ACE inhibitors. What do the numerous and sometimes conflicting trials say? When do these agents work best? Which agents are best tested? Which doses should be used? Which modifications are required when dealing with elderly or pediatric patients? How do these potent agents compare with others, such as the calcium antagonists, which are also highly effective in hypertension but contraindicated in congestive heart failure? When can ACE inhibitors beneficially be combined with other antihypertensives? What are the anticipated side-effects? When the gloss is taken away from the advertisements, what is really left?

FOREWORD TO THE FIRST EDITION

The beginning of the era of hypertension research dates back to 1934, to the classic Goldblatt's experiment on the dog made hypertensive by renal artery stenosis. It may seem surprising, therefore, that antihypertensive therapy had so long ignored the possibility of antagonizing the renin-angiotensin system. The fact is that Goldblatt's experiment was correctly interpreted as a model of renovascular hypertension rather than of the most common form of hypertension, essential hypertension. As a consequence, any attempt to interfere pharmacologically with the renin-angiotensin system was considered to be aimed at the limited field of renovascular hypertension. Even in 1976, discussing the first experiences with antagonists and inhibitors of the renin-angiotensin system, an authority like Franz Gross wrote: "Undoubtedly, the antagonists and inhibitors of the renin-angiotensin system are most useful tools, but their application will be limited to the share of the renin-dependent forms of high blood pressure in the total field of hypertension."

The advent of the angiotensin-converting enzyme (ACE) inhibitors has reversed this widespread viewpoint and has initiated an entirely new approach to the treatment of hypertension. Not only have ACE inhibitors been shown to be active outside the limited field of renovascular and renal hypertension, but they are widely recognized among the first choice agents for treatment of hypertension. Nor have these compounds remained restricted to the specific area of hypertension: ACE inhibitors are now successfully used in congestive heart failure and are actively being investigated in cardioprotection after myocardial infarction and in renal protection in diabetic nephropathy and other types of nephropathies.

Complexity of research requires simplicity of presentation, especially when the outcome of research has to be quickly translated into useful therapeutic applications, as was and is still the case with ACE inhibitors. No one could have accomplished the difficult task of clarifying the scientific basis for the practical use of ACE inhibitors better than Lionel Opie, whose gifts as a scientist and a teacher are testified by the success of his two recent volumes, *Drugs for the Heart* and *The Clinical Use of Calcium Channel Antagonists*. I am sure that this new volume, where a large body of data has been screened by the critical judgment of the investigator and the experience of the clinician, will meet the same indisputable success. From these pages, the readers will be able to perceive how the new therapeutic advances initiated by ACE inhibition have promoted a deeper understanding of the pathophysiology of hypertension, heart failure, cardiac remodeling, vascular and renal disease. Such advances in knowledge are, in turn, leading to a broadening of the therapeutic applications of these compounds. This story is a further example of the fascinating interaction betweeen science and clinical practice in medicine.

A. Zanchetti
Professor of Medicine and Director
Institute of Clinical Medicine and
Center of Clinical Physiology and Hypertension
University of Milan
Italy

Angiotensin-Converting Enzyme Inhibitors: Scientific Basis for Clinical Use

Second Edition

The Renin-Angiotensin-Aldosterone System and Other Proposed Sites of Action of Angiotensin-Converting Enzyme Inhibitors

Persistent stimulation of the renin-angiotensin-aldosterone system is likely to promote hypertension because of the strong vasoconstrictive qualities of angiotensin-II and the sodium retention induced by aldosterone. Thus, when angiotensin-converting enzyme (ACE) inhibitors first became available, it was logical to test the antihypertensive effect in patients with high renin states, such as renovascular hypertension, in which arteriolar constriction was playing a prominent role. Not surprisingly, the ACE inhibitors worked very well in these conditions. In addition, we now know that antihypertensive effects are also found when plasma renin is normal, or even sometimes when it is low, suggesting alternate or additional modes of action for these agents.

Recognition of the reactive arteriolar vasoconstriction in states of severe heart failure next led to the successful testing of ACE inhibitors in patients refractory to conventional anti-failure therapy.

The remarkable therapeutic success of ACE inhibitors in hypertension and in heart failure is based on solid scientific evidence for the role of the renin-angiotensin-aldosterone system in these two common cardiological conditions.

THE RENIN-ANGIOTENSIN-ALDOSTERONE SYSTEM

Angiotensin-II, a potent vasoconstrictor, is an octapeptide. It is formed from its precursor, *angiotensin-I*, a decapeptide, by the activity of the *angiotensin-converting enzyme* (ACE). Such ACE activity, although chiefly found in the vascular endothelium of the lungs, also occurs in the endothelium of other vascular beds and in many other tissues including the myocardium and the coronary arteries.

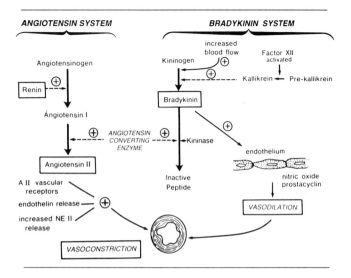

Figure 1–1. ACE inhibitors have dual vasodilatory actions, chiefly on the circulating and tissue renin-angiotensin systems with ancillary effects on the enzymes that inactivate bradykinin. The result of the former action is the inhibition of the vasoconstrictory systems and the result of the latter is the formation of vasodilatory nitric oxide and prostacyclin. AII, angiotensin-II; NE, norepinephrine. Fig. © LH Opie.

Angiotensin-I originates from *angiotensinogen* (Fig. 1–1) under the influence of the enzyme *renin*, a protease. The activity of this enzyme is rate-limiting for the formation of angiotensin-I. This conversion of the angiotensin-I occurs in the liver. Renin in turn is formed in the kidney from the juxtaglomerular cells. Classic stimuli to the release of renin include (1) impaired renal blood flow as in ischemia or hypotension; (2) salt depletion or sodium diuresis; and (3) beta-adrenergic stimulation. When renin formation is enhanced for more than 4 hours, then the rate of synthesis of the precursor, *prorenin*, is also increased in the kidney (Derkx et al., 1983).

The angiotensin-converting enzyme

Also called kininase-II and, technically, EC 3.4.15.1, ACE is a protease with two zinc groups, hence being a metalloprotease. There is, however, only one zinc atom at the high affinity binding site that interacts with angiotensin-II or all the ACE inhibitors (Soubrier et al., 1988). The converting enzyme is nonspecific because it not only converts angiotensin-I to angiotensin-II but inactivates bradykinin, hence the alternate name of *kininase*. The positively charged ions of the zinc atom and of another lower affinity active site interact with terminal negatively charged carboxyl groups of the ACE inhibitor (Ondetti et al., 1977). Inclusion of the -SH group in the structure to replace a -COOH group greatly increases the ACE inhibitory power and thus captopril was born (Ondetti et al., 1977). It is now known, however, that SH groups are not at all essential to achieve ACE inhibition (Fig. 1–2).

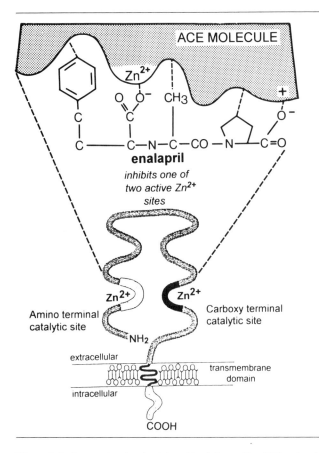

Figure 1–2. Proposed molecular interaction between the ACE molecule and an ACE inhibitor. Note that the zinc-containing inhibitory site lies within the vascular lumen. The structure of the ACE molecule is reproduced by kind permission of Johnston (1994) and the American Heart Association.

Angiotensin-II receptors and intracellular messenger system

Just as there are many intermediate steps between occupation of the beta-adrenoceptor and increased contractile activity of the myocardium, so there are many complex steps between occupation of the angiotensin-II receptor and ultimate mobilization of calcium with a vasoconstrictor effect in vascular smooth muscle. These intervening steps constitute the *signaling system*. There are several interactions between the occupation of the receptor by angiotensin-II and the stimulation of the phosphodiesterase (Fig. 1–3) concerned with the phosphatidylinositol system.

The first component of the phosphatidylinositol system to be discovered was *inositol trisphosphate* (IP_3 or $InsP_3$) formed from the breakdown of inositol phospholipids (Berridge, 1983). The other component formed in this hydrolysis is diacylglycerol, which initiates the activation of a specialized enzyme called protein kinase C that transfers a phosphate group from ATP to a target protein by the pro-

ANGIOTENSIN II: SIGNAL TRANSDUCTION

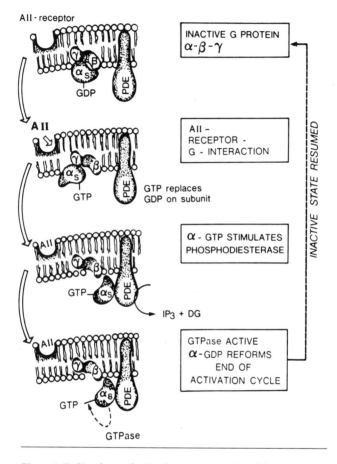

Figure 1–3. Signal transduction between occupation of the angiotensin-II (AII) receptor and stimulation of phosphodiesterase (PDE) also called phospholipase C (PLC). The latter enzyme, when increased in acitvity, leads to activation of the next step in the signaling system, followed by the formation of sequential signals that ultimately lead to vascular contraction (see Fig. 1–4). When angiotensin-II occupies its receptor, then there is an interaction between the receptor and the G-protein in such a way that GTP replaces GDP on the subunit, and the subunit becomes active. The alpha-subunit, thus activated, now stimulates a phosphodiesterase, which leads to formation of inositol trisphosphate (IP_3) and diacylglycerol (DAG) (see Fig. 1–4). Through the activity of GTPase, GTP is broken down to reform GDP, which when it combines with the alpha-subunit of the G-protein inactivates this component of the signaling system. Fig. © LH Opie.

cess of protein phosphorylation (Nishizuka, 1984). Diacylglycerol operates within the plane of the membrane to activate *protein kinase C* without entering the cytosolic space (Berridge and Irvine, 1984). Thus, it is thought that the ultimate messengers of the inositol signaling pathway are, first, IP_3, which liberates calcium from the intracellular sarcoplasmic reticulum by acting on its IP_3 receptor (Berridge, 1993), and, second, protein kinase C, which phosphoryl-

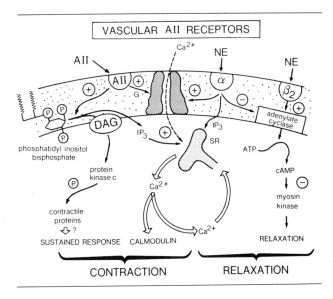

Figure 1–4. Proposed messengers of angiotensin-II receptor stimulation. Activation of this receptor stimulates a phosphodiesterase to split phosphatidylinositol into two messengers: IP_3 (inositol trisphosphate) and DAG (1,2-diacylglycerol). IP_3 promotes the release of calcium from the sarcoplasmic reticulum (SR), and DAG activates protein kinase C, which is thought to act on the contractile apparatus to promote a sustained contractile response. Activity of the angiotensin-II receptor also helps to open the calcium channel through an unknown mechanism possibly involving G-proteins. Fig. © LH Opie.

ates an as-yet-unknown target protein, possibly one of the contractile proteins (Fig. 1–4).

In addition, angiotensin-II enhances the activation of the voltage-dependent calcium channels; that is to say, angiotensin-II makes it easier for the channels to be in the open state in response to a wave of depolarization. This effect of angiotensin-II is probably mediated by a GTP-binding protein. Such channels, whose opening probability is enhanced by G-proteins, are called *G-protein-gated channels* (Brown and Birnbaumer 1988). Alternatively, IP_3 can be changed into the closely related IP_4 (inositol tetraphosphate), which in turn can help open calcium channels (Luckhoff and Clapham, 1992).

When the vascular angiotensin-II receptors are stimulated, it is proposed that two mechanisms lead to an increased release of calcium from the sarcoplasmic reticulum: (1) the formation of IP_3 and (2) the direct G-protein-mediated stimulation of the calcium channel. Such increased release of calcium augments vascular contraction and tone. There is also some evidence for a hypothetical sequence whereby phosphorylation of the contractile proteins by protein kinase C leads to sustained contraction and maintenance of vascular tone (Morgan, 1990).

In the case of the myocardium, there are also angiotensin-II receptors that again, are thought to be coupled to the IP_3 system (Allen et al., 1988). Protein kinase C activation by the nonphysiological experimental agents, the phorbolesters, leads to an increase of myocardial contractile force, supporting the proposal that there is an as-yet-ill-understood phosphorylation of the contractile proteins in response to activation of protein kinase C.

Phosphatidylinositol cycle

There are two limbs to the phosphatidylinositol cycle, the breakdown of phosphatidylinositol to inositol trisphosphate (IP_3) and, thence, to inositol, and the resynthesis of phosphatidylinositol from inositol. Phosphatidylinositol is a compound in which two fatty acid chains, the one predominantly stearic acid and the other predominantly arachidonic acid, are bound by a phosphate group to inositol. Hypothetically, phosphatidylinositol is regarded as the reservoir that supplies the precursor phosphatidylinositol monophosphate to maintain the small intracellular pool of phosphatidylinositol bisphosphate. According to the favored hypothesis (Berridge, 1983), it is the latter substance that responds to occupation of the angiotensin-II receptor by undergoing hydrolysis when an enzyme, a phosphodiesterase, is activated (Fig. 1–5). This enzyme is a phosphodiesterase called *phospholipase C* (Meisenhelder et al., 1989). Just how occupation of the angiotensin-II receptor is coupled to this phosphodiesterase is still not fully understood, but it probably involves a G-protein cycle (Berridge and Irvine, 1984). Once IP_3 has formed, it can in turn undergo hydrolysis via inositol diphosphate and inositol monophosphate to inositol (Fig 1–5). The latter step is inhibited by

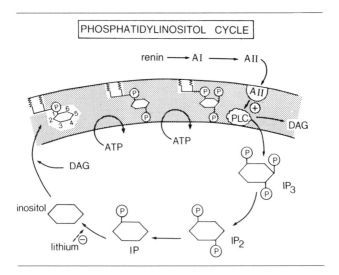

Figure 1–5. *The phosphatidylinositol cycle is shown using the model proposed by Berridge (1983). In vascular tissue, the reservoir compound is phosphatidylinositol, from which phosphatidylinositol bisphosphate is formed, the substrate for the phospholipase C (PLC), which is stimulated in response to occupation of the angiotensin-II receptor. The resulting formation of inositol trisphosphate (IP$_3$), one of the intracellular messengers, precedes the formation of inositol bisphosphate (IP$_2$) and inositol monophosphate (IP). The latter compound is converted to inositol through a reaction inhibited by the antidepressant lithium. Inositol reacts with a derivative of diphosphoglycerol (DAG) to reform phosphatidylinositol (top left). Fig. © LH Opie.*

lithium, which may explain some of the antidepressant effects of that compound on the brain.

The next sequence is the phosphorylation of inositol to phosphatidylinositol phosphate. At this stage inositol interacts with a derivative of diacylglycerol (Berridge, 1983; Nishizuka, 1984). Thereupon follows a further phosphorylation to phosphatidylinositol bisphosphate. Both of these phosphorylations take place under the action of a protein kinase and utilize ATP. Now the phosphatidyl inositol bisphosphate is again ready for hydrolysis in response to angiotensin-II receptor occupation.

This phosphatidylinositol cycle is not confined to vascular tissue, rather it occurs in many different types of cells and has different functions including regulation of cell calcium and secretion (Berridge, 1993). An example of the ubiquitous nature of the system is that platelet-derived growth factor (PDGF) stimulates phospholipase C activity in fibroblasts (Meisenhelder et al, 1989) with mitogenic potential. It is, however, in vascular tissue that the cycling of phosphatidylinositol can clearly be linked to angiotensin-II receptor stimulation and to contraction.

Angiotensin-II receptor subtypes

There is a family of angiotensin-II receptor subtypes, including the AT_1 and AT_2 receptors. For practical purposes, it is the AT_1-receptors that mediate "all the principal responses" to angiotensin-II (Timmermans et al, 1992).

ANGIOTENSIN-II AS GROWTH FACTOR IN VESSELS AND HEART

Neuromodulation in vascular smooth muscle

A dominant factor governing vascular smooth muscle tone is the release of norepinephrine from the terminal neurons into the synaptic space, with stimulation of the postsynaptic vasoconstrictory alpha$_1$- and alpha$_2$-receptors (Fig. 1–6). By altering the rate of norepinephrine release, a large number of hormones and autonomic signals can achieve indirect control of the degree of vasoconstriction. For example, the parasympathetic autonomic messenger, acetylcholine, can decrease release of norepinephrine acting on the presynaptic muscarinic receptor on the terminal neuron (presynaptic receptor). An important neuromodulator is angiotensin-II, which acts to increase the rate of release of norepinephrine from the terminal neuron by its action on the presynaptic angiotensin-II receptor. This action of angiotensin-II is independent from its direct vasoconstrictory effect on the vascular receptor.

Angiotensin-II and vascular endothelium

Yet another dimension to the multiple vasoconstrictory mechanisms of angiotensin-II is formation of endothelin in the vascular endothelium (Luscher, 1993). (For role of endothelin, see Fig. 4–2).

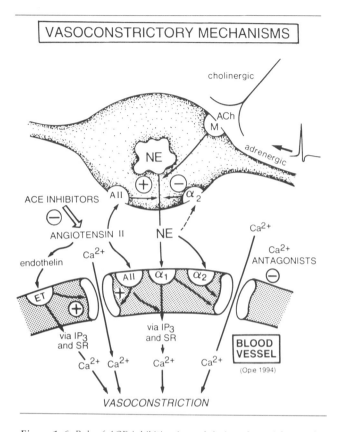

VASOCONSTRICTORY MECHANISMS

Figure 1–6. Role of ACE inhibition in modulation of arterial control. Norepinephrine (NE), released from the storage granules of the terminal neurons, has predominantly vasoconstrictive effects acting via postsynaptic alpha-receptors. In addition, presynaptic alpha$_2$-receptors are stimulated to allow feedback inhibition of its release to modulate any excess release of NE. Parasympathetic cholinergic stimulation releases acetylcholine (ACh), which stimulates the muscarinic (M) receptors to inhibit the release of NE and thereby indirectly to cause vasodilation. Angiotensin-II, formed in response to renin released from the kidneys or locally formed, also is powerfully vasoconstrictive acting (1) to promote release of NE from the terminal neurons, (2) directly on the angiotensin-II receptors, (3) to enhance calcium current influx, and (4) to release endothelin (ET) from the endothelium. The result is that ACE inhibitors cause vasodilation independently of mechanisms responsive to other therapeutic agents such as the alpha$_1$-blockers or the calcium antagonists. For IP$_3$, see Fig. 1–5. Fig. © LH Opie.

Angiotensin-II as growth signal

An interesting hypothesis can be constructed in relation to factors influencing blood vessel growth (angiogenesis). Both angiotensin-II and alpha-receptor agonists have been shown to promote growth of vascular smooth muscle cells in certain conditions. Both types of stimulation are vaso-constrictory. Because calcium is involved in the regulation of muscle growth, a reasonable speculation would be that factors which act as vasoconstrictors in the short term, by temporarily increasing the level of cytosolic calcium, may during long continued stimulation of vascular smooth mus-

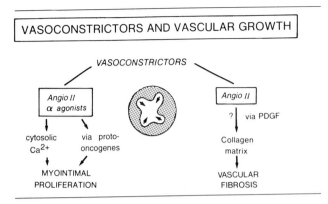

Figure 1–7. A speculative proposal drawing attention to the possiblity that angiotensin-II (Angio II) has an important role in regulating vascular growth. PDGF, platelet-derived growth factor. Fig. © LH Opie.

cle lead to myointimal proliferation. Supporting this hypothesis is the finding that angiotensin-II increases the turnover of the phosphatidylinositol cycle, and the expression of growth-stimulating proto-oncogenes (Lyall et al., 1992). Furthermore, there is evidence that angiotensin-II may stimulate growth of the vascular matrix and in particular collagen formation. These proposals are summarized in Fig. 1–7. Because increased arteriolar growth leads to a decreased ratio between the lumen and the media of the arterioles, which increases the systemic vascular resistance, such a growth promoting potential of angiotensin-II can have an important effect on systemic arteriolar resistance and hence on blood pressure (Chapter 10). Furthermore, a similar growth system may link angiotensin-II to left ventricular hypertrophy.

Myocardial growth

Evidence for an important role of angiotensin-II in promoting cardiac hypertrophy is provided in Chapter 4.

Renal and Adrenal Interactions

Renin release

The major factors stimulating release of renin from the juxtaglomerular cells of the kidney are: (1) increased $beta_1$-sympathetic activity, (2) a low arterial blood pressure, and (3) decreased sodium reabsorption in the distal tubule, as when dietary sodium is low or during diuretic therapy. On the other hand, renin release is inhibited by angiotensin-II activity (Fig. 1–8). The consequences of renin release are not limited to increased conversion of circulating angiotensinogen to angiotensin-I, but probably exert an important intrarenal effect. Components of the renin-angiotensin system are present in the kidney and local formation of angiotensin-II is thought to be the explanation for efferent arteriolar vasoconstriction following renin release (Fig. 1–8). Thus, for example, during a state of arterial hypotension,

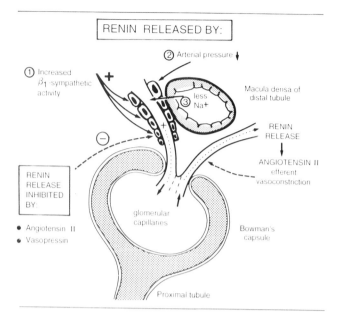

Figure 1–8. Mechanisms for release of renin from juxtaglomerular cells of kidney: (1) beta$_1$-sympathetic activity, (2) hypotension or decreased renal blood flow, and (3) decreased tubular reabsorption of sodium, as for example during a low-sodium diet or diuretic therapy. Note that renin, by forming angiotension-II, maintains efferent arteriolar vasoconstriction and, therefore, the intraglomerular pressure. Fig. © LH Opie.

the increased efferent arteriolar vasoconstriction resulting from increased angiotensin-II will help to preserve renal function by maintaining the intraglomerular pressure.

Stimulation of aldosterone by angiotensin-II

Besides acting as a vasoconstrictor, angiotensin-II also stimulates the formation of the sodium-retaining hormone *aldosterone*. Hence ACE inhibition has potential indirect natriuretic effects. As angiotensin-II levels fall during acute ACE inhibition, so do those of aldosterone (MacGregor et al, 1981; Wilkes, 1984). However, aldosterone formation does not stay blocked during prolonged ACE inhibitor therapy. By 3 months of therapy, aldosterone levels start to rise again and continue to do so for 1 year (Staessen et al., 1981). While this late rise of aldosterone level does not appear to compromise the antihypertensive effects achieved by ACE inhibitors, nonetheless it may detract from the benefit of ACE inhibition in heart failure. The proposed explanation for this late rise of aldosterone, resistant to ACE inhibitor therapy, may be that the early phase natriuresis promotes the production of aldosterone by the adrenal cortex (Oelkers et al, 1974). Alternatively, the late rise in aldosterone formation may merely reflect the rebound formation of circulating angiotensin-II, despite continued ACE inhibition (see later in this chapter).

Feedback inhibition of renin by angiotensin-II

A third action of angiotensin-II is a feedback inhibition of renin secretion (Fig. 1–8). Therefore renin release is suppressed both directly by angiotensin-II and indirectly by the sodium retention associated with the increased aldosterone levels.

SODIUM STATUS, RENIN AND ACE INHIBITOR EFFICACY

During conditions of sodium loading, renin secretion from the juxtaglomerular cells is suppressed. The result is that ACE inhibition, in general, has less hypotensive effect (Hollenberg et al., 1981). Therefore, in the therapy of hypertension, ACE inhibitors are often combined with either a diuretic or a low-sodium diet or both.

Observations in anephric patients

The basic observations of Man in 't Veld et al. (1979) on an anephric patient drew attention to the potential effects of ACE inhibitors on systems other than the renin-angiotensin-aldosterone system activated by release of renin from the kidneys. One possible explanation is the existence of a tissue renin-angiotensin system. Another explanation is the possible importance of the bradykinin-prostaglandin system.

Observations in normotensive subjects

It was originally thought that ACE inhibitors would be effective antihypertensive agents only in high-renin hypertension—especially in unilateral renal artery disease (Ondetti et al., 1977). Then it became clear that effects of ACE inhibition could also be acutely achieved in normotensive subjects and on a normal sodium intake in whom the blood pressure fell as did plasma ACE activity and the levels of angiotensin-II and aldosterone, while renin levels rose (MacGregor et al., 1981). Hence the renin-angiotensin system plays a role in the control of normal blood pressure, even in individuals with normal renin levels. It follows that ACE inhibitors are likely to be effective antihypertensive agents even in the absence of high circulating renin levels.

Nonmodulation and pattern of response to sodium intake

This important proposal by Hollenberg and Williams (1990) suggests why it is that certain individuals react adversely to a high salt intake by increasing the arterial blood pressure. In normal "modulating" subjects, a high salt intake inhibits the formation of renin so that there is less activity of angiotensin-II with an increased renal blood flow, which helps to promote sodium excretion. In addition, in modu-

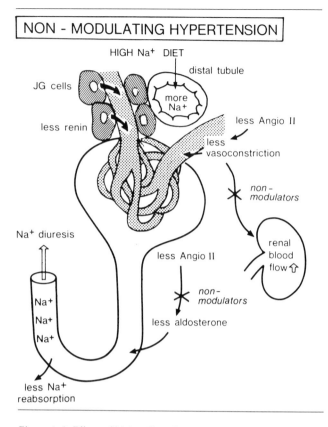

Figure 1–9. *Effects of high-sodium diet in normal subjects and in "nonmodulators." In normal subjects, a high-sodium diet leads to increased tubular reabsorption of sodium, which inhibits renin release, which decreases efferent arteriolar vasoconstriction, so that renal blood flow increases. Furthermore, less formation of angiotensin-II (Angio II) leads to a lower level of aldosterone, which leads to increased sodium diuresis. In nonmodulating hypertensive patients, the above sequence does not happen in response to sodium, so these patients do not modulate this control mechanism the way they should. Nonmodulation is an attractive concept to explain why certain subjects with hypertension are salt-sensitive. It is also proposed that such subjects may respond well to monotherapy by ACE inhibitors because decreased formation of angiotensin-II within the renal vasculature restores the renal blood flow response to the high sodium diet. JG, juxtaglomerular (Fig. 1–8). For concept, see Hollenberg and Williams (1990). Fig. © LH Opie.*

lators, increased angiotensin-II suppresses formation of aldosterone which, in turn, also promotes a sodium diuresis. In "nonmodulators," there is inadequate inhibition of aldosterone in response to a high salt intake (Fig. 1–9). Hollenberg and Williams (1990) propose that "nonmodulation" could be an important mechanism in a subset of the hypertensive population. The hypothesis is that such individuals are salt-sensitive, and that irrespective of the circulating renin level (whether low or high renin), they cannot call forth the required increase in renal perfusion as a result of a sodium challenge.

This hypothesis of "nonmodulation" becomes particularly interesting in view of the proposed specific response of hypertension in such patients to ACE inhibitors. Hollenberg and Williams (1990) suggest that subjects who respond well to ACE inhibitors as monotherapy may all be nonmodulators. The hypothetical reason why ACE inhibitors may be specifically beneficial to nonmodulators is decreased intrarenal formation of angiotensin-II. Therefore the renal blood flow can increase as it should in response to a sodium load.

Renin profiling in hypertension

Circulating levels of plasma renin activity vary widely in patients with hypertension. On the one hand, as expected, high values are found in renovascular hypertension. On the other hand, much lower values are found in essential hypertension, with most falling within the normal range (Kaplan, 1977). Certain population groups, such as black subjects or the elderly, are known to have relatively low renin levels for the group as a whole, although there are still marked individual variations. Logically, ACE inhibitors should work best in high-renin states (Case et al, 1977) and diuretics should work best in low-renin states, as suggested by Laragh on the basis of his concept of renin-profiling (Laragh, 1989). These predictions work well for black subjects with their lower renin levels, and explain why they have a relatively poor response to ACE inhibitor therapy (Chapter 2). In black elderly patients, ACE inhibition is almost totally ineffective (Chapter 2). Despite some defects, the concept of renin profiles explains ethnic differences. Also, high-renin values raise suspicion of renovascular hypertension, and really low values suggest primary aldosteronism. In the individual patient with essential hypertension, the normal renin value usually found is not helpful in predicting whether or not there would be a therapeutic response to ACE inhibitor therapy.

AUTONOMIC INTERACTIONS

Permissive anti-adrenergic effects of ACE inhibitors

Angiotensin-II promotes the release of norepinephrine from adrenergic terminal neurons, and also enhances adrenergic tone by central activation and by facilitation of ganglionic transmission (Antonaccio and Kerwin, 1981). Furthermore, angiotensin-II amplifies the vasoconstriction achieved by alpha$_1$-receptor stimulation (Purdy and Weber, 1988). Thus, angiotensin-II has facilitatory adrenergic actions leading to increased activity of vasoconstrictory norepinephrine (Fig. 1–10). This permissive role of angiotensin-II provides an indirect mechanism for the vasodilatory action of ACE inhibitors.

Additional autonomic effects on the parasympathetic nervous system are possible, so that *parasympathetic* tone may be increased (Ajayi et al., 1985) suggesting a vagomimetic effect of ACE inhibition. There may also be changes in the activity of the baroreflexes, which serve to control

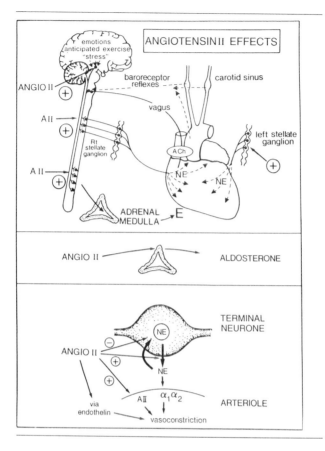

Figure 1–10. Multiple sites of action of angiotension-II (angio II) including central adrenergic activation, facilitation of ganglionic transmission, release of aldosterone from the adrenal medulla, release of norepinephrine (NE) from terminal sympathetic varicosities with inhibition of re-uptake, and direct stimulation of vascular angiotensin-II receptors. Angiotensin-II also releases vasoconstrictory endothelin from the endothelium. The major net effect is powerful vasoconstriction. Fig. © LH Opie.

the blood pressure. In response to ACE inhibition, *down-regulation of baroreflexes* may develop, which means that the baroreceptors respond less well to incoming signals (Guidicelli et al, 1985). Such effects on baroreceptors and on the parasympathetic tone could explain why tachycardia is absent in response to peripheral vasodilation achieved by ACE inhibition.

KALLIKREIN-KININ SYSTEM AND BRADYKININ

Foremost among possible alternate sites of action of ACE inhibitors is bradykinin (Wiemer et al., 1991). This nona-peptide originally described as causing slow contractions in the gut (*brady,* slow; *kinin,* movement) is of increasing cardiovascular importance (Lüscher 1993; Schror, 1992). Bradykinin is formed from *kininogen* by the action of the enzyme *kallikrein,* which in turn is derived from *pre-kallikrein.*

Bradykinin is, in turn, inactivated by two *kininases*, kininase 1 and 2, the latter being identical with ACE. Therefore, ACE inhibition should logically lead to increased local formation of bradykinin (Hajj-ali and Zimmerman, 1991), which has major vasodilatory properties (Fig. 1–1). Formation of bradykinin may be a new cardioprotective mechanism (Scicli, 1994).

Formation of bradykinin

There are two main stimuli to the formation of bradykinin, a process that occurs in the endothelium. Of prime physiologic importance may be the effect of an increased blood flow, probably acting by shear forces on the endothelium (Lüscher, 1993). Thus, hypothetically, during exercise the increased blood flow achieved by an increased cardiac output can help promote local formation of bradykinin. The latter further increases arteriolar diameter and muscle blood flow. Second, when the endothelium is damaged, as by inflammation, tissue factor XIIA increases formation of kallikrein (Fig. 1–1).

Properties of bradykinin

Bradykinin acts on bradykinin receptors in the vascular endothelium to promote the release of two vasodilators. First, there is increased formation of nitric oxide which may mediate vascular protection (Farhy et al., 1993). Second, there is increased conversion of arachidonic acid to vasodilatory prostaglandins, such as prostacyclin and PGE_2 (Schror, 1992).

Bradykinin receptors

Thus, bradykinin is formed locally in the vascular endothelium in response to specific stimuli (Farhy et al., 1993). The bradykinin acts locally on bradykinin receptors of the B_2-subtype (Sung et al., 1988). The result is increased formation in the endothelial cells of nitric oxide and prostaglandins.

Bradykinin inhibitors

Bradykinin does not contribute to the overall regulation of blood pressure, as shown by the injection of a B_2-inhibitor to normotensive rats (Madeddu et al., 1992). During ACE inhibition, however, the situation may change. The potential vasodilatory role of bradykinin during ACE inhibitor therapy could theoretically be followed by changes in blood bradykinin levels (Williams, 1988), which, however, are unlikely to reflect changes in the local rates of formation and degradation of bradykinin. The hypotensive effect of ACE inhibition is reduced by the agent apoprotinin, which inhibits the conversion of prekallikrein to kallikrein (Mimran et al., 1980). In the specific situation of regional ischemia in the dog, bradykinin release into the coronary vein is increased many-fold after coronary occlusion; in addition, the release rate is further enhanced by captopril (Noda et al., 1993). Thus, the current concept is that bradykinin formation, occurring locally and thus not easily measured, can participate in the hypotensive effect of ACE inhibitors.

Prostaglandins and hypotensive effects of ACE inhibitors

During ACE inhibition there is increased local synthesis of the active bradykinin nonapeptide, bradykinin-(1–9), in the kidney (Campbell et al., 1993). Such bradykinin stimulates the conversion of arachidonic acid into vasodilatory prostacyclin (PGI_2) and PGE_2 (McGiff et al., 1972; Schror, 1992). Indomethacin, which inhibits prostaglandin synthesis, reduces the hypotensive effect of ACE inhibitors (Moore et al., 1981). In patients with congestive heart failure, the vasodilatory effects of ACE inhibition are also blunted by indomethacin pretreatment (Nishimura et al., 1989). However, these studies do not give conclusive evidence for the role of vasodilatory prostaglandins in the effects of ACE inhibitors, because indomethacin has some additional actions such as blunting the rise of plasma renin activity after ACE inhibitor therapy (Witzgall et al., 1982).

Bradykinin and anti-ischemic effect of ACE inhibitors

In the heart, it is proposed that increased bradykinin during ACE inhibition protects against ischemic reperfusion damage at least in part by formation of protective nitric oxide and prostacyclin (Linz et al., 1989; 1992).

TISSUE RENIN-ANGIOTENSIN SYSTEMS

Although the acute hypotensive effects of ACE inhibition can clearly be linked to decreased circulating levels of angiotensin-II, during chronic ACE inhibition there is a reactive hyperreninemia linked to re-emergence of circulating angiotensin-II (Mooser et al., 1990; MacFadyen et al., 1991). Furthermore, ACE inhibition can be effective even in low renin states (Chatterjee and Opie, 1987). There is also a discrepancy between hemodynamic effects and circulating levels of ACE inhibitors, possibly due to binding of ACE inhibitors to tissue sites (Sakaguchi et al., 1988; MacFadyen et al., 1991). An increasingly important question is whether angiotensin can be formed in crucial tissues (it can) and whether tissue ACE is a potential or even major site of action for the ACE inhibitors (MacFadyen et al., 1991).

All the components of the renin-angiotensin system are found in vascular tissue including the coronary vessels (Dostal and Baker, 1993)(Fig. 1–11). In a number of vascular beds, local production is the major source of angiotensin-I and angiotensin-II found in the veins (Campbell, 1987; Schalekamp et al., 1989). Tissue ACE activity is found in the lungs, myocardium, brain, kidneys, and testes (MacFadyen et al., 1991). An especially striking finding is the degree to which renal ACE activity is depressed to very low levels by ACE inhibitor therapy given to animals (Veltmar et al., 1991). Furthermore, during chronic ACE inhibitor treatment when plasma ACE activity increases as a result of compensatory induction, there are still low levels of free tissue ACE in kidney, adrenals, and aorta of rats (Kohzuki et al., 1991). Evidence for an intracardiac renin-angiotensin

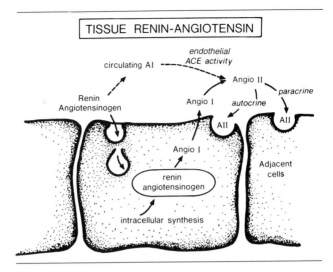

Figure 1–11. *Proposed role of tissue renin-angiotensin systems. Renin and angiotensin from the extracellular space may enter the cell by means of receptor endocytosis. Intracellular renin-angiotensin can be derived either from such endocytosis or from local intracellular synthesis. Angiotensin-I, thus formed, is released from the cell and converted to angiotensin-II either by circulating ACE or by such enzyme attached externally to the cell. Extracellular angiotensin-II can then act on the same cell from which the angiotensin-I was derived, an autocrine effect. Alternatively, the angiotensin-II can be conveyed to the circulation to other cells to exert effects on the angiotensin-II receptor, a paracrine action. Fig. © LH Opie.*

system is reviewed by Dostal and Baker (1993), and criticized by von Lutterotti et al. (1994).

The implication of the discovery of these tissue components of the renin-angiotensin system means that angiotensin-II can be locally formed in or around blood vessels with possible vasoconstrictory effects (Dzau, 1987). ACE can be made in the endothelium, with the major part of the enzyme protruding into the vascular lumen. The result is that angiotensin-II is always generated at this site, and it does not matter whether the precursor angiotensin-I is locally made or derived from the circulation (Gohlke et al., 1992). Local angiotensin-II formation accounts for the autocrine-paracrine effects of the renin-angiotensin system (*autocrine*, local action on the same cells that produce the angiotensin-II; *paracrine*, effects on neighboring cells). According to the concept of local endothelial production of angiotensin-II, there is "no need to postulate tissue penetration by ACE inhibitors to explain their inhibitory effect" on organs such as the heart or brain (Unger and Gohlke, 1993).

An important observation now made in several pharmacokinetic studies in rats is that, when an ACE inhibitor is given to spontaneously hypertensive rats (SH rats), the fall in blood pressure correlates better with the inhibition of the tissue than the circulating renin-angiotensin system (Cohen and Kurz, 1982; Unger et al., 1984; Weishaar et al., 1991). Hence, it is now increasingly believed that tissue systems are of at best some importance in the blood pressure lowering effects of ACE inhibitors, which would explain why antihypertensive effects can be maintained despite the later reactive increase of circulating angiotensin-II (Mac-Fadyen et al., 1991). Nonetheless, decisive studies to prove the significance of local tissue ACE inhibition in humans are still lacking.

Interaction with atrial natriuretic peptide (atriopeptin-II)

Natriuresis induced by atrial natriuretic peptide (ANP) occurs in two phases (peak and shoulder pattern), only the first of which is potentiated by ACE inhibition (Spinelli et al., 1986). These data suggest a possible interactive link between the sodium-retaining renin-angiotensin system (susceptible to ACE inhibition) and the sodium-losing ANP system (not susceptible to ACE inhibition). For example, endothelin can be produced by angiotensin-II stimulation and is probably a stimulus to the release of ANP.

Alternate modes of angiotensin-II generation

Not all angiotensin-II is generated as a result of the activity of angiotensin-converting enzyme. In the failing human heart, it appears that most angiotensin-II could be formed by a path sensitive to a membrane-bound serine proteinase and not to an ACE inhibitor (Urata et al. 1990). Similar observations have been made in the dog heart after coronary ligation (Noda et al., 1993), where both a serine and a cysteine protease are implicated. Other tissues in which angiotensin-I can be converted to angiotensin-II independently of the ACE activity are the renal arteries (Okamura et al., 1990) and the lungs (Mento and Wilkes, 1987). A major controversy is the extent to which these independent pathways are of pathophysiological importance (Johnston, 1994). Use of specific protease inhibitors suggests that the local formation of angiotensin-II by proteases does not regulate infarct size in dogs (Noda et al., 1993).

SUMMARY

There is no doubt that ACE inhibitors have multiple sites of action on the circulation. The chief and best understood mechanism is inhibition of the renin-angiotensin system, not only of the circulating components but very probably also those found in the various tissues, including the heart, particularly in the vascular bed. Although there is as yet no proof in humans that the tissue renin-angiotensin system plays any decisive role as a site of action of ACE inhibitors, that it does play a role is supported by more and more data. Formation of protectory vasodilatory bradykinin and prostaglandins as a result of ACE inhibition seems to be important. An indirect anti-adrenergic effect is experimentally well established. An effect on renal blood flow may be crucial in some hypertensive subjects. Increasing attention is now focused on the role of the renin-angiotensin system in the regulation of vascular and myocardial growth. Of these sites of action, the peripheral vasodilation is the proposed basis of the major antihypertensive effect as well as of the benefit in congestive heart failure.

The chapters to follow will evaluate in more detail the effects of the ACE inhibitors on (1) hypertension, (2) the kidneys and their role not only in hypertension but also in diabetes, (3) the heart in health and in failure, (4) the circulation in congestive heart failure, and (5) the central nervous system. Thereafter the important pharmacokinetic properties will be examined in detail followed by side-effects and drug interactions. Finally, the possible vascular and cardioprotective role of these agents will be evaluated, taking an optimistic look into the future.

REFERENCES

Ajayi AA, Campbell BC, Meredith PA, et al. The effect of captopril on the reflex control heart rate: possible mechanisms. *Br J Clin Pharmacol* 1985; 20: 17–25.

Allen IS, Cohen NM, Dhallan RS, et al. Angiotensin-II increases spontaneous contractile frequency and stimulates calcium current in cultured neonatal rat heart myocytes: insights into the underlying biochemical mechanisms. *Circ Res* 1988; 62: 524–534.

Antonaccio MJ, Kerwin L. Pre- and postjunctional inhibition of vascular sympathetic function by captopril in SHR: implication of vascular angiotensin-II in hypertension and antihypertensive actions of captopril. *Hypertension* 1981; 3 (Suppl 1): I-54–I-62.

Berridge MJ. Rapid accumulation of inositol triphosphate reveals that agonists hydrolyse polyphosphoinositides instead of phosphatidylinositol. *Biochem J* 1983; 212: 849–858.

Berridge MJ. Inositol trisphosphate and calcium signalling. *Nature* 1993; 361: 315–325.

Berridge MJ, Irvine RF. Inositol triphosphate, a novel second messenger in cellular signal transduction. *Nature* 1984; 312: 315–321.

Brown AM, Birnbaumer L. Direct G-protein gating of ion channels. *Am J Physiol* 1988; 254: H401–H410.

Campbell DJ. Circulating and tissue angiotensin systems. *J Clin Invest* 1987; 79: 1–6.

Campbell DJ, Kladis A, Duncan A-M. Bradykinin peptides in kidney, blood, and other tissues of the rat. *Hypertension* 1993; 21: 155–165.

Case DB, Wallace JM, Keim HJ, et al. Possible role of renin in hypertension as suggested by renin-sodium profiling and inhibition of converting enzyme. *N Engl J Med* 1977; 296: 641–646.

Chatterjee K, Opie LH. Angiotensin inhibitors and other vasodilators with special reference to congestive heart failure. *Cardiovasc Drugs Ther* 1987; 1: 1–8.

Cohen ML, Kurz KD. Angiotensin converting enzyme inhibition in tissues from spontaneously hypertensive rats after treatment with captopril or MK-421. *J Pharmacol Exp Ther* 1982; 220: 63–69.

Derkx FHM, Tan-Thong L, Wenting GJ, et al. Asynchronous changes in prorenin and renin secretion after captopril in patients with renal artery stenosis. *Hypertension* 1983; 5: 244–256.

Dostal DE, Baker KM. Evidence for a role of an intracardiac renin-angiotensin system in normal and failing hearts. *Trends Cardiovasc Med* 1993; 3: 67–74.

Dzau VJ. Implications of local angiotensin production in cardiovascular physiology and pharmacology. *Am J Cardiol* 1987; 59: 59A–65A.

Farhy RD, Carretero OA, Ho K-L, Scicli AG. Role of kinins and nitric oxide in the effects of angiotensin-converting enzyme inhibitors on neointima formation. *Circ Res* 1993; 72: 1202–1210.

Gohlke P, Bunning P, Unger T. Distribution and metabolism of angiotensin-I and II in the blood vessel wall. *Hypertension* 1992; 20: 151–157.

Guidicelli JF, Berdeaux A, Edouard A, et al. The effect of enalapril on baroreceptor mediated reflex function in normotensive subjects. *Br J Clin Pharmacol* 1985; 20: 211–218.

Hajj-ali AF, Zimmerman BG. Kinin contribution to renal vasodilator effect of captopril in rabbit. *Hypertension* 1991; 17: 504–509.

Hollenberg NK, Williams GH. Abnormal renal function, sodium-volume homeostasis, and renin system behavior in normal-renin essential hypertension. In: Laragh JH, Brenner BM (eds), *Hypertension: Pathophysiology, Diagnosis, and Management*. Raven Press, New York, 1990, 1349–1370.

Hollenberg NK, Meggs LG, Williams GH, et al. Sodium intake and renal responses to captopril in normal man and in essential hypertension. *Kidney Int* 1981; 20: 240–245.

Johnston CI. Tissue angiotensin-converting enzyme in cardiac and vascular hypertrophy, repair, and remodeling. *Hypertension* 1994; 23: 258–268.

Kaplan NM. Renin profiles. The unfulfilled promises. *JAMA* 1977; 238: 611–613.

Kohzuki M, Johnston CI, Chai SY, et al. Measurement of angiotensin converting enzyme induction and inhibition using quantitative in vitro autoradiography: issue selective induction after chronic lisinopril treatment. *J Hypertens* 1991; 9: 579–587.

Laragh JH. Issues, goals, and guidelines in selecting first-line drug therapy for hypertension. *Hypertension* 1989; 13 (Suppl I): I-103–I-112.

Linz W, Scholkens BA, Kaiser J, et al. Cardiac arrhythmias are ameliorated by local inhibition of angiotensin formation and bradykinin degradation with the converting-enzyme inhibitor ramipril. *Cardiovasc Drugs Ther* 1989; 3: 873–882.

Linz W, Wiemer G, Scholkens BA. ACE inhibition induces NO-formation in cultured bovine endothelial cells and protects isolated ischemic rat hearts. *J Mol Cell Cardiol* 1992; 24: 909–919.

Luckhoff A, Clapham A. Inositol 1,3,4,5-tetrakisphosphate activates an endothelial Ca^{2+}-permeable channel. *Nature* 1992; 355: 356–358.

Lüscher TF. Angiotensin, ACE inhibitors and endothelial control of vasomotor tone. *Basic Res Cardiol* 1993; 88: Suppl 1, 15–24.

Lyall F, Dornan ES, McQueen J, et al. Angiotensin-II increases proto-oncogene expression and phosphoinositide turnover in vascular smooth muscle cells via the angiotensin-II AT_1 receptor. *J Hypertens* 1992; 10: 1463–1469.

MacFadyen RJ, Lees KR, Reid JL. Tissue and plasma angiotensin converting enzyme and the response to ACE inhibitor drugs. *Br J Clin Pharmacol* 1991; 31: 1–13.

MacGregor GA, Markandu ND, Bayliss J, et al. Non-sulfhydryl-containing angiotensin-converting enzyme inhibitor (MK421): evidence for role of renin system in normotensive subjects. *Br Med J* 1981; 283: 401–403.

Madeddu P, Anania V, Parpaglia PP, et al. Effects of HOE 140, a bradykinin B_2-receptor antagonist, on renal function in conscious normotensive rats. *Br J Pharmacol* 1992; 106: 380–386.

Man in 't Veld AJ, Wenting GJ, Schalekamp MADH. Does captopril lower blood pressure in anephric patients? *Br Med J* 1979; ii: 1110.

McGiff JC, Terragno NA, Malik KU, Lonigro AJ. Release of a prostaglandin E-like substance from canine kidney by bradykinin. *Circ Res* 1972; 31: 36–43.

Meisenhelder J, Suh P-G, Rhee SG, Hunter T. Phospholipase C-y is a substrate for the PDGF and EGF receptor protein-tyrosine kinases in vivo and in vitro. *Cell* 1989; 57: 1109–1122.

Mento PS, Wilkes BM. Plasma angiotensins and blood pressure during converting enzyme inhibition. *Hypertension* 1987; 9 (Suppl III): 32–48.

Mimran A, Targhetta R, Laroche B. The antihypertensive effect of captopril: evidence for an influence of kinins. *Hypertension* 1980; 2: 732–737.

Moore TJ, Crantz FR, Hollenberg NK, et al. Contribution of prostaglandins to the antihypertensive action of captopril in essential hypertension. *Hypertension* 1981; 3: 168–173.

Mooser V, Nussberger J, Juillerat L, et al. Reactive hyperreninemia is a major determinant of plasma angiotensin-II during ACE inhibition. *J Cardiovasc Pharmacol* 1990; 15: 276–282.

Morgan KG. The role of calcium in the control of vascular tone as assessed by the Ca^{2+} indicator aequorin. *Cardiovasc Drugs Ther* 1990; 4: 1355–1362.

Nishimura H, Kubo S, Ueyama M, et al. Peripheral hemodynamic effects of captopril in patients with congestive heart failure. *Am Heart J* 1989; 117: 100–105.

Nishizuka Y. Turnover of inositol phospholipids and signal transduction. *Science* 1984; 222: 1365.

Noda K, Sasaguri M, Ideishi M, et al. Role of locally formed angiotensin-II and bradykinin in the reduction of myocardial infarct size in dogs. *Cardiovasc Res* 1993; 27: 334–340.

Oelkers W, Brown JJ, Fraser R, et al. Sensitization of the adrenal cortex to angiotensin-II in sodium-deplete man. *Circ Res* 1974; 34: 69–77.

Okamura T, Okunishi H, Ayajiki K, Toda N. Conversion of angiotensin I to angiotensin II in dog isolated renal artery: Role of two different angiotensin II-generating enzymes. *J Cardiovasc Pharmacol* 1990; 15: 353–359.

Ondetti MA, Rubin B, Cushman DW. Design of specific inhibitors of angiotensin-converting enzyme: new class of orally active antihypertensive agents. *Science* 1977; 196; 441–444.

Purdy RE, Weber MA. Angiotensin-II amplification of alpha-adrenergic vasoconstriction: role of receptor reserve. *Circ Res* 1988; 63: 748–757.

Sakaguchi K, Jackson B, Chai SY, et al. Effects of perindopril on tissue angiotensin-converting enzyme activity demonstrated by quantitative in vitro autoradiography. *J Cardiovasc Pharmacol* 1988; 12: 710–717.

Schalekamp MADH, Admiraal PJJ, Derkx FHM. Estimation of regional metabolism and production of angiotensins in hypertensive subjects. *Br J Clin Pharmacol* 1989; 28: 105S–113S.

Schror K. Role of prostaglandins in the cardiovascular effects of bradykinin and angiotensin-converting enzyme inhibitors. *J Cardiovasc Pharmacol* 1992; 20 (Suppl 9): S68–S73.

Scicli AG. Increases in cardiac kinins as a new mechanism to protect the heart. *Hypertension* 1994; 23: 419–421.

Soubrier F, Alhenc-Gelas F, Hubert C, et al. Two putative active centers in human angiotensin-I converting enzyme revealed by molecular cloning. *Proc Natl Acad Sci* 1988; 85: 9386–9390.

Spinelli F, Kamber B, Schnell C. Observations on the natriuretic response to intravenous infusions of atrial natriuretic factor in water-loaded anaesthetized rats. *J Hypertens* 1986; 4 (Suppl 2): S25–S29.

Staessen J, Lijnen P, Fagard R, et al. Rise in plasma concentration of aldosterone during long-term angiotensin-II suppression. *J Endocr* 1981; 91: 457–465.

Sung C-P, Arleth AJ, Shikano K, Berkowitz BA. Characterization and function of bradykinin receptors in vascular endothelial cells. *J Pharmacol Exp Ther* 1988; 247: 8–13.

Timmermans PBMWM, Benfield P, Chiu AT, et al. Angiotensin-II receptors and functional correlates. *Am J Hypertens* 1992; 5: 221S–235S.

Unger T, Gohlke P. Converting enzyme inhibitors in cardiovascular therapy: current status and future potential. *Cardiovasc Res* 1994; 28: 146–158.

Unger T, Ganten D, Lang RE, Scholkens BA. Is tissue converting enzyme inhibition a determinant of the antihypertensive efficacy of converting enzyme inhibitors? Studies with the two different compounds, HOE 498 and MK 421, in spontaneously hypertensive rats. *J Cardiovasc Pharmacol* 1984; 6: 872–880.

Urata H, Healy B, Stewart RW, et al. Angiotensin-II-forming pathways in normal and failing human hearts. *Circ Res* 1990; 66: 883–890.

Veltmar A, Gohlke P, Unger T. From tissue angiotensin converting enzyme inhibition to antihypertensive effect. *Am J Hypertens* 1991; 4: 263S–269S.

von Lutterotti N, Catanzaro DF, Sealey JE, Laragh JH. Renin is not synthesized by cardiac and extrarenal vascular tissues. A review of experimental evidence. *Circulation* 1994; 89: 458–470.

Weishaar RE, Panek RL, Major TC, et al. Evidence for a functional tissue renin-angiotensin system in the rat mesenteric vasculature and its involvement in regulating blood pressure. *J Pharmacol Exp Ther* 1991; 256: 568–574.

Wiemer G, Scholkens BA, Becker RHA, Busse R. Ramiprilat enhances endothelial autacoid formation by inhibiting breakdown of endothelium-derived bradykinin. *Hypertension* 1991; 18: 558–563.

Wilkes BM. Evidence for a vasodepressor effect of the angiotensin-converting enzyme inhibitor, MK421 (enalapril), independent of blockade of angiotensin-II formation. *J Cardiovasc Pharmacol* 1984; 6: 1036–1042.

Williams GH. Converting-enzyme inhibitors in the treatment of hypertension. *N Engl J Med* 1988; 319: 1517–1525.

Witzgall H, Hirsch F, Scherer B, Weber PC. Acute haemodynamic and hormonal effects of captopril are diminished by indomethacin. *Clin Sci* 1982; 62: 611–615.

CHAPTER 2

ACE Inhibitors for Hypertension

"ACE inhibitors once reserved for refractory hypertension, especially when renal in origin, have edged their way into a prime position" (Kaplan and Opie, 1991)

MECHANISMS FOR ANTIHYPERTENSIVE EFFECTS OF ACE INHIBITORS

Essential hypertension is often regarded as a multifactorial disease, resulting from a number of diverse genetic and environmental factors. Physiologically, the blood pressure (BP) is given by:

$$BP = CO \times SVR$$

where CO = cardiac output and SVR = systemic vascular resistance (Table 2–1). When the cardiac output rises acutely, as during sympathetic adrenergic stimulation, baroreflex adjustments tend to decrease the systemic vascular resistance, so that normal blood pressure values are regained. However, in predisposed individuals, the baroreflex control is inadequate, or the tendency to peripheral vasoconstriction is excessive, so that temporary hypertension becomes permanent. In such circumstances, sustained hypertension will result (1) when the cardiac output is excessive, as in excessive emotional stress, especially when associated with a tachycardia and (2) when the systemic vascular resistance is too high. The latter can result from increased activity of vasoconstrictive regulatory factors such as alpha-adrenergic drive, or renin-angiotensin overactivity, or there can be enhanced sensitivity of the peripheral arterioles to normally acting vasoconstrictive mechanisms.

Excess vasoconstriction may be an important mechanism in salt-sensitive hypertension, in which it is thought that a relatively minor defect in the renal handling of sodium can lead to sodium retention in various cells of the body, including vascular smooth muscle (Campese, 1994). Consequent on such intracellular sodium retention would follow increased activity of the sodium-calcium exchange,

TABLE 2–1 PHYSIOLOGIC-BASED APPROACH TO
MECHANISMS FOR ESSENTIAL HYPERTENSION

---

1. Excess cardiac output

- Beta-adrenergic drive as in excessive emotional stress with tachycardia

2. Excess peripheral vascular resistance

(i) Enhanced vasoconstrictor activity

- Alpha-adrenergic drive

- Renin-angiotensin II

- Endothelial dysfunction with increased endothelin and/or decreased nitric oxide

(ii) Enhanced response of vascular smooth muscle to normal vasoconstrictor activity

a) sodium-retaining states

- salt-sensitive hypertension (common)

- aldosterone excess (rare)

b) defective sodium regulation by cell membrane

- possible genetic defect in black subjects

Note: Because BP = CO × SVR, abnormalities in either of the entities controlling BP could only cause sustained hypertension in the presence of inadequate baroreceptor control.

thereby leading to an increased cytosolic calcium ion concentration in the smooth muscle cell with vasoconstriction and elevation of the blood pressure. Abnormalities of cell membrane pumps and exchanges regulating sodium have been described in black subjects, which may explain their greater tendency to a type of hypertension responding better to diuretic therapy. Furthermore, sodium retention inhibits renin secretion, which could help to explain why low-renin hypertension appears to be more common in black subjects. These physiologic-based proposals are summarized in Table 2–1.

Antihypertensive mechanisms of ACE inhibitors

At least six antihypertensive mechanisms may be involved (Table 2–2). First, the major and self-evident effect of angiotensin-converting enzyme (ACE) inhibitors is to decrease circulating angiotensin-II levels and thereby to have a vasodilatory and antihypertensive effect. A second and possibly major site of action is on the tissue renin-angiotensin system including ACE activity in vascular cells. A third potential antihypertensive mechanism is by modulation and downregulation of the adrenergic activity and in particular the release of norepinephrine from terminal neurons. A fourth antihypertensive mechanism is by a lessened release of vasoconstrictory endothelin from the vascular endothelium. A fifth mechanism is by an increased formation of bradykinin and vasodilatory prostaglandins. Sixth, natriuresis may be achieved or minor degrees of sodium reten-

TABLE 2–2 POSSIBLE ANTIHYPERTENSIVE MECHANISMS OF ACE INHIBITORS

1. Inhibition of circulating renin-angiotensin II system

2. Inhibition of tissue and vascular renin-angiotensin system

3. Decreased release of norepinephrine from terminal neurons

4. Decreased formation of endothelin from endothelium

5. Increased formation of bradykinin and vasodilatory prostaglandins

6. Decreased sodium retention from lessened secretion of aldosterone and/or increased renal blood flow

tion countered by decreased release of aldosterone and increased renal blood flow (Fig. 2–1).

Because it is not presently possible to predict which of these various mechanisms is the major one contributing to the blood pressure elevation in any given patient, there is no logical choice for first-line therapy. Accordingly, the initial choice of antihypertensive agent is governed by the anticipated efficacy and side-effects of the agent concerned. The purpose of this chapter is to review all available data on the ACE inhibitors, analyze their comparative properties in relation to diuretics, beta-blockers, and calcium antago-

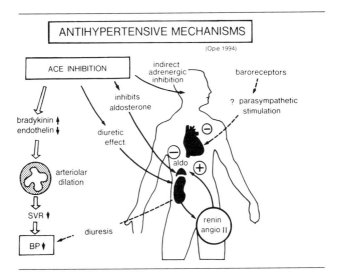

Figure 2–1. Proposed mechanisms whereby ACE inhibitors as a class may exert their antihypertensive effects. Note that the major effect is on the peripheral arterioles causing vasodilation and a fall in the systemic vascular resistance (SVR), also called the peripheral vascular resistance. Indirect inhibition of adrenergic activity also promotes arteriolar dilation. Decreased angiotensin-II levels may also act by increased formation of bradykinin and vasodilatory prostaglandins as well as by inhibition of central effects of angiotensin-II. Parasympathetic activity appears to be stimulated (Boni et al., 1990). Fig. © LH Opie.

nists, and provide recommendations on practical therapy with these agents in hypertension.

Sodium status

As sodium depletion is a major stimulus to the release of renin, it follows that variations in the sodium content of the diet have potentially a major effect on the efficacy of ACE inhibitors in antihypertensive therapy because of the high renin status following sodium depletion. In most studies, the sodium content of the diet has not been controlled. The ACE inhibitors have a natriuretic effect evident even in subjects on a moderate sodium intake of 80 mmol/day (Sanchez et al., 1985). A very low sodium diet abolishes this natriuretic effect (Taylor et al., 1984).

Thus, the antihypertensive effect of ACE inhibitors could be expected to vary. In patients on a low-sodium intake and with high circulating renin levels, the antihypertensive effect is likely to be more evident because decreased peripheral vasoconstriction would follow decreased circulating levels of angiotensin-II (Jenkins and McKinstry, 1979). An important additional beneficial mechanism could be the increased renal blood flow in salt-restricted subjects (Fig. 2–2). In contrast, patients on a high-sodium intake with low circulating renin levels are less likely to respond with an antihypertensive effect. *Hence a low sodium diet should be standard advice to all patients receiving ACE inhibitor therapy for hypertension* (MacGregor et al., 1987; Singer et al., 1991).

Renin status

The plasma renin activity of the patient may also influence the response to ACE inhibition. In high-renin patients, for example those with renal artery stenosis, the response to ACE inhibition is consistent and often marked. In "average" patients with hypertension, the blood pressure fall after captopril could be related to the pretreatment plasma renin activity (MacGregor et al., 1982), which in most patients was low. The concept of high versus low renin states is, however, more complex than just the level of plasma renin activity; the renin level should be related to the sodium intake to give the renin-sodium profile (Case et al., 1977).

Black patients and elderly patients are thought to be *low-renin hypertension groups,* which should theoretically not respond to ACE inhibitors. In the case of black patients, there are indeed several studies suggesting that ACE inhibitor therapy on its own is not likely to be effective (Materson et al., 1993). In elderly white patients, however, increasing evidence shows that ACE inhibitor therapy can be effective as monotherapy, as will be discussed later in this chapter. The role of circulating renin activity in determining the response to ACE inhibitors is, therefore, not clearcut. Rather, the mechanism of the antihypertensive effect of ACE inhibitors is probably multifactorial and only partially dependent on the renin and sodium status.

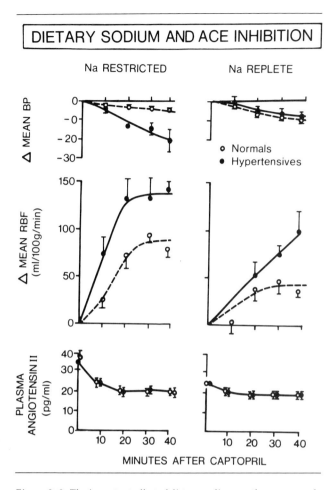

DIETARY SODIUM AND ACE INHIBITION

Figure 2–2. The important effect of dietary sodium on the response of normotensive and hypertensive patients to acute administration of captopril. Despite an identical fall and time course of changes in plasma angiotensin-II concentration in the normotensive and hypertensive patients, the renal vascular response (RBF, renal blood flow) is greater in the hypertensive patients than in the normal subjects. Note particularly that in sodium restriction the fall in the blood pressure is much more marked in hypertensive patients than in states of sodium repletion. Part of the difference may be due to the greater increase in renal blood flow achieved in sodium-restricted hypertensive patients. Reproduced from Hollenberg et al. (1981) with permission.

ACE Inhibitors as Monotherapy in Hypertension

Captopril was the first ACE inhibitor clinically used in the therapy of hypertension. Initially its severe side-effects, including neutropenia and renal damage, led to its use only when other agents had failed. Gradually, as the dose given dropped, so did the side-effects, and it became evident that captopril could be effective even as initial monotherapy. In 1985, Jenkins et al. reviewed the use of captopril in nearly 7,000 hypertensive patients, with a mean entry blood pressure of 183/111 mmHg. Captopril in a mean dose of 150 mg, usually together with a diuretic, was often effective therapy. However, at about the same time, eminent leaders in the area of hypertension, such as Zanchetti (1985), mooted the possibility of using an ACE inhibitor as first-line monotherapy. The basis for this recommendation was concurrent work with the ACE inhibitor enalapril, which did not contain an SH-group, had not provided evidence of renal or hematologic toxicity (at least not to the same extent as captopril), and had been used as monotherapy in several small studies (Brunner et al., 1983; Bauer and Jones, 1984).

In larger groups of patients, enalapril was shown to bring down mean blood pressure values in patients with mild to moderate hypertension when used in doses of 2.5 to 40 mg/day (Bergstrand et al., 1985). In 116 patients with uncomplicated essential hypertension, a randomized crossover study comparing three doses of enalapril given daily with a placebo showed a "flat" dose-response curve with a major antihypertensive effect at 10 mg daily and a small added effect at 40 mg daily (Salvetti and Arzilli, 1989).

More recently a host of ACE inhibitors have become available, including lisinopril, perindopril, ramipril, quinapril, cilazapril, and many others. They all have in common the capacity to reduce blood pressure when given as monotherapy in patients with mild to moderate hypertension. There is no reason to suppose that the mechanism of antihypertensive effect differs between these agents.

Response rates

Precisely because of the multifactorial causation of hypertension and the multimechanism mode of action of ACE inhibitors, it is not easy to predict whether or not ACE inhibitor monotherapy would be effective in a given patient, although an acute test may be useful (Meredith et al., 1990). In general, a good response to monotherapy can be obtained in only 35% to 70% of patients depending on the dose and criteria used (Williams, 1988). In some series, even higher response rates are reported (Morlin et al., 1987). The concept of response rates is not easy to define, because generally the sodium status of the patients is not reported. The salt intake and the race of the patient may be crucial factors in determining the response to ACE inhibitors. There is an important difference between the response to ACE inhibitor therapy in the individual patient and in a group of patients. In the group as a whole, the mean blood pressure is almost certain to fall because there will be a mixture of excellent, good, and poor responders. A good example of this situation is with ramipril in which the mean intra-arterial blood pressure fell significantly in 12 patients over 24 hours, yet only 7 of the 12 were really responders (Heber et al., 1988).

New end-points

Increasingly, physicians are asking not whether a drug simply lowers blood pressure but a host of more sophisticated questions. What is the quality of life? Are there effects on organ damage, such as ventricular and vascular hypertrophy? What are the effects on renal function? Are the drugs metabolically neutral with reference to blood lipids and glucose, or even beneficial? Are there pharmacokinetic benefits to any particular drug (see Chapter 7)? Are there effects on hard end-points such as mortality, stroke, and heart attacks? While more and more of these questions can now be positively answered for the ACE inhibitors, it must be admitted that proof of reduction of hard end-points must still be obtained. This important aim is being addressed in the Captopril Prevention Project (The CAPPP Group, 1990).

COMPARATIVE STUDIES WITH ACE INHIBITORS IN MILD TO MODERATE HYPERTENSION

ACE inhibitors versus placebo

In a number of studies, there have been careful dose-response observations made with a wide range of doses of the ACE inhibitor used (Table 2–3). The study with the widest range of doses, a 64-fold variation, is that of Gomez et al. (1989) with lisinopril. This study perhaps gives the clearest indication of the apparently "flat" dose-response with ACE inhibitor therapy for hypertension, although the fact that the response was still better at the highest dose used might mean that the top of the range was not studied. The ideal protocol is that in which patients are randomized in a double-blinded manner to one of several doses of a drug and also to concurrent placebo therapy, in a parallel manner. The fall in blood pressure with ACE inhibitor therapy is much more marked when no allowance is made for the concurrent placebo effect (Fig. 2–3) than when allowance is made for the concurrent placebo effect (Fig. 2–4). In every case there is a relatively "flat" dose-response effect from which some "average" antihypertensive doses can be suggested, such as captopril 37.5 to 75 mg daily, enalapril 10 to 20 mg daily, lisinopril 20 to 40 mg daily, perindopril 4 to 8 mg daily, and ramipril 2.5 to 5 mg daily. In attempting to compare these studies, it should be considered that several aspects were not standardized. For example, in none was the salt intake stated. Although the diastolic blood pressure values were taken with the patients supine in most studies, in one the subjects were seated, and in another the posture was not stated. Hence these studies cannot easily be compared.

Antihypertensive effects of ACE inhibitors versus each other

Enalapril and captopril have been extensively compared. Equipotency is given by an enalapril dose about one-fifth or even slightly less than that of captopril (Walker et al., 1984; Chrysant et al., 1985; Lewis et al., 1985; Thind et al., 1985). In one 16-week study, that of Thind et al. (1985), enalapril was claimed to be significantly more effective than captopril, but the blood pressure reductions were very similar.

TABLE 2–3 DOSE-RESPONSE STUDIES OF ACE INHIBITORS IN HYPERTENSION

Drug	Author	Dose range	Initial BP (mmHg)	Number of patients	Study design	Duration (weeks)	Results
Captopril	Veterans Administrtion Co-operative Study Group (1982b)	37.5–150 mg daily in 3 divided doses	146/98 (position not stated)	722	DB, R, parallel, concurrent Pl	7	Increasing dose-response
Enalapril	Bergstrand et al. (1985)	2.5–40 mg in 2 divided doses	156/96 (supine)	91	DB, R, Pl, part parallel part CO	3	Increasing response over the range 5–40 mg daily
Enalapril	Salvetti et al. (1989)	10–40 mg once daily	164/10 (seated)	116	DB, R, PRI, CO, concurrent Pl	4	Similar hypotensive effect over the range 10–40 mg, slightly better effect at 40 mg
Enalapril	Enalapril Study Group (1984)	10–40 mg in 2 divided doses	165/102	28	DB, PRI, parallel	16	Mean daily dose required 20 mg
Fosinopril	Anderson et al. (1991)	10–40 mg once daily	155/100 (supine)	220	DB, R, parallel, concurrent Pl	8	SDBP fall in absence of diuretic (4 weeks): Pl −6, 10 mg −6, 40 mg −11, 80 mg −12 mmHg. Diuretic added if needed at 4 weeks and total results at 8 weeks Pl −10, 10 mg −12, 40 mg −14 and 80 mg −17 mmHg

Drug	Reference	Dose	Baseline BP	n	Design	Weeks	Comments
Lisinopril	Gomez et al. (1989)	1.25–80 mg once daily	161/100 (supine)	216	DB, R, parallel, concurrent Pl	6	Increasing dose-response
Perindopril	Luccioni et al. (1989)	2–8 mg daily	168/106	40	DB, PRI, concurrent Pl	4	Dose-related BP fall over the range, 2 mg similar to placebo
Perindopril	Chrysant et al. (1993)	4–16 mg daily	157/100 (supine)	289	DB, R, parallel, concurrent Pl	16	Increasing dose-response
Ramipril	Heber et al. (1988)	10–40 mg daily	Not stated	12	Intra-arterial 24-hour BP	8	Dose used not stated. 7/12 good responders, 5/12 non-responders
Ramipril	Walter et al. (1987)	1.25–5 mg once daily	173/106 (sitting)	174	DB, R, parallel, no Pl	6	Increasing dose-response cannot exclude placebo effect. DBP fell by 16, 17 and 20 mmHg for doses of 1.25, 2.5 and 5 mg
Ramipril	Vasmant and Bender (1989)	1.25–10 mg once daily	149–154/99–101 (supine)	187	DB, R, parallel, concurrent Pl	12	2.5 mmHg minimum effective dose. Maximum BP fall with 10 mg dose

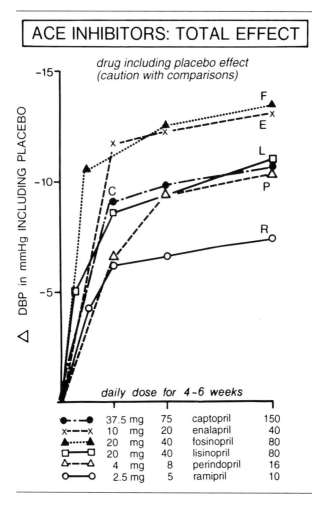

Figure 2–3. *Dose-response studies for differences in diastolic blood pressure (DBP) in response to a variety of ACE inhibitors (as shown in Table 2–3). Fig. © LH Opie.*

In a number of these early studies, for example that by Vlasses et al. (1986), the captopril top dose was rather high, reaching 400 mg daily (in two doses), and the enalapril dose was also high, being 40 mg daily (in two doses). Both agents brought down the blood pressure to a similar extent, and the addition of 50 mg daily of hydrochlorothiazide reduced the blood pressure further by the same amount in each group.

An obvious advantage of enalapril over captopril is the longer half-life and, hence, the presumed requirement for less frequent dosage. In fact, in almost all the comparative studies, enalapril has been given twice daily and captopril three times daily. Claims for differential effects of captopril and enalapril on the quality of life seem to be conflicting (Steiner et al., 1990; Testa et al., 1993). In the study of Lewis et al. (1985), enalapril was given twice daily as was the captopril, and they were equieffective. In an interesting study, Garanin (1986) showed that captopril 50 to 100 mg once-daily was the approximate equivalent of enalapril 10 to 20

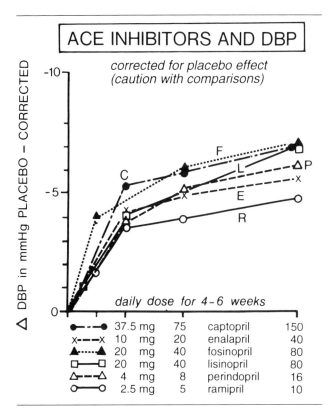

ACE INHIBITORS AND DBP

corrected for placebo effect (caution with comparisons)

daily dose for 4-6 weeks

●——●	37.5 mg	75	captopril	150
x——x	10 mg	20	enalapril	40
▲······▲	20 mg	40	fosinopril	80
□——□	20 mg	40	lisinopril	80
△——△	4 mg	8	perindopril	16
○——○	2.5 mg	5	ramipril	10

Figure 2–4. By excluding concurrent placebo effect, the antihypertensive benefit of ACE inhibitors becomes less striking. A similar placebo effect could probably be found with every other class of antihypertensive agent. In clinical practice, in a correctly treated patient, the real blood pressure response will correspond to that shown in Fig. 2–3. Note that in none of the studies is the salt intake stated, and some studies contain black patients. Hence comparisons of dose-responses between agents are invalid. Fig. © LH Opie.

mg once-daily and that the lower dose of each agent achieved satisfactory blood pressure reduction in about 50% of patients, with the higher dose giving a further 25% blood pressure reduction.

Perindopril and captopril have also been compared. In the Glasgow double-blinded study, 80 patients on perindopril 4 mg daily had a greater fall of diastolic blood pressure than 79 patients on captopril 25 mg twice daily (Lees et al., 1989); side-effects were not significantly different. In patients with inadequate responses, the dose could be doubled and then a diuretic added. In the end, 75% of those initially receiving perindopril achieved satisfactory blood pressure reduction versus 57% of the captopril group.

Perindopril and enalapril had approximately similar effects in a small series of elderly males (Morgan and Anderson, 1992) with equivalent doses being perindopril 4 mg and enalapril 10 mg, or perindopril 8 mg and enalapril 20 mg. Nonetheless, the blood pressure control 24 hours after the dose was better with the longer-acting agent, perindopril (Morgan and Anderson, 1992), as were the trough/peak ratios of efficacy.

Ramipril and captopril are approximately equieffective at daily doses of 10 mg and 100 mg, respectively, as also are *ramipril and enalapril* with doses of 5 to 10 mg ramipril corresponding to 10 to 20 mg enalapril (Todd and Benfield, 1990).

Ramipril and lisinopril. Lisinopril 10 mg daily was not quite as good as ramipril 2.5 mg daily with respective blood pressure reductions of 23/11 mmHg for lisinopril and 27/15 mmHg for ramipril (Koenig, 1992).

Lisinopril and enalapril. In 110 patients randomized to either lisinopril 10 mg or enalapril 10 mg daily, the mean ambulatory blood pressure fell equally (Whelton et al., 1992). Lisinopril did, however, give better control 24 hours after the dose.

ACE inhibitors versus or combined with diuretic therapy

There have been numerous studies showing that ACE inhibitor therapy becomes more effective in the presence of concurrent diuretic therapy (Weinberger, 1982; MacGregor et al., 1982; Weinberger, 1983; Vlasses et al., 1983; Thind et al., 1983; Vidt, 1984; Bauer and Jones, 1984; Freier et al., 1984; Croog et al., 1986; Merrill et al., 1987; Muiesan et al., 1987; Shapiro et al., 1987; Frishman et al., 1987; Kayanakis and Baulac, 1987; Kochar et al., 1987; Zezulka et al., 1987; Gums et al., 1988; Sassano et al., 1989; Zanchetti and Desche, 1989; Brown et al., 1990), or sodium restriction (Morgan and Anderson, 1992). Addition of a diuretic to a standard dose of ACE inhibitor gives a better response than increasing the dose of the ACE inhibitor (Sassano et al., 1989). The combination of captopril 50 mg daily and hydrochlorothiazide 25 mg daily reduced both blood pressure and plasma lipids (Lacourciere and Gagne, 1993). The rationale for the combination is shown in Fig. 2–5. In the case of hydrochlorothiazide, a low dose (12.5 mg daily) can be as effective as a standard dose (25 mg daily) in obtaining better blood pressure control when added to enalapril 20 mg daily (Dahlof et al., 1985). The importance of the so-

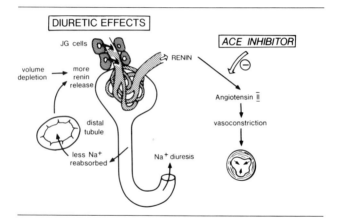

Figure 2–5. Rationale for combination of ACE inhibitors with diuretics. JG, juxtaglomerular. Fig. © LH Opie.

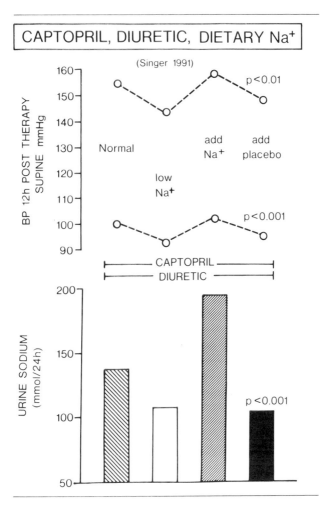

CAPTOPRIL, DIURETIC, DIETARY Na⁺

Figure 2–6. In patients already treated by captopril 50 mg twice daily and a diuretic, hydrochlorothiazide 25 mg once daily, a low-salt diet further reduces the blood pressure and the urine sodium. When sodium is added in the form of Slow-Sodium tablets, blood pressure increases, and urine sodium rises. When Slow-Sodium placebo tablets are given, blood pressure reverts to that found with a low-sodium diet, as does urine sodium. Note highly significant fall in urine sodium and diastolic blood pressure with sodium restriction (righthand column, Slow-Sodium placebo). These data, taken from Singer et al. (1991), show that even in patients who are diuretic treated in addition to receiving an ACE inhibitor a low sodium diet should be advised. The figure is redrawn from the data of Singer et al. (1991) with permission.

dium status in the effect of ACE inhibitor therapy is shown by the *added hypotensive effect of a low sodium diet even in patients already treated by captopril and a diuretic* (Fig. 2–6).

Ethnic effect. Compared with thiazide diuretics, ACE inhibitors are slightly more effective antihypertensive agents in white patients (Perry and Beevers, 1989), especially in younger patients (Materson et al, 1993). Yet in black patients, whether younger or older groups are considered, diuretics are much better especially in the older age group

(Materson et al., 1993). The combination ACE inhibitor plus diuretic gives a better response than ACE inhibitor alone in black patients (Vidt et al., 1984; Pool et al., 1987).

Comparison of metabolic effects of thiazide and captopril: insulin resistance. In an influential study, Pollare et al. (1989) achieved equal blood pressure reduction in a group of patients with initial values of about 165/100 mmHg, using approximately a mean dose of captopril 80 mg daily and of hydrochlorothiazide 40 mg daily. Over the 4 month treatment period, captopril appeared to increase the sensitivity to infused insulin, whereas hydrochlorothiazide appeared to decrease it. Hydrochlorothiazide also increased serum cholesterol and triglyceride levels. No outcome data were presented to indicate that these adverse metabolic effects had hard end-points such as a greater incidence of diabetes mellitus or coronary heart disease. Nonetheless, on first principles, the changes found during thiazide therapy could with justification be regarded as disadvantageous.

A major reservation attached to the Pollare study is that the dose of hydrochlorothiazide (mean daily dose about 40 mg) is considerably higher than that currently recommended for thiazide monotherapy, which should begin at 12.5 mg and be no more than 25 mg daily (Opie and Kaplan, 1990).

ACE inhibitor versus beta-blockade therapy

Many studies have been undertaken to show how various ACE inhibitors compare with beta-blockers (Table 2–4).

Captopril versus propranolol. In the "quality of life" study (Croog et al., 1986), captopril 50 mg twice daily (total dose 100 mg daily) was the approximate equivalent of propranolol 80 mg twice daily (total dose 160 mg daily) on diastolic blood pressure. Systolic values were not reported. It is well known that the study found that captopril caused fewer side-effects than did propranolol and, in fact, improved the quality of life, whereas propranolol did not. It is less well known that added diuretic therapy by hydrochlorothiazide 25 to 50 mg daily was required to control the blood pressure in 33% of captopril-treated patients and only 22% of propranolol-treated patients ($p < 0.02$). The inescapable conclusion must be that, for monotherapy in hypertension, captopril is less effective than propranolol, but propranolol induces more side-effects. Thus, patients felt better on captopril alone than on propranolol, but their blood pressure values were higher.

Captopril versus atenolol. These two drugs were approximately equipotent at fixed doses of captopril 25 mg twice daily and atenolol 50 mg daily, and the quality of life was similar (Palmer et al., 1992).

Enalapril compared with propranolol. The major comparison made by the Enalapril in Hypertension Study Group (1984) was between enalapril 10 to 40 mg daily and propranolol 80 to 240 mg daily with better blood pressure reduction achieved over 12 weeks by enalapril. The mean daily doses used were enalapril 20 mg and propranolol 180 mg. In another study of almost similar size and design (Simon et al., 1984), enalapril was only marginally better than propranolol. Similar results were found in a smaller study by de Leeuw et al. (1983).

Enalapril versus atenolol or metoprolol. In comparison with *atenolol,* enalapril doses of 20 to 40 mg gave better reduction of systolic blood pressure than did atenolol 50 to 100 mg (Gabriel et al., 1985; Webster et al., 1986). In a triple comparison between enalapril, atenolol, and hydrochlorothiazide in a double-blind randomized parallel study, Helgeland et al. (1986) found better systolic blood pressure reduction with enalapril (20 to 40 mg daily) than with atenolol (50 to 100 mg daily). Furthermore, about double the number of patients withdrew from using atenolol as did from enalapril. Whereas enalapril decreased the fasting blood sugar by a small amount, atenolol increased it, also by a small amount. Among the more common side-effects that the atenolol patients had were muscular weakness and cold extremities with an incidence approximately twice that of the enalapril group. Compared with a mean daily dose of 26 mg of *metoprolol,* 309 mg of enalapril was more effective (O'Connor et al., 1984).

Enalapril versus celiprolol. Celiprolol, a new highly selective beta-blocker with vasodilating properties, was the antihypertensive equivalent of enalapril (doses: celiprolol 400 mg daily, enalapril 20 mg daily) in a 2 week trial on only 20 patients with mild to moderate hypertension (Ghiringhelli et al., 1988). However, during exercise the blood pressure increase with celiprolol was much less.

Lisinopril versus atenolol or metoprolol. In a large multicenter study (Bolzano et al., 1987), lisinopril 20 to 80 mg daily was the approximate equivalent of atenolol 50 to 200 mg daily (mean doses not stated). Lisinopril was better at reducing the systolic blood pressure ($p < 0.01$), and fewer patients taking lisinopril required additional diuretic. In a further analysis of the same study, the greater efficacy of lisinopril on systolic blood pressure was chiefly in elderly white patients (Pannier et al., 1991). In yet another study on 144 patients, once again lisinopril reduced systolic blood pressure more than did atenolol (Beevers et al., 1991). In a much smaller study by Thind (1986), lisinopril (mean daily dose 50 mg) reduced blood pressure more than atenolol (mean daily dose 106 mg).

Lisinopril 40 to 80 mg daily was the equivalent of metoprolol 100 to 200 mg, although lisinopril reduced the systolic blood pressure more (Zachariah et al., 1987).

Thus the somewhat surprising finding emerges that lisinopril has a consistently better effect on the systolic blood pressure than atenolol or metoprolol. Similar comparisons in favor of ACE inhibitor therapy come from comparisons of enalapril or perindopril with atenolol (Gabriel et al., 1985; Webster et al., 1986; Zanchetti and Desche, 1989). Hypothetically, the explanation may lie in a specific vascular effect of the ACE inhibitors as considered in Chapter 10.

Cilazapril versus propranolol. A mean cilazapril dose of 2.5 mg daily was compared with propranolol 120 mg daily in a cross-over design of 3 weeks' duration (Belz et al., 1989). Aiming at a diastolic blood pressure response of 90 mmHg or less, only 4 of 13 patients responded to cilazapril

TABLE 2–4 ACE Inhibition Compared with Beta-Blockade in the Therapy of Patients with Mild to Moderate Essential Hypertension

Author	ACE inhibitor	Beta-blocker	Trial design	Duration	Patient number	Percentage response	Daily drug dose	Antihypertensive result
Croog et al. (1986)	Captopril	Propranolol	RDB, parallel	24 weeks	C = 213, P = 212	— —	50 mg 2×, 80 mg 2×, Add HCTZ if needed	C = P but (i) more diuretic for C and (ii) better quality of life on C. *NB.* Cough not evaluated
Belz et al. (1989)	Cilazapril	Propranolol	RDB, PRI, CO	3 weeks	13 (CO design)	Low rates	C 2.5 mg, P 120 mg	C = P
Enalapril Study Group (1984)	Enalapril	Propranolol	RDB, PRI, parallel	12 weeks	E = 26, P = 24	65%, 54%	E 5–20 mg 2×, P 40–120 mg 2×	E>P, Mean doses: E 20 mg, P 180 mg
Simon et al. (1984)	Enalapril	Propranolol	RDB, PRI, parallel	12 weeks	E = 25, P = 21	72%, 67%	E 5–20 mg 2×, P 40–120 mg 2×	E = P, Mean doses: E 21 mg, P 164 mg
de Leeuw et al. (1983)	Enalapril	Propranolol	RDB, PRI, parallel	12 weeks	E = 12, P = 12	— —	E 5–20 mg 2×, P 40–120 mg 2×	E = P
Helgeland et al. (1986)	Enalapril	Atenolol	RDB, PRI, parallel	16 weeks	E = 140, A = 145	— —	E 20–40 mg 1×, A 50–100 mg 1×	E = A DBP, E>Af SBP

Study	Drug	Comparator	Design	Duration	N	%	Doses	Results
Webster et al. (1986)	Enalapril ± HCTZ	Atenolol ± HCTZ	RDB, PRI, parallel	26 weeks	E = 51 A = 43	— —	E 20–40 mg A 50–100 mg	E = A DBP E > A SBP Mean doses: E 37 mg + HCTZ 49 mg A 92 mg + HCTZ 53 mg
Canadian Enalapril Study Group (1987)	Enalapril	Atenolol	RDB, PRI, parallel	14 weeks	E = 86 A = 94	— —	E 10–40 mg 1× A 50–100 mg 1×	E = A Mean doses: E 26 mg, A 80 mg
O'Connor et al. (1984)	Enalapril	Metoprolol	RDB, PRI, parallel	5–7 weeks	E = 12 M = 11	— —	E titrated M titrated	E > M Mean doses: E 26 mg, M 309 mg
Ghiringhelli et al. (1988)	Enalapril	Celiprolol	RSB, PRI, parallel	2 weeks	E = 10 C = 10	— —	E 20 mg 1× C 400 mg 1×	E = C except during exercise when C is greater than E
Bolzano et al. (1987); Pannier et al. (1991)	Lisinopril	Atenolol	RDB, PRI, parallel	8 weeks	L = 284 A = 203	30–70%	L 20–80 mg 1× A 50–200 mg 1×	L = A DBP L > A SBP Mean doses: L 50 mg, A 105 mg
Beevers et al. (1991)	Lisinopril	Atenolol	RDB, PRI, parallel	8 weeks	L = 75 A = 69	L 47% A 55%	L 10–40 mg 1× A 50–100 mg 1×	L = A DBP L > A SBP Mean doses: L 23 mg, A 64 mg

TABLE 2–4 ACE INHIBITION COMPARED WITH BETA-BLOCKADE IN THE THERAPY OF PATIENTS WITH MILD TO MODERATE ESSENTIAL HYPERTENSION (*CONTINUED*)

Author	ACE inhibitor	Beta-blocker	Trial design	Duration	Patient number	Percentage response	Daily drug dose	Antihypertensive result
Thind (1986)	Lisinopril	Atenolol	RDB, PRL, parallel	10 weeks	L = 8 A = 8	—	L 20–60 mg 1× A 50–200 mg 1×	L>A Mean doses: L 50 mg, A 106 mg
Zachariah et al. (1987)	Lisinopril	Metoprolol	RDB, PRL, parallel	8 weeks	L = 118 M = 61	L 63% M 65%	L 40–80 mg 1× M 100–200 mg 1×	L = M DBP L>M SBP
Morgan (1990)	Perindopril	Atenolol	RDB, PRL, parallel	8 weeks	P = 86 A = 86	P 67% A 63%	P 2–8 mg A 25–100 mg	P = A Mean doses: P 5.4 mg, A 63 mg
Zanchetti and Desche (1989)	Perindopril	Atenolol	RDB, PRL, parallel	12 weeks	P = 78 A = 81	P 55% A 48%	P 4–8 mg A 50–100 mg	P = A or P>A (with diuretic) Mean doses: P 4.9 mg, A 67 mg
Hoechst, data on file, quoted by Todd and Benfield (1990)	Ramipril	Atenolol	RDB, PRL, parallel	6 weeks	R = 69 A = 70	R 71% A 71%	R 10 mg 1× A 100 mg 1×	R = A

Abbreviations - as for Table 2–3
HCTZ, hydrochlorothiazide

and 2 of 13 to propranolol, hence the doses chosen were probably too low.

Perindopril versus atenolol. In the Australian Multicenter Study, perindopril 2 to 8 mg daily was the approximate equivalent of atenolol 25 to 100 mg daily (Morgan, 1990). Side-effects were similar in the two groups except that cough, a class side-effect of ACE inhibitors, was more common in the perindopril group. However, it was not established whether the lowest doses of either agent used (2 mg perindopril and 25 mg atenolol, each once daily) were better than placebo. In another study, perindopril 4 to 8 mg was compared with atenolol 50 to 100 mg daily, with hydrochlorothiazide added to each agent if needed (Zanchetti and Desche, 1989). In the end, perindopril controlled hypertension in more patients than did atenolol.

Ramipril versus atenolol. In an unpublished study, cited by Todd and Benfield (1990), ramipril 10 mg once daily was the antihypertensive equivalent of atenolol 100 mg once daily.

Combination of ACE inhibitor and beta-blocker therapy. If ACE inhibitor therapy is most effective for hypertension that is associated with a high plasma renin level and if beta-blockade tends to reduce plasma renin level, then it follows that beta-blockade and ACE inhibition should not be a good antihypertensive combination. However, there are few good studies to test this proposition. In three studies, captopril doses were very much higher than those currently used. First, in 24 patients with moderate to severe hypertension, treated by captopril 150 mg three times daily, the blood pressure fell as the plasma renin activity rose (MacGregor et al., 1982). The addition of hydrochlorothiazide 25 mg twice daily further reduced the blood pressure and increased the plasma renin, whereas the addition of propranolol 20 to 40 mg three times daily decreased plasma renin but did not alter blood pressure. The dose of propranolol at 60 to 120 mg/day is lower than is generally accepted. In a second study, captopril (mean daily dose 350 mg) and propranolol (144 mg) were additive in effect (Pickering et al., 1982). In a third study, again on high-dose captopril up to 450 mg daily, the addition of propranolol up to 360 mg (Jenkins and McKinstry, 1979) showed there was no additional benefit obtained by the combination. In the case of perindopril, the combination with a diuretic is better than with atenolol, yet the latter combination seemed to have some benefit (Zanchetti, 1990). In a small short-term cross-over study, the addition of propranolol 120 mg daily to cilazapril 2.5 mg nearly doubled the fall in diastolic blood pressure and increased the number of responders from 4 of 13 with cilazapril or 2 of 13 with propranolol to 10 of 13 (Belz et al., 1989).

In a large multicenter parallel group study on 100 patients, the addition of lisinopril 10 to 20 mg daily was more effective than placebo in reducing the blood pressure of patients previously inadequately controlled on atenolol 50 mg daily (Soininen et al., 1992).

Clearly the question of combination therapy with ACE inhibitor and beta-blocker needs much further study in prospective carefully designed trials. The small study on cilazapril suggests that the combination could be more promising than previously thought.

Evaluation of ACE inhibitor versus beta-blocker therapy. Review of 15 comparative studies on over 2,000 patients (Table 2–4) reveals that ACE inhibitor monotherapy is almost always as good as beta-blocker monotherapy and sometimes better, particularly in relation to reduction of systolic blood pressure. There are, however, no long-term outcome studies available with ACE inhibitors as there are in the case of beta-blockers. The side-effects of these two types of agents are comparable in incidence although different in nature (Table 2–5). The quality of life is better with ACE inhibitor therapy than with propranolol, and approximately equivalent or slightly better when ACE inhibitors are compared with atenolol or metoprolol (Table 2–5). However, combination with a diuretic may be required more often with ACE inhibitor therapy than with beta-blockade. To achieve optimal response with ACE inhibitor monotherapy requires a low sodium diet. Although the benefits of the combination of ACE inhibition with beta-blockade are controversial, few good studies exist so that the combination warrants further appraisal.

ACE inhibitors compared with or combined with calcium antagonists

Although ACE inhibitors have not been so well compared with calcium antagonists as with beta-blockers, a number of studies testify to the approximate equivalence of the antihypertensive effects of both types of agents (Table 2–6). The different antihypertensive mechanisms involved are shown in Fig. 2–7.

Captopril versus or combined with nifedipine. One of the first studies to compare captopril with nifedipine was that by Guazzi et al. (1984) which was detailed in its design in that patients were admitted to hospital and blood pressure values taken every 6 hours. Even though only a small number of patients (14) was studied, the data showed an antihypertensive effect after 1 week of nifedipine use (blood pressure fell from 178/114 mmHg to 152/103 mmHg at the end of the week) and a further effect with combination with captopril (mean blood pressure by the end of the week was 141/91 mmHg), yet the data for the initial treatment by captopril are not presented in figures but only visually. From the figure it can be estimated that the systolic blood pressure reduction with nifedipine was much better than with captopril (the doses used were 10 mg every 4 hours for nifedipine and 25 mg every 4 hours for captopril). Clearly the combination therapy was better, but again the data must be judged visually.

In another study in patients with moderately severe essential hypertension (initial mean blood pressure at entry 168/107 mmHg), captopril 25 mg three times daily reduced the mean blood pressure by 12 mmHg and the further addition of nifedipine (20 mg tablet form twice daily) reduced the blood pressure by an additional 10 mmHg (Singer et al., 1987). Conversely, in patients initially treated by nifedipine, the blood pressure fell by 17 mmHg, and with the addition of captopril, there was a further fall of 11 mmHg. A defect of the combined therapy used in this study was its relatively short duration of action, and 12 hours after therapy the blood pressure was nearly back to pretreatment values with captopril alone, but there was still a detectable reduction when captopril was combined with nifedipine. Thus the combined therapy was effectively longer acting than monotherapy (Singer et al., 1987).

Captopril versus nitrendipine. Captopril has also been compared with and then combined with nitrendipine by Gennari et al. (1989). In a single-blind randomized placebo-controlled study, 24 patients were divided into two groups (12 in each group) receiving either 20 mg nitrendipine as a single oral daily dose or 50 mg captopril twice daily for 4 weeks. Captopril 100 mg daily reduced the mean supine blood pressure from 174/109 mmHg to 163/98 mmHg. Nitrendipine 20 mg daily reduced the blood pressure from 174/109 mmHg to 160/95 mmHg. Thereafter a placebo washout period of 4 weeks followed, and then the patients were continued on a combination of half of the initial doses, i.e., nitrendipine 10 mg daily and captopril 50 mg daily, whereupon the final blood pressure was 155/92 mmHg, i.e., better than with the higher dose of each agent separately.

Enalapril versus nifedipine. In a double-blind parallel-group study, 65 patients receiving enalapril 10 to 40 mg once daily were compared with 63 receiving nifedipine retard 10 to 40 mg twice daily (MacLean et al., 1990). Doses were titrated to achieve blood pressure values of below 150 mmHg systolic and below 90 mmHg diastolic, taken about 3 hours post-dose. Such values were achieved in only about 45% of patients with either treatment. Mean daily doses are not given, but in the case of enalapril can be deduced from another report to be 33 mg daily (Yeo et al., 1991). Although standing blood pressure was lower on nifedipine, symptomatic orthostatic hypotension was more frequent in enalapril treated patients, whereas flushing, edema, and palpitations occurred more commonly with nifedipine. Enalapril seemed to be better tolerated, in that 7% of the enalapril group and 22% of the nifedipine group were withdrawn because of adverse effects. Also, compliance was better in the enalapril group.

Enalapril versus isradipine. In a dose-titrated randomized double-blind parallel-group study (Eisner et al., 1991), enalapril (mean daily dose 20.5 mg in two doses) was the approximate equivalent of isradipine (6.5 mg daily in two doses); diastolic blood pressure fell more with isradipine but since half the patients were black, a group known not to respond so well to the ACE inhibitors, this study will need further analysis to separate out the effects of these two agents according to ethnic group.

Lisinopril versus nifedipine. Lisinopril 20 to 80 mg daily was regarded as the equivalent of nifedipine retard 40 to 80 mg daily in two studies with, however, the lisinopril somewhat better tolerated in that 13 to 21% of patients reported an adverse effect with lisinopril and 50 to 57% with nifedipine (p < 0.01 in both studies)(Morlin et al, 1987; Richardson et al., 1987). Lisinopril-treated patients more often

TABLE 2–5 COMPARATIVE STUDIES ON QUALITY OF LIFE AND SIDE-EFFECTS OF ACE INHIBITORS VERSUS BETA-BLOCKERS

Author	Drugs compared	Trial duration	Mean daily doses (mg)	Patient number	Effects on BP	Effects on quality of life	Side-effects
Croog et al. (1986)	Captopril Propranolol	24 weeks	C 100 P 160	213 212	Equal but more diuretic required with C	C>P for general wellbeing, sexual function, and physical symptoms	Withdrawals C8%, P13%, NS Fatigue P>C
Palmer et al. (1992)	Captopril Atenolol	6 weeks	C 50 A 50	144 152	Equal, but added diuretic doses not stated	C = A	A caused sleepiness and blocked nose; C caused cough
Lichter et al. (1986)	Enalapril Atenolol	16 weeks	E 20–40 A 50–100	12 13	Equal but diuretic added in 45% of E and 33% of A	E>A for memory	Incidence of adverse effects similar (Webster et al, 1986)

Study	Drugs	Duration	Doses	n		Comments
Steiner et al. (1990)	Captopril Enalapril Propranolol Atenolol	8 weeks	C 50–210 (94) E 5–40 (12) P 80–240 (133) A 50–100 (56)	69 80 73 78	E>C E>P (SBP)	E=C=A and all better than P	Adverse experiences: C52%, E57%, P64%, A56% Dropouts (any reason): C25%, E10%, P19%, A11%
Dietrich and Herrmann (1989)	Cilazapril Metoprolol	2 weeks	C 2.5 M 200 (Both plus diuretic)	23 23 (CO)	Normal patients	C = M for memory C>M for sleep	(Normal subjects)

Abbreviations - as for Table 2–3

TABLE 2–6 ACE INHIBITORS COMPARED WITH CALCIUM ANTAGONISTS IN PATIENTS WITH MILD TO MODERATE HYPERTENSION

Author	ACE inhibitor	Calcium antagonist	Trial design	Duration	Patient number	Daily drug dose	Antihypertensive result	Tolerability and other effects
Guazzi et al. (1984)	Captopril	Nifedipine capsules	R, Pl, CO	1 week	C = 14 N = 14 (CO)	C 25 mg 4× N 10 mg 4×	C = N, C + N = best	C > N (foot volume lower)
Singer et al. (1987)	Captopril	Nifedipine retard	R, no Pl, parallel	4 weeks	C = 10 N = 9	C 25 mg 3× N 20 mg 2×	N > C, N + C = best	Equal
Gennari et al. (1989)	Captopril	Nitrendipine	SBR, PRI, parallel	14 weeks	C = 12 N = 12	C 50 mg 2× N 20 mg 1×	N > C, N + C = best (Combination C50, N10)	Equal
MacLean et al. (1990)	Enalapril	Nifedipine retard	DBR, PRI, parallel	8 weeks	E = 65 N = 63	E 10–40 mg 1× N 10–40 mg 2×	N > E, standing BP N = E, sitting BP	E > N (more N withdrawals)
Maharaj and van der Byl (1993)	Enalapril	Isradipine SRO	DBR, PRI, parallel	8 weeks	E = 27 I = 25 (all black)	E 10–29 mg 1× I 2.5–5 mg 1× (mean doses: E 18, I 4.7)	I > E supine I = E erect	

Study	ACE inhibitor	Comparator	Design	Duration	N	Doses	BP result	Notes
Eisner et al. (1991)	Enalapril	Isradipine	DBR, PRI, parallel	10 weeks	E = 8 I = 78 (50–65% black)	E 2.5–20 mg 2× I 1.25–5 mg 2× (mean doses: I 6.5, E 20.5)	I>E DBP I = E SBP	Equal
Morlin et al. (1987)	Lisinopril	Nifedipine retard	DBR, PRI, parallel	12 weeks	L = 89 N = 47	L 20–80 mg 1× N 20–40 mg 2×	L = N	L>N (more N withdrawals, more N side-effects)
Os et al. (1991)	Lisinopril	Nifedipine (? retard)	DBR, PRI, parallel	10 weeks	L = 412 N = 416	L 10–40 mg 1× N 10–40 mg 2× (mean doses: L 19, N 37)	L>N	L>N (more N withdrawals more N side-effects)
Richardson et al. (1987)	Lisinopril	Nifedipine retard	DBR, PRI, parallel	12 weeks	L = 30 N = 15	L 20–80 mg 1× N 20–40 mg 2× (mean doses: L 36, N 48)	L = N	L>N (more N adverse side-effects)
Schulte et al. (1992)	Perindopril	Nifedipine retard	DBR, PRI, parallel	24 weeks	P = 20 N = 20	P 4–8 mg 1× N 20–40 mg 2×	P = N or P>N	LV mass fell with both

Abbreviations - as for Table 2–3

SB, single-blind; SRO, modified slow release oral preparation.

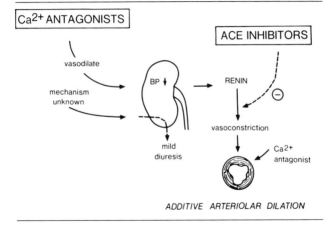

Figure 2–7. Rationale for combination of calcium antagonists with ACE inhibitor therapy. Both agents are arteriolar dilators acting through different mechanisms and therefore additive. Calcium antagonists by vasodilation tend to raise plasma renin and also act as mild diuretics. Both of these effects should sensitize the patient to the combination of these two agents. Fig. © LH Opie.

needed an added diuretic than the nifedipine group (Richardson et al., 1987). In contrast, in a large Norwegian study on 828 patients, lisinopril (titrated 10 to 40 mg daily, mean dose 19 mg) was better than titrated nifedipine (mean dose 37 mg) and also had fewer side-effects (Os et al., 1991).

Lisinopril versus amlodipine, felodipine, and diltiazem. In small groups of patients studied at different times, lisinopril titrated to a mean dose of 25 mg was the approximate equivalent of amlodipine 9 mg, felodipine 15 mg, and diltiazem 278 mg (Omvik and Lund-Johansen, 1993). Judging by the degree of reduction of blood pressure at rest, lisinopril was better than these three other agents; however, it seemed as if a diuretic or low-salt diet was often added.

Perindopril versus nifedipine. In a small study, perindopril 4 to 8 mg daily was the approximate equivalent of nifedipine 40 to 80 mg daily (Schulte et al., 1992).

Combination of ACE inhibitors and calcium antagonists. In the studies of both Guazzi et al. (1984) and Singer et al. (1987), captopril plus nifedipine gave better blood pressure reduction than either agent alone. In 16 patients with moderately severe hypertension, monotherapy with a calcium antagonist (verapamil or nitrendipine) did not satisfactorily reduce the diastolic blood pressure, but the combination of captopril and a calcium antagonist (verapamil 500 mg daily or nitrendipine 70 mg daily) was successful in 15 of 16 patients (Brouwer et al., 1985).

Isradipine monotherapy (1.25 or 2.5 mg twice daily) brought down diastolic blood pressure from a mean of 100 mmHg to below 95 mmHg in 64% of patients (Yodfat and Cristal, 1993), whereas further addition of captopril increased the response rate to 90%.

The combination of nitrendipine (10 mg once daily) and captopril (25 mg twice daily) reduced blood pressure more than double the dose of either agent alone (Gennari et al., 1989).

The combination of nitrendipine and cilazapril in patients with mild chronic renal failure produced larger blood pressure reductions than either agent alone (Kloke et al., 1989).

Evaluation of ACE inhibitor therapy compared with or combined with calcium antagonists. Compared with calcium antagonists, ACE inhibitors are approximately equieffective antihypertensive agents, often with fewer side-effects. The ACE inhibitors are more likely to be effective at lower blood pressure levels, with an estimated threshold of efficacy at 120/80 mmHg compared with that of calcium antagonists at 135/85 mmHg (Herpin et al., 1992). Yet an optimal response to ACE inhibitors requires a low sodium diet and, fairly frequently, the addition of a diuretic. ACE inhibitors are much less likely to be effective in black patients (Materson et al., 1993). Regarding the calcium antagonist-ACE inhibitor combination, there are only a relatively small number of studies. Yet the attraction of these agents in combination is that neither has any negative central effects nor adverse effects on blood lipid profile nor on metabolic parameters, such as plasma potassium or uric acid. Both types of agents act peripherally without any central nervous component, as far as is known. Both agents may have beneficial effects on renal function. Therefore, the combination calcium antagonist-ACE inhibitor is likely to be studied more frequently in the future and to be used more often. The only defect of this combination, as far as is known, is cost. An additional problem that must be emphasized is that there are no long-term outcome studies in hypertension with this combination, nor for that matter with either of the components.

ACE inhibitors versus centrally acting agents

Captopril versus clonidine. Captopril (mean daily dose 75 mg) was the approximate equivalent of clonidine (mean daily dose 0.43 mg) in the VA study (Materson et al., 1993). In whites, captopril was somewhat better, whereas in blacks, clonidine was better. Only patients receiving clonidine, however, had significantly more side-effects during the titration phase than patients receiving captopril or placebo. Thus clonidine had many more side-effects.

Captopril versus methyldopa. Both agents reduced blood pressure, but captopril gave a much better quality of life (Croog et al., 1986).

LARGE MULTIDRUG STUDIES

Two recent large studies on male subjects have compared an ACE inhibitor with a calcium antagonist, a beta-blocker, a diuretic and an alpha-blocker as first-line therapy (Table 2–7). In very mildly hypertensive patients with a mean blood pressure of only 140/91 mmHg and all receiving lifestyle advice and a low salt diet, there was no difference in the hypotensive potencies of the various drugs used, all in low doses (TOHM study, 1993). Metabolically, the diuretic increased the plasma total cholesterol at 1 but not 4 years (TOHM study, 1991), whereas the beta-blocker unexpectedly decreased LDL-cholesterol and, as expected, triglyceride levels. It should be recalled that acebutolol has

TABLE 2-7 COMPARISON OF TWO LARGE MULTIDRUG TRIALS IN MALES. EACH TRIAL INVOLVED FIVE OR MORE TYPES OF DRUGS

	TOHM study (1993)	Materson (VA)(1993)
ACE inhibitors (ACE)	enalapril (5 mg)	captopril (75 mg)
Alpha-blocker (α)	doxazosin (2 mg)	prazosin (13 mg)
Beta-blocker (β)	acebutolol (400 mg)	atenolol (64 mg)
Calcium antagonist (Ca)	amlodipine (5 mg)	diltiazem (272 mg)
Diuretic (D)	chlorthalidone (15 mg)	hydrochlorothiazide (48 mg)
Number of patients (approx per group)	125	180
Duration of study	4 years	1 year
Mean initial BP	140/91 (mmHg)	152/99 (mmHg)
SBP fall, range	11–15 (mmHg)[+]	9–16 (mmHg)

DBP fall, range	10–14 (mmHg)[+]	10–14 (mmHg)
Side-effects[+]	lightheaded ACE, α; SOB α; impotent D	fatigue α; sleepiness α; dizziness α
Blood lipids	D, transient (1 year) rise	rise in D vs fall in α
Blood potassium	fall D	no data
Blood glucose	unchanged	rise in D
Blood uric acid	rise, D	no data
White, younger group (mean age 51)	no data	ACE > β > α > Ca > D
White, older group (mean age 66)	no data	β > Ca > ACE > D > α
Black, younger group (mean age 49)	no data	Ca > β > D > α > ACE
Black, older group (mean age 66)	no data	Ca > D > α > β ACE no effect

(), fixed dose in TOHM study, mean dose in VA study; >, better than; BP, blood pressure; S, systolic; D, diastolic; SOB, shortness of breath + Drugs added to nutritional measures and weight loss.

specific qualities, namely cardioselectivity and intrinsic sympathomimetic activity (ISA). The diuretic also increased plasma uric acid and decreased potassium values. Most parameters judging the quality of life were unchanged in all groups, except that the "general functioning index" improved slightly with the beta-blocker and with the diuretic, whereas it fell with the alpha-blocker. In virtually all aspects, the ACE inhibitor had similar side-effects to placebo. Paradoxically, the diuretic *increased* the incidence of impotence, whereas the alpha-blocker gave the lowest incidence of impotence. It follows that at least some of the male patients "functioned" better if they had impotence (sexual intercourse is a strain?).

Whereas the TOHM study was largely on whites (80%), the second had 42% blacks (Materson et al., 1993). Although each of the five categories of drugs used in the TOHM report was also used, none of the drugs were the same. A sixth drug, clonidine, was also used and gave good antihypertensive results, yet with unacceptable side-effects. The incidence of sleepiness increased 5-fold, dry mouth 6-fold, and fatigue 2-fold. Hence, clonidine is left out of further evaluation. The hypotensive effects of the drugs differed according to race and age. In younger whites (mean age 50 years) the ACE inhibitor captopril was most effective, with 55% of patients responding. Then came the beta-blocker atenolol, then the alpha-blocker prazosin, then the calcium antagonist diltiazem, and lastly the diuretic. In older whites, the ACE inhibitor only came third. In younger blacks, the ACE inhibitor came last, and in older blacks, it was no better than placebo. There was no information on salt intake, which could have differed between the races and the age groups. As in the TOHM study, the diuretic gave rise to most metabolic disturbances. Side-effects were worse for the alpha-blocker. This study shows the major impact of race and to a lesser extent of age on the use of ACE inhibitors for hypertension.

Hemodynamic effects. In a unique study, Omvik and Lund-Johansen (1993) sequentially undertook hemodynamic studies on 171 white patients in non-matched groups, using nine different drugs, the tenth group receiving a low salt diet. There was also an untreated control group. Each patient was subject to outpatient drug titration for 6 to 12 months before the second hemodynamic study. Lisinopril (mean daily dose 25 mg) gave the second best pressure reduction at rest, exceeded only by the combined alpha-beta blocker carvedilol (mean daily dose 52 mg). Of importance is that, when lisinopril was accompanied by a low salt diet or by hydrochlorothiazide 12.5 to 25 mg daily, it reduced the total peripheral resistance as much as did carvedilol or the calcium antagonists.

ACE INHIBITOR THERAPY FOR SEVERE OR REFRACTORY HYPERTENSION

Acute therapy

Of the ACE inhibitors, captopril, which is not a prodrug, has one of the most rapid onsets of action and has been used in the therapy of acute severe hypertension. In the study of Tschollar and Belz (1985), the initial mean blood pressure of 6 patients was 233/132 mmHg; 30 minutes after sublingual captopril the values were very much lower. However, the data are only reported in Letter form, so that it is difficult to assess this study critically. In another acute study by Biollaz et al. (1983), in 9 previously untreated patients with severe hypertension, the mean blood pressure decreased from 239/134 mmHg to 204/118 mmHg 30 minutes following captopril 25 mg. These patients were previously untreated and needed urgent blood pressure reduction because of symptoms and signs of neurologic/cardiologic complications. A point of interest is that the maximal hypotensive effect of captopril only occurred 4 hours after administration; however, by that time 5 of the 9 patients had been given additional intravenous furosemide, so it is not possible to conclude whether the total hypotensive effect was due to captopril or the combination captopril-furosemide.

An intravenous preparation of captopril can be given to promote a smooth blood pressure reduction (Padfield et al, 1985); an initial mean blood pressure of 199/115 mmHg came down to 143/86 mmHg over several hours after a very low dose of captopril, which was associated with a plasma level of only 15 ng/ml.

Whereas acute oral therapy of a hypertensive emergency by captopril is one of several promising therapeutic approaches, it should be noted that it is difficult in the emergency situation to exclude bilateral renal artery stenosis or severe unilateral renal artery stenosis, either of which could result in an excess precipitous fall in blood pressure or even serious prolonged renal failure.

ACE inhibitor therapy combined with other agents for apparently refractory hypertension

In the early phases of its use, captopril appeared to achieve miracles, since many apparently resistant patients did in fact have high renin states with marked angiotensin-induced vasoconstrictor tone. In such patients, often with renal artery stenosis, the response to captopril was dramatic (Studer et al., 1981).

In "standard" resistant hypertension, the efficacy of *combined ACE inhibitor and diuretic therapy* can be striking. In patients with severe uncontrolled hypertension with a mean arterial pressure exceeding 140 mmHg and the majority with accelerated hypertension, there was a good response to captopril combined with furosemide; nonetheless, it should be noted that the captopril dose was very high—up to 450 mg daily—and likewise the furosemide dose went up to 1 g daily (White et al., 1980).

In patients with less severe hypertension and mean initial values of about 200/120 mmHg, captopril combined with hydrochlorothiazide reduced the blood pressure by about 15% with a slightly lesser fall during exercise (12%)(Omvik and Lund-Johansen, 1984).

Other workers have not been so enthusiastic about the combination captopril-loop diuretic (Swales et al., 1982). Of

15 patients with severe hypertension in that study, 9 achieved acceptable blood pressure control but there were 6 treatment failures. On the other hand, satisfactory blood pressure control was achieved in a somewhat comparable group of patients by the combination diuretic plus beta-blocker plus hydralazine plus prazosin.

When comparing captopril with hydralazine or nifedipine as third-line agent after a beta-blocker plus diuretic combination, captopril was marginally better in these white patients of mean age 55 years (Bevan et al., 1993). Mean daily doses were captopril 119 mg, hydralazine 135 mg, and nifedipine retard 68 mg. An unexpected benefit of hydralazine was reduction of blood lipid levels.

Although not well documented, practical experience at the Groote Schuur Hospital Hypertension Clinic is that patients with really severe hypertension almost always require quadruple drug therapy consisting of ACE inhibitor plus diuretic plus calcium antagonist plus beta-blocker and often also an alpha-blocker. This combination, if conscientiously applied, usually obviates the need for minoxidil, a very useful agent (Swales et al., 1982) but with unfavorable effects, such as hirsutism and skin thickening.

Scleroderma crisis

In patients with scleroderma (progressive systemic sclerosis), there may be the combination of a rapid fall-off in renal function together with malignant hypertension. At least some of these patients respond to captopril therapy, and the suggestion is that early captopril therapy will lessen severe renal impairment (Brogden et al., 1988).

ACE Inhibitors in Special Groups of Patients

In general, ACE inhibitors can be used in most clinical situations that are associated with hypertension. In the presence of aortic stenosis, caution is required to avoid excess blood pressure falls, thereby increasing the gradient across the valve, and in bilateral renal artery stenosis these drugs are contraindicated.

Diabetic hypertension

Because of the neutral or possibly favorable effects of ACE inhibitors and carbohydrate metabolism (Pollare et al., 1989) and the consistent reports showing a decrease in microalbuminuria, it has been proposed that ACE inhibitors should be preferential therapy for diabetic hypertensive patients (Perry and Beevers, 1989). Captopril improves hard end-points in diabetic nephropathy (Lewis et al., 1993).

Chronic pulmonary disease

In some patients, ACE inhibitors may improve pulmonary function by decreasing hypoxic vasoconstriction (Bertoli et al., 1986); nonetheless, the high incidence of cough as a side-effect is disturbing. Although it is reasonably well established that ACE inhibitors do not precipitate asthma and in this way are completely different from beta-blockers, an irritating cough in a patient with pulmonary disease can be disabling and distressing.

Hypertensive heart failure

In view of the great efficacy of ACE inhibitors in heart failure, the combination ACE inhibitor-diuretic should be prime therapy for such patients presenting with congestive heart failure.

Hypertension and peripheral vascular disease

In a placebo-controlled cross-over study, continuing over 6 months, captopril 25 mg twice daily was compared with atenolol 100 mg once daily, labetalol 200 mg twice daily or pindolol 10 mg twice daily (Roberts et al., 1987). Each active agent was given for 1 month. At equieffective blood pressure lowering doses, only captopril did not reduce walking distance. Postexercise calf blood flow was impaired by all the beta-blockers but not by captopril. Thus, beta-blockers, even those with added alpha-blockade or intrinsic sympathomimetic activity, were less effective than captopril in maintaining walking distance in patients with intermittent claudication. Therefore, ACE inhibitors can be regarded as better therapy.

Hypertension and coronary artery disease

In such patients ACE inhibitors can be expected to have neutral or possibly mildly beneficial effects. In contrast to beta-blockers, ACE inhibitors cannot be expected to have a consistent antianginal effect unless they act to relieve the increased oxygen demand induced by left ventricular wall dilation in left ventricular failure or unless they act by an antihypertensive effect (see also Chapter 4).

Postinfarct hypertension

There are no formal studies on such patients. Beta-blockers remain one of the agents of choice because of their known effect in improving postinfarct mortality. On the other hand, ACE inhibitors may be freely used, particularly in view of their beneficial effects on postinfarct prognosis in patients with left ventricular dysfunction. Therefore, it would be logical to combine ACE inhibitors with beta-blockers should the beta-blocker therapy be ineffective or to prefer ACE inhibitors should there be a risk of developing heart failure.

Hypertension and renal disease

This group is reviewed in Chapter 3. Although ACE inhibitors are generally regarded as safe in patients with chronic renal failure, occasionally deterioration of renal function takes place (see Chapter 8). In patients with renovascular hypertension, ACE inhibitor therapy is the cornerstone of the medical management. Although renal failure is a risk in patients with bilateral renal artery stenosis or stenosis of a solitary kidney, Hollenberg (1983) found only 6% of such patients developed renal failure.

The elderly

Current indications are that ACE inhibitors can be almost as effective as monotherapy in the elderly as in younger whites, despite the low renin status of most elderly patients. In a large multicenter study, lisinopril (mean daily dose 50 mg) was as effective in elderly patients as in those whose age was below 65 years (Pannier et al., 1991). In 12 elderly patients, with chiefly systolic hypertension (initial blood pressure 189/89 mmHg sitting), a mean dose of captopril of 50 mg twice daily reduced the blood pressure to 172/83 mmHg (Cox et al., 1989). Captopril monotherapy was also effective in another small group of elderly patients (Katz, 1986). In 34 elderly patients, perindopril reduced blood pressure from a mean of 185/95 mmHg to 164/87 mmHg (Forette et al., 1989). In the study on six possible first-line antihypertensive drugs, captopril was the best for younger whites (mean age 50), third best in older whites (mean age 66), but strikingly ineffective in older blacks (Materson et al., 1993).

Hypertension in black patients

Here it seems as if ACE inhibitors are not as effective as in white patients, so that concurrent diuretic therapy is often required to achieve a benefit (Veterans Administration Cooperative Study Group, 1982a). Thus, in that study, white patients had a mean seated blood pressure decrease of 14.7/10.7 mmHg in response to captopril, whereas the blood pressure of black patients fell by 9.1/7.9 mmHg. After administration of hydrochlorothiazide, equal blood pressure decreases were found in the two racial groups. In the case of enalapril, hydrochlorothiazide addition rendered the drug equally effective in black and white patients (Vidt, 1984). In the case of lisinopril, there were similar racial differences in the response (Pannier et al., 1991), and even the addition of hydrochlorothiazide did not achieve as great a blood pressure fall in black patients as in white patients (Pool et al., 1987). In the recent VA study, older black males did not respond at all to captopril (Materson et al., 1993). In a much smaller study on South African blacks aged 18 to 65 (no mean given), enalapril was partially effective (Table 2–6).

As a group, black patients are thought to have low-renin hypertension (Savage et al., 1990), which logically should respond less well to ACE inhibitors. Logically too, a low-salt diet and/or diuretic therapy should increase renin levels and make the patients more susceptible to ACE inhibitor therapy. It should be recalled, though, that despite the general trend to lower renin values in black patients, in one large series on 371 subjects, 42% had low-renin hypertension, 46% had normal renin values, and 12% had high values (Mroczek et al., 1973).

Left ventricular hypertrophy

The proposed molecular mechanisms whereby ACE inhibitors could affect left ventricular hypertrophy are reviewed in Chapter 4. There are several studies showing that ACE inhibitors improve left ventricular hypertrophy (Dunn et al., 1984; Pfeffer 1985). In a prospective randomized trial comparing the effects of ACE inhibitor therapy with beta-blockade, enalapril (mean daily dose 31 mg) in 28 patients gave the same antihypertensive effect as did bisoprolol (mean daily dose 17 mg) in 21 patients, and both reduced left ventricular mass over 6 months (Gosse et al., 1990). Perindopril and nifedipine were equally effective in achieving left ventricular regression over 6 months (Schulte et al., 1992).

In a meta-analysis of 109 studies on 2,357 patients, ACE inhibitors, beta-blockers, and calcium antagonists all induced left ventricular regression (Dahlof et al., 1992). Of these, ACE inhibitors were the most effective (about 15% loss of left ventricular mass) with beta-blockers and calcium antagonists each reducing left ventricular mass by about 10%.

High blood uric acid

Diuretics may cause hyperuricemia and predispose to gout by inducing renal retention of urate. In contrast, ACE inhibitors increase renal urate excretion in normal volunteers and in hypertensive patients (Leary and Reyes, 1987). The mechanism of this uricosuric effect is not known, but it does indicate that ACE inhibitor therapy could be a prime choice for patients with gout and hypertension or for hypertensive hyperuricemic patients. However caution is required in that a vigorous uricosuric effect may precipitate gouty stones so that the ACE inhibitors should be instituted gradually (Leary and Reyes, 1987).

Pregnancy

Since the initial reports linking captopril usage to possible skull defects and oligohydramnios, and the finding of toxicity in animal studies, captopril has been regarded as an embryopathic drug that should be avoided or used with great caution in pregnancy. By analogy, other ACE inhibitors have the same restriction, and recently the Food and Drugs Administration in the United States has required a prominent warning against the use of all ACE inhibitors during the second and third trimesters of pregnancy (see Chapter 8). If, therefore, there is a specific indication for an ACE inhibitor in pregnancy hypertension, the agent of choice should be used carefully and in the lowest possible dose. An example would be unilateral renal artery stenosis discovered in pregnancy and not responding to other types of therapy.

ACUTE TESTING OF ACE INHIBITORS

Not all patients respond to one specific type of drug given as first-line monotherapy. In the case of ACE inhibitors, an acute test may predict long-term response (Meredith et al., 1990). Unfortunately, a full therapeutic dose cannot be routinely used as a test dose because patients with high-renin hypertension are at risk of excessively decreasing the blood pressure when given standard doses of the ACE inhibitor (Webster et al,, 1985). A reasonable practical policy might be to give a low initial test dose of captopril (6.25 mg) and to wait for 30 minutes. If there is no excessive response sensitivity to the ACE inhibitor, another 25 mg of captopril can be given. If the blood pressure comes down within another hour, then the patient is potentially responsive to ACE inhibition and the agent of choice can then be given long-term. This approach does not, however, exclude a placebo response. The patient should be on a low sodium diet for optimal response. Alternatively, low-dose diuretic therapy may be added as needed. Although this policy has no documentation in the literature, it seems reasonable and practicable.

COMPARATIVE EVALUATION OF ACE INHIBITORS AS ANTIHYPERTENSIVE AGENTS

General comparison

The data available show that ACE inhibitors are acceptable first-line antihypertensive agents, and that there are relatively few contraindications in comparison with other agents. ACE inhibitors can be used in a variety of co-existing disease states (Stumpe and Overlack, 1993). Although expensive, they do not precipitate diseases, such as diabetes or gout, as in the case of diuretics nor do they pose respiratory problems nor exaggerate congestive heart failure as in the case of beta-blockers. Any such precipitation of a co-existing disease can dramatically increase the cost of antihypertensive therapy. Situations specifically favoring the use of ACE inhibitors as first-line antihypertensive agents include (Table 2–7) patients with high-renin hypertension or low-renin hypertension on a low salt diet; when optimal intellectual and physical activity is essential; and when maintenance of normal metabolic status is crucial. As a group, white males with a mean age of 50 years respond very well to the ACE inhibitor captopril (Materson et al., 1993). Certain co-existing disease states favor the use of ACE inhibitor therapy, including large vessel vascular disease, left ventricular hypertrophy, diabetic nephropathy, and the presence of left ventricular failure. On the other hand, there are a number of situations suggesting caution or reserve in the use of ACE inhibitors as first-line antihypertensive agents (Table 2–7). These include patients on a high salt diet, black patients, when expense is crucial, and when there is a pre-existing dry cough. In addition, there are a number of uncommon absolute or relative contraindications including bilateral renal artery stenosis, stenosis in a single kidney, unilateral renal artery stenosis in the presence of excess diuresis, and sodium-depleted patients with severe congestive heart failure.

Comparison of ACE inhibitors with diuretic therapy (Table 2–8)

The following factors favor ACE inhibitors as first choice agents: type-II noninsulin-requiring diabetes or family history of diabetes, gout or family history of gout, hyperlipidemia or a borderline lipid profile, or when the salt intake is low. On the other hand, diuretics should be considered as first-line agents when cost is crucial, when the salt intake is high and cannot easily be reduced, when there is renal disease with sodium retention, or when the patient is black. In obese patients, there is some evidence favoring the use of diuretics and ACE inhibitors are not specifically reported as being beneficial.

Comparison of ACE inhibitors with beta-blockers (Table 2–9)

As first-line therapy, the initial use of ACE inhibitors should be favored when there is left ventricular failure, when peak physical and mental activity is required, when there is hyperlipidemia or a borderline lipid profile, when there is borderline glucose tolerance, in the presence of diabetes mellitus especially with nephropathy, when there is peripheral vascular disease, when the hypertension is predominantly systolic, and when there are contraindications to beta-blockade therapy. On the other hand, favoring the use of beta-blockers is the co-existence of ischemic heart disease, angina or the postinfarct state unaccompanied by left ventricular dilation; co-existing anxiety or tachycardia; pre-existing dry cough; and pregnant hypertensive patients. Neither type of agent is suited for first-line therapy of black hypertensive patients.

TABLE 2–8 HYPERTENSION: ACE INHIBITOR THERAPY VERSUS DIURETICS

Favoring ACE inhibitors as first choice

1. Type-II diabetes or family history of diabetes or diabetic nephropathy

2. Gout or family history of gout

3. Hyperlipidemia or borderline lipid profile

4. When salt intake is low

5. When there is left ventricular hypertrophy

Favoring diuretics as first choice

1. When cost is crucial

2. When salt intake is high and cannot easily be reduced

3. When there is renal disease with sodium retention

4. In blacks

5. Possibly in obese patients

6. When ACE inhibitors are contraindicated

TABLE 2–9 HYPERTENSION: COMPARATIVE PROPERTIES OF ACE INHIBITORS VERSUS BETA-BLOCKERS

Situations favoring initial use of ACE inhibitors

1. Left ventricular failure or postinfarct left ventricular dysfunction

2. When optimal or peak physical and mental activity is required

3. Hyperlipidemia or borderline lipid profile

4. Borderline glucose tolerance

5. Diabetes mellitus especially with nephropathy

6. Peripheral vascular disease

7. Systolic hypertension

8. Early postinfarct patients to avoid left ventricular remodeling

9. Contraindications to beta-blockade (asthma, left ventricular failure, conduction disturbances, psychogenic depression, active peripheral vascular disease)

Situations favoring beta-blockade

1. Ischemic heart disease, angina, postinfarct prophylaxis

2. Co-existing anxiety or tachycardia

3. Pregnant hypertensive patients

4. Patients with dry cough or contraindications to ACE inhibitors (bilateral renal artery stenosis and related conditions)

Note: Neither type of agent is indicated for first-line therapy of black hypertensive patients

Comparison of ACE inhibitors with calcium antagonists (Table 2–10)

Both agents have numerous similar positive arguments as first-line therapy. For example, both ACE inhibitors and calcium antagonists are claimed to maintain optimal physical and mental activity, to be lipid neutral, not to alter insulin tolerance, to revert left ventricular hypertrophy, to inhibit experimental atherosclerosis, to improve arterial compliance, to treat diabetic nephropathy, and to benefit Raynaud's phenomenon. ACE inhibitors are preferred therapy in the presence of left ventricular systolic failure when calcium antagonists are contraindicated, and when there is combination therapy with diuretics (because calcium antagonists have some diuretic properties of their own). Calcium antagonists are preferred in combination with beta-blockers where the evidence is that at least some ACE inhibitors do not show a fully additive antihypertensive effect when combined with beta-blockers. Calcium antagonists are preferred in black patients and when there is co-existing angina especially on a vasospastic basis. In severe urgent hypertension, both agents can be shown to work, but there must always be some risk of occult renal artery stenosis, which is a relative contraindication to ACE inhibitors. There is a strong contraindication when the stenosis is bilateral.

TABLE 2–10 COMPARATIVE ASSESSMENT OF ACE INHIBITORS WITH CALCIUM ANTAGONISTS

Both are claimed to:

1. Maintain optimal physical, mental and sexual activity, with no central side-effects (ACE inhibitors better documented for quality of life.

2. Be lipid neutral.

3. Leave insulin tolerance unchanged or possibly improved (ACE inhibitors better documented).

4. Revert left ventricular hypertrophy (ACE inhibitors may be better).

5. Inhibit experimental atherosclerosis (calcium antagonists better documented).

6. Improve arterial wall compliance (ACE inhibitors better documented especially perindopril).

7. Improve diabetic nephropathy (ACE inhibitors better documented).

8. Improve Raynaud's phenomenon (calcium antagonists much better documented).

ACE inhibitors preferred initial therapy:

1. When there is co-existing left ventricular systolic failure (calcium antagonists contraindicated).

2. In combination with diuretics.

3. When the salt intake is low.

4. In postinfarct left ventricular dysfunction.

Calcium antagonists preferred:

1. In combination with beta-blockers.

2. In blacks.

3. When salt intake is high.

4. When angina is associated especially on a vasospastic basis.

5. In severe urgent hypertension.

Summary of first-line therapy

The particular properties of a given patient can define whether that patient is a strong candidate for first-line ACE inhibitor therapy (Table 2–10) or whether there should be caution or reserve (Table 2–11). The minimal side-effects of these agents (often limited to cough), the simplicity of use, a flat dose-response curve, the virtual absence of contraindications except for bilateral renal artery stenosis and some related types of renal impairment, and ready combination with other modalities of treatment, as well as acceptability by the elderly, are all factors promoting the increasing use of these agents. However, use in pregnancy is contraindicated. Whether, in addition, ACE inhibitors have a superior capacity to normalize vascular abnormalities in hypertension still remains to be proven although this is an increasingly considered possibility.

TABLE 2–11 SITUATIONS FAVORING THE USE OF
ACE INHIBITORS AS FIRST-LINE
ANTIHYPERTENSIVE AGENTS

1. High-renin hypertension or low-renin hypertension on low
   salt diet

2. When maintenance of optimal "quality of life" is crucial
   • Exercise capacity
   • Intellectual activity
   • Sexual function

3. When maintenance of normal metabolic status is crucial with
   the following aims:
   • Avoiding insulin resistance
   • Unaltered diabetic control
   • Lipid-neutrality

4. Presence of large vessel vascular disease
   • Loss of aortic compliance
   • Peripheral vascular disease

5. Presence of left ventricular hypertrophy

6. Diabetic nephropathy (with or without hypertension)
   • Microalbuminuria
   • Proteinuria
   • Type I insulin-requiring diabetes (Chapter 12)

7. Presence of congestive heart failure (low test dose essential
   especially if over-diuresed)

8. Postinfarct left ventricular dysfunction

SUMMARY

The picture that emerges is that ACE inhibitors are a group
of agents effective in blood pressure reduction in most patient groups except when given as monotherapy to blacks.
There is a relatively low cost in terms of side-effects and
contraindications. Although ACE inhibitors are highly effective in high-renin patients, yet in elderly whites, a low-
renin group, these agents work well as monotherapy. In
general, they are about as effective as other potential first-
line agents, such as the diuretics, beta-blockers, and calcium antagonists. In white males, mean age 51 years, ACE
inhibitors are better than five other types of drugs. Regarding combination therapy, a particularly attractive combination is that with diuretics, because diuretics increase circulating renin activity and angiotensin-II levels, which ACE
inhibitors counterregulate by inhibiting the conversion of
angiotensin-I to angiotensin-II. Adding a low dose diuretic
to a standard dose of ACE inhibitor seems more effective
than increasing the ACE inhibitor dose and sensitizes black
patients to the antihypertensive effects of ACE inhibitors.
In addition, an oft neglected point is dietary sodium restriction should be advised for all patients receiving ACE inhib-

itor monotherapy or ACE inhibitor plus diuretic therapy. A drug combination now receiving increasing attention is that of ACE inhibitor with calcium antagonist. Both types of drugs are metabolically neutral and preserve the quality of life.

REFERENCES

Anderson RJ, Duchin KL, Gore RD, et al. Once-daily fosinopril in the treatment of hypertension. *Hypertension* 1991; 17: 636–642.

Bauer JH, Jones LB. Comparative studies: enalapril versus hydrochlorothiazide as first-step therapy for the treatment of primary hypertension. *Am J Kidney Dis* 1984; 4: 55–62.

Beevers DG, Blackwood RA, Garnham S, et al. Comparison of lisinopril versus atenolol for mild to moderate essential hypertension. *Am J Cardiol* 1991; 67: 59–62.

Belz GG, Essig J, Erb K, et al. Pharmacokinetic and pharmacodynamic interactions between the ACE inhibitor cilazapril and beta-adrenoceptor antagonist propranolol in healthy subjects and in hypertensive patients. *Br J Clin Pharmacol* 1989; 27: 317S–322S.

Bergstrand R, Herlitz H, Johansson S, et al. Effective dose range of enalapril in mild to moderate essential hypertension. *Br J Clin Pharmacol* 1985; 19: 605–611.

Bertoli L, Lo Cicero S, Busnardo I, et al. Effects of captopril on hemodynamics and blood gases in chronic obstructive lung disease with pulmonary hypertension. *Respiration* 1986; 49: 251–256.

Bevan EG, Pringle SD, Waller PC, et al. Comparison of captopril, hydralazine and nifedipine as third drug in hypertensive patients. *J Human Hypertens* 1993; 7: 83–88.

Biollaz J, Waeber B, Brunner HR. Hypertensive crisis treated with orally administered captopril. *Eur J Clin Pharmacol* 1983; 25: 145–149.

Bolzano K, Arriaga J, Bernal R, et al. The antihypertensive effect of lisinopril compared to atenolol in patients with mild to moderate hypertension. *J Cardiovasc Pharmacol* 1987; 9 (Suppl 3): S43–S47.

Boni E, Alicandri C, Fariello R, et al. Effect of enalapril on parasympathetic activity. *Cardiovasc Drugs Ther* 1990; 4: 265–268.

Brogden RN, Todd PA, Sorkin EM. Captopril. An update of its pharmacodynamic and pharmacokinetic properties, and therapeutic use in hypertension and congestive heart failure. *Drugs* 1988; 36: 540–600.

Brouwer RML, Bolli P, Erne P, et al. Antihypertensive treatment using calcium antagonists in combination with captopril rather than diuretics. *J Cardiovasc Pharmacol* 1985; 7: S88–S91.

Brown CL, Backhouse CI, Grippat JC, Santoni JP. The effect of perindopril and hydrochlorothiazide alone and in combination on blood pressure and on the renin-angiotensin system in hypertensive subjects. *Eur J Clin Pharmacol* 1990; 39: 327–332.

Brunner HR, Waeber B, Nussberger J, et al. Long-term clinical experience with enalapril in essential hypertension. *J Hypertens* 1983; 1 (Suppl 1): 103–107.

Campese VM. Salt sensitivity in hypertension. Renal and cardiovascular implications. *Hypertension* 1994; 23: 531–550.

Canadian Enalapril Study Group. Comparison of monotherapy with enalapril and atenolol in mild to moderate hypertension. *Can Med Assc J* 1987; 137: 803–808.

The CAPPP group. The Captopril Prevention Project: a prospective intervention trial of angiotensin converting enzyme inhibition in the treatment of hypertension. *J Hypertens* 1990; 8: 985–990.

Case DB, Wallace JM, Keim HJ, et al. Possible role of renin in hypertension as suggested by renin-sodium profiling and inhibition of converting enzyme. *N Engl J Med* 1977; 296: 641–646.

Chrysant SG, Singh BI, Johnson B, McPherson M. A comparative study of captopril and enalapril in patients with severe hypertension. *J Clin Pharmacol* 1985; 25: 149–151.

Chrysant SG, McDonald RH, Wright JT, et al. for the Perindopril Study Group. Perindopril as monotherapy in hypertension: a multicenter comparison of two dosing regimens. *Clin Pharmacol Ther* 1993; 53: 479–484.

Cox JP, Duggan J, O'Boyle CA, et al. A double-blind evaluation of captopril in elderly hypertensives. *J Hypertens* 1989; 7: 299–303.

Croog SH, Levine S, Testa MA, et al. The effect of antihypertensive therapy on the quality of life. *N Engl J Med* 1986; 314: 1657–1664.

Dahlof B, Andren L, Eggertsen R, et al. Potentiation of the antihypertensive effect of enalapril by randomized addition of different doses of hydrochlorothiazide. *J Hypertens* 1985; 3 (Suppl 3): S483–S486.

Dahlof B, Pennert K, Hansson L. Reversal of left ventricular hypertrophy in hypertensive patients. A meta-analysis of 109 treatment studies. *Am J Hypertens* 1992; 5: 95–110.

de Leeuw PW, Hoogma RPLM, van Soest GAW, et al. Physiological effects of short-term treatment with enalapril in hypertensive patients. *J Hypertens* 1983; 1 (Suppl 1): 87–91.

Dietrich B, Herrmann WM. Influence of cilazapril on memory functions and sleep behaviour in comparison with metoprolol and placebo in healthy subjects. *Br J Clin Pharmacol* 1989; 27: 249S–261S.

Dunn FG, Oigman W, Ventura HO, et al. Enalapril improves systemic and renal hemodynamics and allows regression of left ventricular mass in essential hypertension. *Am J Cardiol* 1984; 53: 105–108.

Eisner GM, Johnson BF, McMahon FG, et al. A multicenter comparison of the safety and efficacy of isradipine and enalapril in the treatment of hypertension. *Am J Hypertens* 1991; 4: 154S–157S.

Enalapril in Hypertension Study Group. Enalapril in essential hypertension: a comparative study with propranolol. *Br J Clin Pharmacol* 1984; 18: 51–56.

Forette F, McClaran J, Delesalle MC, et al. Value of angiotensin converting enzyme inhibitors in the elderly: the example of perindopril. *Clin Exper Theory Pract* 1989; A11 (Suppl 2): 587–603.

Freier PA, Wollam GL, Hall WD, et al. Blood pressure, plasma volume, and catecholamine levels during enalapril therapy in blacks with hypertension. *Clin Pharmacol Ther* 1984; 36: 731–737.

Frishman WH, Goldberger J, Sherman D. Enalapril, hydrochlorothiazide, and combination therapy in patients with moderate hypertension. *J Clin Hypertens* 1987; 3: 520–527.

Gabriel MA, Tscianco MC, Kramsch DM, Moncloa F. Once-a-day enalapril compared with atenolol in hypertension (abstr). *Clin Pharmacol Ther* 1985; 37: 198.

Garanin G. A comparison of once-daily antihypertensive therapy with captopril and enalapril (abstr). *Curr Ther Res* 1986; 40: 567.

Gennari C, Nami R, Pavese G, et al. Calcium-channel blockade (nitrendipine) in combination with ACE inhibition (captopril) in the treatment of mild to moderate hypertension. *Cardiovasc Drugs Ther* 1989; 3: 319–325.

Ghiringhelli S, Cozzi E, Tsialtas D. Hemodynamic effects of celiprolol at rest and during exercise; a comparison with enalapril. *Cardiovasc Drugs Ther* 1988; 2: 211–218.

Gomez HJ, Cirillo VJ, Sromovsky JA, et al. Lisinopril dose-response relationship in essential hypertension. *Br J Clin Pharmacol* 1989; 28: 415–420.

Gosse P, Roudaut R, Herrero G, Dallocchio M. Beta-blockers vs angiotensin-converting enzyme inhibitors in hypertension: effects on left ventricular hypertrophy. *J Cardiovasc Pharmacol* 1990; 16 (Suppl 5): S145–S150.

Guazzi MD, De Cesare N, Galli C, et al. Calcium-channel blockade with nifedipine and angiotensin-converting enzyme inhibition with captopril in the therapy of patients with severe primary hypertension. *Circulation* 1984; 70: 279–284.

Gums JG, Lopez MN, Quay GP, et al. Comparative evaluation of enalapril and hydrochlorothiazide in elderly patients with mild to moderate hypertension. *Drug Intell Clin Pharmacol* 1988; 22: 680–684.

Heber ME, Brigden GS, Caruana MP, et al. First dose response and 24-hour antihypertensive efficacy of the new once-daily angiotensin converting enzyme inhibitor, ramipril. *Am J Cardiol* 1988; 62: 239–245.

Helgeland A, Strommen R, Hagelund CH, Tretli S. Enalapril, atenolol and hydrochlorothiazide in mild to moderate hypertension. A comparative multicentre study in general practice in Norway. *Lancet* 1986; 1: 872–875.

Herpin D, Vaisse B, Pitiot M, et al. Comparison of angiotensin-converting enzyme inhibitors and calcium antagonists in the treatment of mild to moderate systemic hypertension, according to baseline ambulatory blood pressure level. *Am J Cardiol* 1992; 69: 923–926.

Hollenberg NK. Medical therapy of renovascular hypertension: efficacy and safety of captopril in 269 patients. *Cardiovasc Rev Rep* 1983; 4: 852–876.

Hollenberg NK, Meggs LG, Williams GH, et al. Sodium intake and renal responses to captopril in normal man and in essential hypertension. *Kidney Int* 1981; 20: 240–245.

Jenkins AC, McKinstry DN. Review of clinical studies of hypertensive patients treated with captopril. *Med J Aust* 1979; 2 (Suppl): 32–37.

Jenkins AC, Dreslinski GR, Tadros SS, et al. Captopril in hypertension: seven years later. *J Cardiovasc Pharmacol* 1985; 7: S96-S101.

Kaplan NM, Opie LH. Antihypertensive drugs. In: Opie LH (ed), *Drugs for the Heart*, Third Edition. WB Saunders Company, Philadelphia, 1991, 155–179.

Katz LA. Captopril for geriatric hypertensives. *J Hypertens* 1986; 4 (Suppl 5): S426–S428.

Kayanakis JG, Baulac L. The comparative study of once-daily administration of captopril 50 mg, hydrochlorothiazide 25 mg and their combination in mild to moderate hypertension. *Br J Clin Pharmacol* 1987; 23: 89S–92S.

Kloke HJ, Huysmans FThM, Wetzels JFM, et al. Antihypertensive effects of nitrendipine and cilazapril alone, and in combination in hypertensive patients with chronic renal failure. *Br J Clin Pharmacol* 1989; 27: 289S–296S.

Kochar MS, Bolek G, Klabfleisch JH, et al. A 52 week comparison of lisinopril, hydrochlorothiazide and their combination in hypertension. *J Clin Pharmacol* 1987; 27: 373–377.

Koenig W, on behalf of the Multicentre Study Group. Ramipril vs lisinopril in the treatment of mild to moderate primary hypertension—a randomised double-blind multicentre trial. *Drug Invest* 1992; 4: 450–457.

Lacourciere Y, Gagne C. Influence of combination of captopril and hydrochlorothiazide on plasma lipids, lipoproteins and apolipoproteins in primary hypertension. *J Human Hypertens* 1993; 7: 149–152.

Leary WP, Reyes AJ. Angiotensin-I converting enzyme inhibitors and the renal excretion of urate. *Cardiovasc Drugs Ther* 1987; 1: 29–38.

Lees KR, Reid JC, Scott MG, et al. Captopril versus perindopril: a double-blind study in essential hypertension. *J Human Hypertens* 1989; 3: 17–22.

Lewis EJ, Hunsicker LG, Bain RP, Rohde RD for the Collaborative Study Group. The effect of angiotensin-converting enzyme inhibition on diabetic nephropathy. *N Engl J Med* 1993; 329: 1456–1462.

Lewis RA, Baker KM, Ayers CR, et al. Captopril versus enalapril maleate: a comparison of antihypertensive and hormonal effects. *J Cardiovasc Pharmacol* 1985; 7 (Suppl 1): S12–S15.

Lichter I, Richardson PJ, Wyke MA. Differential effects of atenolol and enalapril on memory during treatment for essential hypertension. *Br J Clin Pharmacol* 1986; 21: 641–645.

Luccioni R, Frances Y, Gass R, Gilgenkrantz JM. Evaluation of the dose-effect relationship of perindopril in the treatment of hypertension. *Clin Exper Theory Prac* 1989; A11 (Suppl 2): 521–534.

MacGregor GA, Markandu ND, Banks RA, et al. Captopril in essential hypertension; contrasting effects of adding hydrochlorothiazide or propranolol. *Br Med J* 1982; 284: 693–696.

MacGregor GA, Markandu ND, Singer DA, et al. Moderate sodium restriction with angiotensin converting enzyme inhibitor in essential hypertension: a double blind study. *Br Med J* 1987; 294: 531–534.

MacLean D, Ramsay LE, Richardson PJ. Enalapril and nifedipine in the treatment of mild to moderate essential hypertension: a 6 month comparison. *Br J Clin Pharmacol* 1990; 30: 203–211.

Maharaj B, van der Byl K. A comparative study of isradipine SRO and enalapril in black patients with mild-to-moderate hypertension. *Am J Hypertens* 1993; 6: 80S–81S.

Materson BJ, Reda DJ, Cushman WC, et al. Single-drug therapy for hypertension in men. A comparison of six antihypertensive agents with placebo. *N Engl J Med* 1993; 328: 914–921.

Meredith PA, Donnelly R, Elliott HL, et al. Prediction of the antihypertensive response to enalapril. *J Hypertens* 1990; 8: 1085–1090.

Merrill DD, Byymy RL, Carr A, et al. Lisinopril/HCTZ in essential hypertension (abstr). *Clin Pharmacol Ther* 1987; 41: 227.

Morgan TO. Australian Multicenter Study of perindopril compared with atenolol in the management of hypertension. *JAMA* 1990; 6 (Suppl): 18–22.

Morgan T, Anderson A. Clinical efficacy of perindopril in hypertension. *Clin Exp Pharmacol Physiol* 1992; 19 (Suppl 19): 61–65.

Morlin C, Baglivo H, Boeijinga JK, et al. Comparative trial of lisinopril and nifedipine in mild to severe essential hypertension. *J Cardiovasc Pharmacol* 1987; 9 (Suppl 3): S48–S52.

Mroczek WJ, Finnerty FA, Catt KJ. Lack of association between plasma-renin and history of heart attack or stroke in patients with essential hypertension. *Lancet* 1973; 2: 464–469.

Muiesan G, Agabiti-Rosei E, Buoninconti R, et al. Antihypertensive efficacy and tolerability of captopril in the elderly: comparison with hydrochlorothiazide and placebo in a multicentre double-blind study. *J Hypertens* 1987; 5 (Suppl 5): S599–S602.

O'Connor DT, Mosley CA, Cervenka J, Bernstein KN. Contrasting renal haemodynamic responses to the angiotensin converting enzyme inhibitor enalapril and the beta-adrenergic agonist metoprolol in essential hypertension. *J Hypertens* 1984; 2 (Suppl 2): 89–92.

Omvik P, Lund-Johansen P. Combined captopril and hydrochlorothiazide therapy in severe hypertension: long-term haemodynamic changes at rest and during exercise. *J Hypertens* 1984; 2: 73–80.

Omvik P, Lund-Johansen P. Long-term hemodynamic effects at rest and during exercise of newer antihypertensive agents and salt restriction in essential hypertension: review of epanolol, doxazosin, amlodipine, felodipine, diltiazem, lisinopril, dilevalol, carvedilol, and ketanserin. *Cardiovasc Drugs Ther* 1993; 7: 191–206.

Opie LH, Kaplan NM. Diuretics. In: Opie LH (ed). *Drugs for the Heart*, Third Edition. WB Saunders, Philadelphia, 1990, 74–99.

Os I, Bratland B, Dahlof B, et al. Lisinopril or nifedipine in essential hypertension. A Norwegian multicenter study on efficacy, tolerability and quality of life in 828 patients. *J Hypertens* 1991; 9: 1097–1104.

Padfield PL, Rademaker M, Atherden SM, et al. Inhibition of the renin-angiotensin-aldosterone axis by low dose intravenous captopril as a treatment for accelerated phase hypertension. *J Hypertens* 1985; 3 (Suppl 3): S475–S477.

Palmer AJ, Fletcher AE, Rudge PJ, et al. Quality of life in hypertensives treated with atenolol or captopril: a double-blind crossover trial. *J Hypertens* 1992; 10: 1409–1416.

Pannier BE, Garabedian VG, Madonna O, et al. Lisinopril versus atenolol: decrease in systolic versus diastolic blood pressure with converting enzyme inhibition. *Cardiovasc Drugs Ther* 1991; 5: 775–782.

Perry IJ, Beevers DG. ACE inhibitors compared with thiazide diuretics as first-step antihypertensive therapy. *Cardiovasc Drugs Ther* 1989; 3: 815–819.

Pfeffer JM. Role of afterload reduction by angiotensin converting enzyme inhibition in the regression of cardiac hypertrophy in hypertension. *ACE Report* 18; 1985; 1–4.

Pickering TG, Case DB, Sullivan PA, Laragh JH. Comparison of antihypertensive and hormonal effects of captopril and propranolol at rest and during exercise. *Am J Cardiol* 1982; 49: 1566–1568.

Pollare T, Lithell H, Berne C. A comparison of the effects of hydrochlorothiazide and captopril on glucose and lipid metabolism in patients with hypertension. *N Engl J Med* 1989; 321: 868–873.

Pool JL, Gennari J, Goldstein R, et al. Controlled multicentre study of antihypertensive effects of lisinopril, hydrochlorothiazide, and lisinopril plus hydrochlorothiazide in the treatment of 394 patients with mild to moderate essential hypertension. *J Cardiovasc Pharmacol* 1987; 9 (Suppl 3): S36–S42.

Richardson PJ, Meany B, Breckenridge AM, et al. Lisinopril in essential hypertension: a six month comparative study with nifedipine. *J Human Hypertens* 1987; 1: 175–179.

Roberts DH, Tsao Y, McLoughlin GA, Breckenridge A. Placebo-controlled comparison of captopril, atenolol, labetalol, and pindolol in hypertension complicated by intermittent claudication. *Lancet* 1987; 2: 650–653.

Salvetti A, Arzilli F. Chronic dose-response curve of enalapril in essential hypertensives. An Italian Multicenter Study. *Am J Hypertens* 1989; 2: 352–354.

Sanchez RA, Marco E, Gilbert HB, et al. Natriuretic effect and changes in renal haemodynamics induced by enalapril in essential hypertension. *Drugs* 1985; 30 (Suppl 1): 49–58.

Sassano P, Chatellier G, Billaud E, et al. Comparison of increase in the enalapril dose and addition of hydrochlorothiazide as second-step treatment of hypertensive patients not controlled by enalapril alone. *J Cardiovasc Pharmacol* 1989; 13: 314–319.

Savage DD, Watkins LO, Grim CE, Kumanyika SK. Hypertension in black populations. In: Laragh JH, Brenner BM (eds), *Hypertension, Pathophysiology, Diagnosis, and Management.* Raven Press, New York, 1990, 1837–1852.

Schulte K-L, Meyer-Sabellek W, Liederwald K, et al. Relation to regression of left ventricular hypertrophy to changes in ambulatory blood pressure after long-term therapy with perindopril versus nifedipine. *Am J Cardiol* 1992; 70: 468–473.

Shapiro DL, Liss CL, Walker JF, et al. Enalapril and hydrochlorothiazide as antihypertensive agents in the elderly. *J Cardiovasc Pharmacol* 1987; 10 (Suppl 7): S160–S162.

Simon AL, Levenson JA, Bouthier JD, et al. Comparison of oral MK-421 and propranolol in mild to moderate essential hypertension and their effects on arterial and venous vessels of the forearm. *Am J Cardiol* 1984; 53: 781–785.

Singer DRJ, Markandu ND, Shore AC, MacGregor GA. Captopril and nifedipine in combination for moderate to severe essential hypertension. *Hypertension* 1987; 9: 629–633.

Singer DRJ, Markandu ND, Sugden AL, et al. Sodium restriction in hypertensive patients treated with a converting enzyme inhibitor and a thiazide. *Hypertension* 1991; 17: 798–803.

Soininen K, Gerlin-Piira L, Suihkonen J, et al. A study of the effects of lisinopril when used in addition to atenolol. *J Human Hypertens* 1992; 6: 321–324.

Steiner SS, Friedhoff AJ, Wilson BL, et al. Antihypertensive therapy and quality of life: a comparison of atenolol, captopril, enalapril and propranolol. *J Human Hypertens* 1990; 4: 217–225.

Studer A, Luscher T, Siegenthaler W, Vetter W. Captopril in various forms of severe therapy-resistant hypertension. *Klin Wochenschr* 1981; 59: 59–67.

Stumpe KO, Overlack A, on behalf of the Perindopril Therapeutic Safety Study Group (PUTS). A new trial of the efficacy, tolerability, and safety of angiotensin-converting enzyme inhibition in mild systemic hypertension with concomitant diseases and therapies. *Am J Cardiol* 1993; 71: 32E–37E.

Swales JD, Bing RF, Haegerty A, et al. Treating refractory hypertension. *Lancet* 1982; 1: 894–896.

Taylor T, Moore TJ, Hollenberg NK, Williams GH. Converting-enzyme inhibition corrects the altered adrenal response to angiotensin-II in essential hypertension. *Hypertension* 1984; 6: 92–99.

Testa MA, Anderson RB, Nackley JF, Hollenberg NK, and the Quality-of-Life Hypertension Study Group. Quality of life and antihypertensive therapy in men. A comparison of captopril with enalapril. *N Engl J Med* 1993; 328: 907–913.

Thind GS. Lisinopril versus atenolol alone and with hydrochlorothiazide in the treatment of mild to moderate hypertension. *J Hypertens* 1986; 4 (Suppl 5): S423–S425.

Thind GS, Mahapatra RK, Johnson A, Coleman RD. Low-dose captopril titration in patients with moderate-to-severe hypertension treated with diuretics. *Circulation* 1983; 67: 1340–1346.

Thind GS, Johnson A, Bhatnagar D, Henkel TW. A parallel study of enalapril and captopril and 1 year of experience with enalapril treatment in moderate-to-severe essential hypertension. *Am Heart J* 1985; 109: 852–858.

Todd PA, Benfield P. Ramipril. A review of its pharmacological properties and therapeutic efficacy in cardiovascular disorders. *Drugs* 1990; 1: 110–135.

TOHM study—Treatment of Mild Hypertension Research Group (TOMH). The treatment of mild hypertension study. A randomized, placebo-controlled trial of a nutritional-hygienic regimen along with various drug monotherapies. *Arch Intern Med* 1991; 151: 1413–1423.

TOMH study—Neaton JD, Grimm RH, Prineas RJ, et al. for the Treatment of Mild Hypertension Study Research Group. Treatment of mild hypertension study. Final results. *JAMA* 1993; 270: 713–724.

Tschollar W, Belz GG. Sublingual captopril in hypertensive crises (Letter). *Lancet* 1985; 2: 34–35.

Vasmant D, Bender N. The renin-angiotensin system and ramipril, a new converting enzyme inhibitor. *J Cardiovasc Pharmacol* 1989; 14 (Suppl 4): S46–S52.

Veterans Administration Co-operative Study Group. Racial differences in response to low-dose captopril are abolished by the addition of hydrochlorothiazide. *Br J Clin Pharmacol* 1982a; 14: 97S–101S.

Veterans Administration Cooperative Study Group on Antihypertensive Agents. Captopril: evaluation of low doses, twice-daily doses and the addition of diuretic for the treatment of mild to moderate hypertension. *Clin Sci* 1982b; 63 (Suppl 8): 443S–445S.

Vidt DG. A controlled multiclinic study to compare the antihypertensive effects of MK-421, hydrochlorothiazide, and MK-421 combined with hydrochlorothiazide in patients with mild to moderate essential hypertension. *J Hypertens* 1984; 2 (Suppl 2): 81–88.

Vlasses PH, Rotmensch HH, Swanson BN, et al. Comparative antihypertensive effects of enalapril maleate and hydrochlorothiazide, alone and in combination. *J Clin Pharmacol* 1983; 23: 227–233.

Vlasses PH, Conner DP, Rotmensch HH, et al. Double-blind comparison of captopril and enalapril in mild to moderate hypertension. *J Am Coll Cardiol* 1986; 7: 651–660.

Walker JF, Kulaga SF, Kramsch DM. The efficacy and safety of enalapril in moderate to severe essential hypertension. *J Hypertens* 1984; 2 (Suppl 2): 107–111.

Walter U, Forthofer R, Witte PU. Dose-response relation to angiotensin converting enzyme inhibitor ramipril in mild to moderate essential hypertension. *Am J Cardiol* 1987; 59: 125D–132D.

Webster J, Newnham DM, Petrie JC. Initial dose of enalapril in hypertension. *Br Med J* 1985; 290: 1623–1624.

Webster J, Petrie JC, Robb OJ, et al. Enalapril in moderate to severe hypertension: a comparison with atenolol. *Br J Clin Pharmacol* 1986; 21: 489–495.

Weinberger MH. Comparison of captopril and hydrochlorothiazide alone and in combination in mild to moderate essential hypertension. *Br J Clin Pharmacol* 1982; 14: 127S–131S.

Weinberger MH. Influence of an angiotensin-converting enzyme inhibitor on diuretic-induced metabolic effects in hypertension. *Hypertension* 1983; 5 (Suppl III): 132–138.

Whelton A, Dunne B, Glazer N, et al. Twenty-four hour blood pressure effect of once-daily lisinopril, enalapril, and placebo in patients with mild to moderate hypertension. *J Human Hypertens* 1992; 6: 325–331.

White NJ, Rajagopalan B, Yahaya H, Ledingham JGG. Captopril and frusemide in severe drug-resistant hypertension. *Lancet* 1980; 2: 108–110.

Williams GH. Converting-enzyme inhibitors in the treatment of hypertension. *N Engl J Med* 1988; 319: 1517–1525.

Yeo WW, MacLean D, Richardson PJ, Ramsay LE. Cough and enalapril: assessment by spontaneous reporting and visual analogue scale under double-blind conditions. *Br J Clin Pharmacol* 1991; 31: 356–359.

Yodfat Y, Cristal N on behalf of the LOMIR^R-MCT-IL Research Group. A multicenter, double-blind, randomized, placebo-controlled study of isradipine and methyldopa as monotherapy or in combination with captopril in the treatment of hypertension. *Am J Hypertens* 1993; 6: 57S–61S.

Zachariah PK, Bonnet G, Chrysant SG, et al. Evaluation of antihypertensive efficacy of lisinopril compared to metoprolol in moderate to severe hypertension. *J Cardiovasc Pharmacol* 1987; 9 (Suppl 3): S53–S58.

Zanchetti A. A re-examination of stepped-care: a retrospective and a prospective. *J Cardiovasc Pharmacol* 1985; 7 (Suppl 1): S126–S131.

Zanchetti A. First-line treatment in hypertension. Role of perindopril. *Drugs* 1990; 3 (Suppl 1): 71–75.

Zanchetti A, Desche P. Perindopril : first-line treatment for hypertension. *Clin Exper Theory Pract* 1989; A11 (Suppl 2): 555–573.

Zezulka AV, Gill JS, Dews I, et al. Comparison of enalapril and bendrofluazide for treatment of systemic hypertension. *Am J Cardiol* 1987; 59: 630–633.

CHAPTER 3

ACE Inhibitors and the Kidney

"The importance of angiotensin in the regulation of renal vascular resistance is beyond doubt" (Dollery, 1988).

ANGIOTENSIN-II AND RENAL PHYSIOLOGY

Renal hemodynamic effects of angiotensin-II

The importance of the renal circulation as a potential site of action of angiotensin-converting enzyme (ACE) inhibitors is now established. These agents can potentially modulate intraglomerular pressure because it is the angiotensin-II receptors in the proximal part of the renal afferent arterioles that help to control the intraglomerular filtration pressure, as shown by Edwards (1983) who infused angiotensin-II into isolated renal microvessels. The glomerular filtration pressure is the result of the balance between the preglomerular and postglomerular arterial tone (Fig. 3–1). Thus, the relative degree of constriction or relaxation of efferent and afferent arterioles regulates the filtration pressure and the amount of protein excreted. This normal balance between afferent and efferent arteriolar control can be altered in diseased states, such as diabetes mellitus, with an increase of the intraglomerular filtration pressure so that microalbuminuria occurs. Experimental evidence favoring differential regulation of preglomerular and postglomerular arterial tone is provided by measurements of renal vascular resistance during the administration of calcium antagonists or ACE inhibitors to dogs (Navar et al., 1986).

If the major effects of angiotensin-II on the renal circulation are at the level of the efferent arterioles, then it follows that therapy by ACE inhibition could be expected to benefit those conditions in which there is intraglomerular hypertension or glomerular damage, as in diabetes mellitus, a condition that will be considered later in this book (Chapter 12).

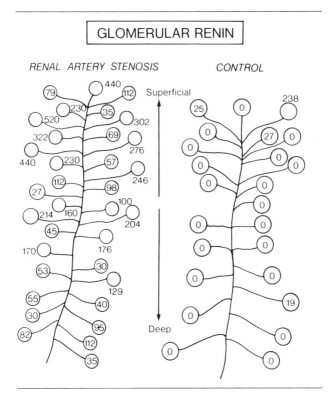

Figure 3–1. Increased intraglomerular formation of renin in experimental unilateral renal artery stenosis shown on the left compared with controls on the right. Each circle represents one glomerulus. The figure inside represents the relative amounts of renin formed. From Brown et al. (1966) with permission.

Effect of angiotensin-II on sodium balance and potential natriuretic effect of ACE inhibitors

The effects of angiotensin-II on the handling of sodium by the kidney can ultimately be traced to three different mechanisms. First, there is the relatively well known stimulation of the release of aldosterone by angiotensin-II. Second, there is the more recently reported effect of angiotensin-II on the renal sodium pump; angiotensin-II is thought to stimulate this pump to enhance the reabsorption of sodium by the kidney and, hence, to promote sodium retention (Wald et al., 1991). Third, there may be additional vascular effects on the vasa recta. These three mechanisms merit further consideration.

First, in conditions in which aldosterone is thought to contribute to sodium retention, such as congestive heart failure, inhibition of its formation following ACE inhibition should lead to a diuretic effect. Nonetheless, various studies with captopril and other ACE inhibitors have not shown a consistent diuretic effect either in patients with hypertension or in those with heart failure. The probable reason is that the aldosterone-mediated component to the exaggeration and progression of heart failure may be overshadowed

by peripheral mechanisms such as arteriolar vasoconstriction and renal vasoconstriction. It may, therefore, be proposed that ACE inhibitors do not consistently exhibit a net
natriuretic effect because it is overwhelmed by other vascular changes induced by the ACE inhibitor. Furthermore,
*the potential natriuretic effect is dependent on the state of sodium
loading.* When there is a low sodium load, which calls forth
a compensatory stimulation of renin secretion and, hence,
formation of angiotensin-II and aldosterone, then ACE inhibitors are more likely to have a diuretic effect.

Second, angiotensin-II at physiological levels has an
antinatriuretic effect by increasing sodium reabsorption in
the proximal tubules (Lang et al., 1992).

Third, besides the effects on efferent arterioles and sodium balance, angiotensin-II has effects on the vasa recta
(Brenner et al., 1982). It also causes contraction of the mesangial cells of the glomerulus and plays a role in the regulation of peritubular vascular pressure (Brenner et al.,
1982).

Thus, acting by these three mechanisms, secretion of
angiotensin-II is of prime importance for maintenance of
normal renal function.

Formation of renin and angiotensin-II by the kidney

Although a considerable amount of conversion of angiotensin-I to angiotensin-II occurs in the vascular endothelium
of the lung, nonetheless there is also an intrarenal renin
system (Fig. 3–2). In the kidney, ACE is found in the vascular endothelium of the juxtaglomerular apparatus and
the efferent arterioles, where angiotensin has a prominent
vascular effect (Edwards, 1983). Phylogenetic evidence suggests that the intrarenal renin system existed for millions of
years before the appearance of amphibia with their lung
tissue. The natural question, asked by Hollenberg and Williams (1990), is what the physiological role of this primitive
renin-angiotensin system might be. They propose that the
intrarenal system is the "original, primitive volume-control
apparatus, acting through its strategic intrarenal location to
control renal perfusion".

These authors propose that people in whom there is a
tendency to excess local production of angiotensin-II would
fail to increase their renal blood flow in response to a large
increase in sodium intake. This inability to change the renal
vascular responsiveness to angiotensin-II has been termed
nonmodulation (see Fig. 1–9) and is thought to correspond
to the group of salt-sensitive hypertensive subjects. In such
subjects, ACE inhibition restores the renal capacity to han-
dle a sodium load (Hollenberg and Williams, 1990).

Angiotensinogen formation by kidney

The renal tissue content of mRNA for angiotensinogen is
increased by a low sodium diet, both in cortical and med-
ullary fractions (Ingelfinger et al., 1986). This finding supports the existence of a local renal renin-angiotensin system
and provides a mechanism for upgrading of the renin-

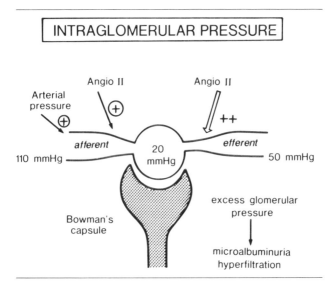

Figure 3–2. Schema for control of intraglomerular pressure by relative degrees of afferent and efferent arteriolar constriction. Fig. © LH Opie.

angiotensin system in response to a low salt diet, because the level of angiotensinogen appears to be the rate limiting substrate of the system.

Renal autoregulation and maintenance of glomerular filtration rate

In response to a low perfusion pressure, angiotenin-II maintains efferent arteriolar tone (Blythe, 1983). It follows that ACE inhibitors should be administered with caution to those patients who already have a low level of renal perfusion as in severe congestive heart failure or those with bilateral renal artery stenosis.

INTRAGLOMERULAR HYPERTENSION AND ACE INHIBITION

Hypertensive renal damage

The prototype experiments for hypertensive renal damage consist of experimental hypertension in which part of one kidney has been removed. There is a corresponding strain on the remaining nephrons, which coupled with the systemic hypertension leads to a intraglomerular hypertension that in turn leads to protein loss, i.e., microalbuminuria. Logically, therefore, it should be possible to prevent renal complications of hypertension in humans by ACE inhibition therapy.

Nonetheless, it should be considered that renal endpoints have never been studied in large trials of antihypertensive agents, i.e., the only end-points have been stroke and cardiac disease. It seems likely that mild to moderate hypertension is seldom complicated by overt renal failure. Some current studies are using microalbuminuria as a trial

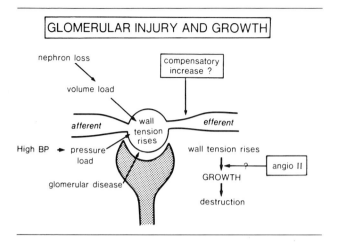

Figure 3–3. Glomerular injury with an increased intraglomerular pressure can evoke mesangial growth with threat of complete glomerular closure. Angiotensin-II may be an important growth signal acting via calcium. Fig. © LH Opie.

end-point. Thus, the real relation between hypertension and renal glomerular vascular disease is not known. It is possible that the association between renal disease and hypertension frequently found is noted in patients in whom the renal disease had first developed. In contrast, in malignant hypertension, deterioration of renal function follows in the wake of excess accelerated hypertension with fibrinoid necrosis of the renal arterioles.

Pathogenic mechanisms in renal vascular disease

On first principles it might be expected that there could be two major mechanisms for inducing glomerular damage. First, an excess intraluminal pressure could both damage the endothelium and the vessel wall and also induce excess vascular growth (Fig. 3–3), thereby setting in train a sequence of events that could end with obliteration of the glomerulus. Second, disease of the glomerular blood vessel wall, even in the presence of a normal intraluminal pressure, could sensitize the glomerulus to what would otherwise be an acceptable intraluminal pressure. An example of the first type of glomerular injury would be one dependent on hypertension. An example of the second type of glomerular injury would be one caused by diabetes mellitus. The combination of the two, as in patients with diabetic nephropathy with hypertension, is particularly likely to cause severe glomerular injury and irreversible damage (Chapter 12).

GLOMERULAR INJURY IN HYPERTENSION

The effects of chronic hypertension on the kidney have been reviewed by Reams and Bauer (1990). In hypertensive renal disease, the renal vascular resistance undergoes a progressive rise as the renal plasma flow falls. On the whole, the glomerular filtration rate is relatively well maintained but falls in about 20% of patients with essential hypertension. Initially the changes are potentially reversible, presumably reflecting vasoconstriction in response to norepinephrine and angiotensin-II. Once structural changes occur, then the process becomes irreversible. A decreased blood flow means that the glomeruli will suffer from ischemia, which brings in its wake the risk of hyaline formation in the capsular space, which is irreversible. There are a number of secondary changes such as tubular atrophy and interstitial fibrosis. Vascular changes are often focal, hence the secondary ischemic changes are also. Only when changes are severe and generalized does the entire kidney undergo ischemic atrophy.

Experimental glomerular injury and hyperfiltration

The normal adaptation to operative removal of renal mass in rats with spontaneous hypertension is dilation of the afferent arterioles to allow a greater filtration in the remaining glomeruli. Such hyperfiltration is accompanied by glomerular changes that can persist even if the systemic blood pressure is apparently well controlled. Experimentally, ACE inhibitor therapy is better than some other modalities in decreasing the hyperfiltration and the injury score of the glomeruli (Raij et al., 1985).

In rats with salt-sensitive hypertension, subject also to 5/6 nephrectomy, captopril and a calcium antagonist were equally able to decrease blood pressure but only captopril reduced proteinuria and the glomerular injury score (Tolins and Raij, 1990).

These data suggest, but of course do not prove, that ACE inhibitor therapy may play a specific role in normalizing intraglomerular hypertension. Thus, the concept would be that ACE inhibitors have a protective effect in averting the hypertrophied hypertensive glomerulus (Dworkin et al., 1993). Even in normotensive rats with renal ablation, ACE inhibitor therapy by perindopril can avert hyperfiltration (Corman and Vienet, 1991).

Microalbuminuria in hypertension

Whereas about 10% of hypertensive patients may manifest proteinuria, a much higher percentage develop microproteinuria, also called microalbuminuria (Bianchi et al., 1992). Drugs reducing blood pressure but not microalbuminuria were nitrendipine 20 mg daily, atenolol 100 mg daily, and chlorthalidone 50 mg daily. Despite apparently similar blood pressure reductions in moderately hypertensive patients (initial blood pressure about 160/105 mmHg), only enalapril 20 mg daily was able to reduce microalbuminuria. An effect of enalapril on intraglomerular pressure and/or glomerular permeability was postulated. Similarly, enalapril (10 to 20 mg daily) but not nicardipine (40 to 80 mg daily) was able to reduce microalbuminuria over 2 years, even though the blood pressure fell slightly more with nicardipine than with enalapril (Bigazzi et al., 1992).

These effects of enalapril are likely to be a class property of ACE inhibitors in view of (1) a short report indicating that captopril rather than beta-blockade reduced microalbuminuria (De Venuto et al., 1985); (2) data on perindopril in a subset of hypertensive patients, some of them, being diabetic, showing reduction of microalbuminuria (Stumpe and Overlack, 1993); and (3) the effect of captopril on diabetic nephropathy (Lewis et al., 1993).

ACE inhibitors versus calcium antagonist therapy in hypertensive patients with renal failure

In a small series of patients with renal hypertension and creatinine clearance values of 20 to 50 ml/min and a mean initial blood pressure of 159/101 mmHg on placebo, the effects of nitrendipine 10 mg once daily were compared with those of cilazapril 1.25 to 2.5 mg daily in a double-blind randomized fashion (Kloke et al., 1990). The active period of treatment was only 1 week for each drug, and such periods were separated by further placebo periods. Eleven patients were studied. Neither agent significantly reduced the blood pressure and only cilazapril reduced albuminuria and renal vascular resistance. Nitrendipine increased the fractional excretion of sodium. Combination therapy was best because it reduced the blood pressure, the filtration fraction fell, urinary albumin decreased, and renal vascular resistance fell, while the fractional excretion of sodium was increased. These data suggest that there would be an advantage to a long-term trial studying the effects of combined ACE inhibitor-calcium antagonist therapy.

NONDIABETIC PROGRESSIVE RENAL FAILURE

In progressive renal failure, from whatever cause, there is a progressive rise in serum creatinine and fall in glomerular function. Another index of the severity of the disease is the degree of proteinuria. Besides dietary protein restriction, a variety of drugs have been used with apparent benefit: ACE inhibitors, calcium antagonists, nonsteroidal anti-inflammatory drugs (NSAIDs), and combination therapy. There are some data suggesting that ACE inhibitors might be better than other agents in limiting the rise in serum creatinine (Mann et al., 1990), and lisinopril appears to be better than methyldopa (Heeg et al., 1989). The effect of lisinopril is highly dependent on the sodium status; it is more effective during a low sodium diet. Thus, there is reasonable but not conclusive evidence that among the therapies of choice for chronic renal failure would be protein restriction with a low sodium diet combined with ACE inhibitor therapy. There appear to be no comparative studies between ACE inhibitors and calcium antagonists, the latter also being effective (Eliahou et al., 1988). Experimentally, these two groups of drugs reduce renal injury by different and possibly additive mechanisms (Dworkin et al., 1993).

Glomerular filtration rate in essential hypertension

It will, therefore, be seen that the potential effects of ACE inhibition on glomerular filtration are complex and potentially conflicting, depending on the pathophysiologic state of the nephron. At least three factors could be operative in essential hypertension. First, by decreasing arterial pressure, ACE inhibition therapy could be expected to prevent further progress of the processes leading to a deterioration in the glomerular filtration rate. Second, by relief of efferent vasoconstriction, ACE inhibitors could be expected to decrease intraglomerular pressure and thereby to decrease the glomerular filtration-rate. Third, by relief of renal arteriolar afferent vasoconstriction, ACE inhibitors could be expected to promote renal blood flow and to increase the glomerular filtration rate. Because of these potentially conflicting mechanisms, it is not surprising that converting enzyme inhibition therapy has been reported to increase the glomerular filtration rate in essential hypertension (patients with initial values down to 66 ml/min per $1.73m^2$; see Hollenberg et al., 1979), to leave the glomerular filtration rate unchanged (Pessina et al., 1982; Chaignon et al., 1988), or even to decrease it (Hollenberg et al., 1981). In patients with albuminuria, it can be expected that ACE inhibitor therapy will decrease the albuminuria and slow the rate at which the renal component of essential hypertension increases, but such long-term data are not available. Hopefully, in time, the factors that can predict a favorable response to ACE inhibitors will become better defined (Opsahl et al., 1990).

ACE Inhibitors and Exaggeration of Circulatory-Induced Renal Failure

The preceding studies outline the situations in which ACE inhibitor therapy can be expected to improve renal damage or to prevent the progression of hypertensive microalbuminuria. Nonetheless, it should be carefully considered that efferent arteriolar vasoconstriction can be expected to be *beneficial* in certain conditions with poor renal blood flow, where the following sequence may operate:

renal ischemia → renin release → angiotensin-II formation → efferent arteriolar vasoconstriction → improved renal function.

Such a sequence could potentially improve the impaired glomerular filtration rate that is the result of a low arterial perfusion pressure. It is, therefore, not unexpected that in conditions such as severe cardiac failure in which renal blood flow is diminished, arteriolar efferent vasoconstriction can help maintain renal function. Instances of marked deterioration in renal function in patients with severe heart failure have been shown, particularly in relation to combination therapy of ACE inhibitor and diuretic (Funck-Brentano et al., 1986). In such patients, it is the degree of diuretic-induced sodium depletion and ACE inhibitor-induced hypotension that appear to play a major

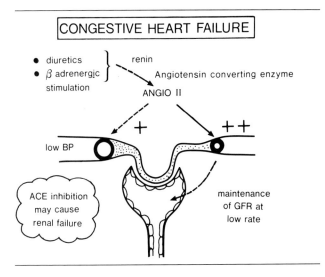

Figure 3–4. In severe congestive heart failure, there is a low renal perfusion pressure that can be further decreased by ACE inhibitor therapy. The danger is precipitation of renal failure, most marked when dealing with a severe sodium depletion state. The mechanism of the potential adverse effects of ACE inhibitors includes relief of efferent arteriolar constriction that is helping to maintain the intraglomerular pressure. The solution is to give a small test dose of the ACE inhibitor and to avoid excess diuresis. Note preliminary evidence that perindopril may avoid first dose hypotension in heart failure. Fig. © LH Opie.

role. The combination of sodium depletion and poor renal perfusion should lead to a greater degree of efferent arteriolar vasoconstriction, a greater dependence on angiotensin-II and, therefore, a more marked effect of ACE inhibition in causing deterioration of renal function. In addition, another factor causing potential deterioration of renal function following ACE inhibitor therapy in congestive heart failure is increasing systemic hypotension, one of the major side-effects of this category of drugs (Fig. 3–4).

Renal insufficiency in renal glomerular disease

Efferent vasoconstriction could also be expected to play an important role in maintaining renal perfusion in patients with chronic renal disease treated by diuretics, in which case the efferent vasoconstriction could be expected to help maintain glomerular filtration. There are isolated case reports of patients with hypertension and chronic glomerular disease receiving diuretic therapy in whom renal function has deteriorated upon addition of ACE inhibitor therapy (Murphy et al., 1984; Brivet et al., 1985).

ACE Inhibitors, Renal Artery Stenosis, and Renovascular Hypertension

Pathophysiology

The mechanism whereby renal artery stenosis leads to renin-dependent hypertension is well established (Fig.

3–5). Increased renin is manufactured especially by the deep glomeruli, which are normally renin-deficient (see Fig. 3–1). When the rate of renin release is chronically elevated, then manufacture of the renin precursor, *pro-renin,* also increases (Derkx et al., 1983). In addition, all the other components of the renin-angiotensin system are present in the kidney as one component of the various tissue renin-angiotensin systems (Robertson, 1985). Hence, there is an increased intrarenal production of angiotensin-II (see p. 73) with its many complex effects besides regulation of efferent arteriole tone. On the whole, this increased secretion of angiotensin-II serves to maintain the function of the kidney affected by unilateral renovascular hypertension.

ACE inhibitor therapy in unilateral renal artery stenosis

Because angiotensin-II by efferent arteriolar constriction helps to maintain intraglomerular pressure in the affected kidney in renovascular hypertension, it may be expected on first principles that ACE inhibitor therapy will almost inevitably adversely influence the already compromised renal function (Robertson, 1985). Because such therapy also lowers total body sodium through inhibition of aldosterone formation, the potentially adverse effects of ACE inhibitor therapy on the unilateral diseased kidney are especially marked in patients who are also being treated by a high diuretic dose or are on a very low sodium diet. Hence, ACE inhibitor therapy should be initiated without diuretics in patients on a normal sodium diet. ACE inhibitor therapy will, at the same time, remove the adverse effects of excess circulating angiotensin-II on the normal contralateral kidney. Thus, the overall effects of ACE inhibitor therapy can

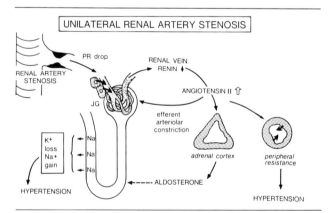

Figure 3–5. In unilateral renal artery stenosis, it is the drop in pressure (PR) that stimulates secretion of renin from the juxtaglomerular (JG) cells to form renin (see also Fig. 3–1). Increased renin leads to increased circulating angiotensin-II, which stimulates aldosterone secretion that in turn promotes hypotension, as does the effect of angiotensin-II on the peripheral arterioles. Angiotensin constriction of efferent renal arterioles helps to maintain renal function on the side of the renal artery stenosis. Fig. © LH Opie.

be expected to be beneficial despite the potentially adverse effects on the ischemic kidney.

Indeed, soon after the introduction of ACE inhibitors, it was noted that they were strikingly effective in the therapy of hypertension associated with renal artery stenosis. *Precipitous falls in blood pressure* were also found leading to the requirement for the more cautious introduction of ACE inhibitors and of prior low test doses to exclude patients with excessive hypotension. The response of the hypertension in patients with renal artery stenosis to ACE inhibitor therapy can be correlated with the response to subsequent corrective surgery (Staessen et al, 1983). Debate continues as to whether sustained ACE inhibitor therapy, or surgical correction, or renal angioplasty is the optimal therapy for renal artery stenosis. An important argument is that if renal artery stenosis is caused by localized atheroma and is left untreated surgically or by angioplasty, complete renal artery obstruction may occur with renal atrophy (Guzman et al., 1994). Nonetheless, the natural history of renal artery stenosis is not well studied.

There are *two separate types of renal artery stenosis,* that caused by renal artery atheroma and increasingly recognized in older patients, and that caused by fibromuscular dysplasia, more often the cause of the problem in younger patients. In neither case are there detailed studies concerning the natural history of the condition, and many decisions regarding therapy are based on incomplete assumptions. Therefore, despite the excellent overall response in the blood pressure that is standard in renal artery stenosis treated by ACE inhibitor therapy, the decision whether to undertake interventional surgery or angioplasty is not easy. There is a current tendency to prefer interventional therapy, but the decision in any individual patient must be carefully considered. Among the points to note are that the function of the affected kidney is unlikely to improve substantially and that there are no detailed studies including measurements of glomerular filtration rate and renal blood flow after surgical intervention or angioplasty. Furthermore, surgical intervention fairly often includes nephrectomy, which may contribute to the short-term control of the blood pressure but takes away residual functioning renal mass. Bearing in mind these complex and conflicting considerations, the long-term management of each patient with renal artery stenosis must be critically evaluated, the local facilities considered, and it may still be that ACE inhibitor therapy is an acceptable long-term option.

ACE inhibitor therapy in bilateral renal artery stenosis

In the therapy of renal artery stenosis by ACE inhibitors, it became apparent that a subset of patients, namely those with bilateral renal artery stenosis, were at high risk of renal failure upon initiation of ACE inhibitor therapy (Fig. 3–6). This hazard is held to be the result of combined preglomerular and postglomerular vasodilation. Not all patients with bilateral renal artery stenosis develop irreversible renal failure; reversible failure is also common.

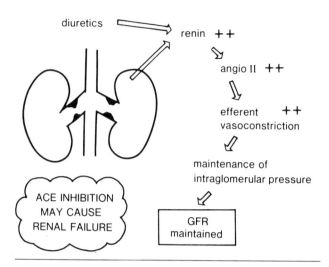

Figure 3–6. In bilateral renal artery stenosis, maintenance of intraglomerular pressure and glomerular filtration rate (GFR) may be critically dependent on formation of angiotensin-II. ACE inhibitor therapy, therefore, may precipitate renal failure so that this condition is generally a contraindication to therapy by ACE inhibitors unless cautiously applied and under careful observation. Fig. © LH Opie.

Furthermore, it is possible to treat bilateral renal artery stenosis cautiously by ACE inhibitor therapy without precipitating renal failure, especially if there is no combined ACE inhibitor-diuretic therapy (Hodsman et al., 1983; Watson et al., 1983). However, when reversible renal failure occurs upon initiation of ACE inhibitor therapy, one of the conditions that must be considered is bilateral renal artery stenosis or, equally probable, renal artery stenosis affecting a solitary kidney (Silas et al., 1983).

Thus, in the presence of severe renovascular hypertension, ACE inhibitor therapy can permanently interfere with renal autoregulation, with marked initial deterioration and subsequent improvement without full recovery of normality (Bender et al., 1984). Severe renal failure occurs in only about 6% (see p. 56).

Other permutations of severe renovascular hypertension

Unilateral stenosis in a single functioning kidney provides a situation very similar to bilateral renal artery stenosis from the functional point of view (Fig. 3–7).

After renal transplantation, renal artery stenosis may also develop. Four patients with *stenosis of the transplanted renal artery* reacted adversely to the introduction of captopril therapy with acute loss of renal excretory function (Curtis et al., 1983).

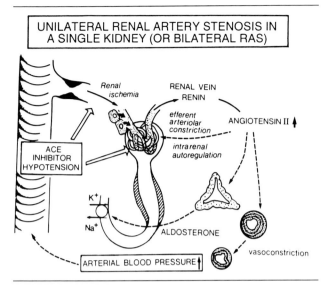

Figure 3–7. In unilateral renal artery stenosis in a single kidney, as in bilateral renal artery stenosis (RAS), there is risk of severe renal failure when the compensatory efferent arteriolar constriction is removed. In this condition, as in bilateral renal artery stenosis, intrarenal autoregulation is maintained by the efferent arteriolar constriction. Therefore, again, ACE inhibitor therapy must be started cautiously and under observation, if at all. Usually, ACE inhibitor therapy is contraindicated. Fig. © LH Opie.

Functional renal insufficiency

The concept emerges that in patients with severe renal perfusion defects, usually a combination of preglomerular and postglomerular abnormalities, the introduction of an ACE inhibitor can lead to functional renal failure, which is usually reversible but sometimes fails to revert to normal upon cessation of therapy (Hricik et al., 1983).

ACE INHIBITORS IN DIAGNOSIS OF RENIN-DEPENDENT HYPERTENSION

An extension of the above principles lies in diagnostic radiology or diagnostic nuclear renography. Because of the acute effect of ACE inhibition in decreasing renal perfusion to the affected side in renal artery stenosis, acute ACE inhibition by captopril (the quickest acting of the currently available oral agents) results in shunting of blood away from the affected kidney and thereby exaggerating the effects of renal artery stenosis. In this way, borderline perfusion abnormalities can be magnified and clarified. For example, the renal cortical activity of injected ^{131}I-hippuran is increased in renovascular hypertension after ACE inhibition because of decreased glomerular filtration and delayed washout of hippuran in the tubules of the affected side (Erbsloh-Moller et al., 1991). This procedure is commonly known as the *captopril renogram* and is highly specific but not very sensitive (Mann et al., 1990); similar principles can be applied before renal arteriography to enhance the difference in the density of dye between the two sides, or before sampling of renal vein renin values to increase the values on the affected side. The test is not specific to captopril, which is used only for its rapidity of action; alternatively, intravenous enalaprilat is suitable and acts even faster than oral captopril (Erbsloh-Moller et al., 1991).

RENAL SIDE-EFFECTS OF ACE INHIBITORS

Captopril toxicity

In the initial phases of the introduction of captopril, when doses that today would be regarded as very high were commonly used (such as 450 mg/day), it was noted that in about 1% of cases a marked proteinuria occurred, and there were occasional reports of captopril-induced renal failure. Such renal deterioration has become increasingly uncommon now that lower doses of captopril (ceiling dose 150 mg/day) are used. Furthermore, it seems likely that it is the association between the SH-group and ACE inhibitor therapy that causes the deterioration in renal function. Thus, ACE inhibitor-induced proteinuria has not been reported when ACE inhibitors other than captopril have been used.

Renal failure

As already outlined, even the absence of any direct drug-induced proteinuria does not preclude complex vascular mechanisms whereby ACE inhibitors could impair renal function in situations such as severe cardiac failure, renal artery stenosis, and during excess diuretic therapy with a pre-existing negative sodium balance. Because it is impossible to predict the overall effects of angiotensin-II in any given pathophysiologic situation in any given patient, it is correct *always to give a small test dose* of an ACE inhibitor before proceeding to long-term therapy and to build up the dose of the ACE inhibitor cautiously, while following indices of renal function.

SUMMARY

Angiotensin-II acts as a marked arteriolar vasoconstrictor in various vascular beds, and the renal vascular bed is no exception. The specific sites of vasoconstriction are preglomerular, that is to say afferent renal arteriolar vasoconstriction, and, second, efferent vasoconstriction. There is evidence that it is particularly efferent arteriolar vasoconstriction that is a major effect of angiotensin-II. Efferent vasoconstriction maintains intraglomerular filtration pressure in a variety of circumstances, such as severe heart failure, bilateral renal artery stenosis, renal artery stenosis treated vigorously with diuretics, and, theoretically, in some cases of hypertension-induced renal damage. Relief of efferent vasoconstriction can be expected to have therapeutic benefits in conditions where intraglomerular hypertension and hyperfiltration is a basic problem, such as hypertensive microalbuminuria, certain other instances of hypertension-induced renal damage, and some patients with progressive renal disease.

The marked therapeutic benefits of ACE inhibitors in renal artery stenosis can be related to the degree of increase of circulating renin, and thereby a general relief of arterial pressure elevation with an increase in preglomerular plasma flow. Nonetheless, these advantages have to be balanced against the potential disadvantage of decreased efferent vasoconstriction in response to ACE inhibitor therapy. Particularly when renal artery perfusion is low, as in bilateral renal artery stenosis, severe heart failure, unilateral renal artery stenosis in a solitary kidney, renal artery stenosis in a transplant kidney, and similar situations, there is the potential for severe temporary renal failure to occur, with in some cases permanent failure.

To prevent temporary or permanent failure, care should be taken to avoid significant or excess concurrent diuretic therapy, because a negative sodium balance stimulates the angiotensin-renin system and, therefore, makes the intraglomerular pressure more reliant on the degree of efferent vasoconstriction. Thus, it can be seen that the benefits of ACE inhibitors in renal disease can be marked in certain instances, for example in hypertensive microalbuminuria. Yet, in renal artery stenosis a complex counterregulation may exist whereby efferent vasoconstriction balances afferent constriction, so that considerable caution must be exercised during the introduction of ACE inhibitor therapy. In severe heart failure with poor renal perfusion, ACE inhibitor therapy must be introduced only when excess diuresis has been avoided and after a low test dose.

References

Bender W, La France N, Walker WG. Mechanism of deterioration in renal function in patients with renovascular hypertension treated with enalapril. *Hypertension* 1984; 6 (Suppl I): I-193–I-197.

Bianchi S, Bigazzi R, Baldari G. Microalbuminuria in patients with essential hypertension: effects of several antihypertensive drugs. *Am J Med* 1992; 93: 525–528.

Bigazzi R, Bianchi S, Baldari D, et al. Long-term effects of a converting enzyme inhibitor and a calcium channel blocker on urinary albumin excretion in patients with essential hypertension. *Am J Hypertens* 1992; 6: 108–113.

Blythe WB. Captopril and renal autoregulation. *N Engl J Med* 1983; 308: 390–391.

Brenner BM, Schor N, Ichikawa I. Role of angiotensin-II in the physiologic regulation of glomerular filtration. *Am J Cardiol* 1982; 49: 1430–1433.

Brivet F, Roulot D, Poitrine A, Dormont J. Reversible acute renal failure during enalapril treatment in patient with chronic glomerulonephritis without renal artery stenosis. *Lancet* 1985; 1: 1512.

Brown JJ, Davies DL, Lever AF, et al. The assay of renin in single glomeruli and the appearance of the juxtaglomerular apparatus in the rabbit following renal artery constriction. *Clin Sci* 1966; 30: 223–235.

Chaignon M, Barrou Z, Ayad M, et al. Effects of perindopril on renal haemodynamics and natriuresis in essential hypertension. *J Hypertens* 1988; 6 (Suppl 3): S61–S64.

Corman B, Vienet R. Converting enzyme inhibition prevents postprandial hyperfiltration in rats with renal mass ablation. *Am J Hypertens* 1991; 4: 253S–257S.

Curtis JJ, Luke RG, Whelchel JD, et al. Inhibition of angiotensin converting enzyme in renal-transplant recipients with hypertension. *N Engl J Med* 1983; 308: 377–381.

Derkx FHM, Tan-Thong L, Wenting GJ, et al. Asynchronous changes in prorenin and renin secretion after captopril in patients with renal artery stenosis. *Hypertension* 1983; 5: 244–256.

De Venuto G, Andreotti C, Mattarei M, Pegoretti G. Long-term captopril therapy at low doses reduces albumin excretion in patients with essential hypertension and no sign of renal impairment. *J Hypertens* 1985; 3 (Suppl 2): S143–S145.

Dollery CT. Concluding remarks. *J Hypertens* 1988; 6 (Suppl 3): S83–S84.

Dworkin LD, Benstein JA, Parker M, et al. Calcium antagonists and converting enzyme inhibitors reduce renal injury by different mechanisms. *Kidney Int* 1993; 43: 808–814.

Edwards RM. Segmental effects of norepinephrine and angiotensin-II on isolated renal microvessels. *Am J Physiol* 1983; 244: F526–F534.

Eliahou HE, Cohen D, Ben-David A, et al. The calcium channel blocker nisoldipine delays progression of chronic renal failure in humans (preliminary communication). *Cardiovasc Drugs Ther* 1988; 1: 523–528.

Erbsloh-Moller B, Dumas A, Roth D, et al. Furosemide-^{131}I-hippuran renography after angiotensin-converting enzyme inhibition for the diagnosis of renovascular hypertension. *Am J Med* 1991; 90: 23–29.

Funck-Brentano C, Chatellier G, Alexandre J-M. Reversible renal failure after combined treatment with enalapril and frusemide in a patient with congestive heart failure. *Br Heart J* 1986; 55: 596–598.

Guzman RP, Zierler E, Isaacson JA. Renal atrophy and arterial stenosis. A prospective study with duplex ultrasound. *Hypertension* 1994; 23: 346–350.

Heeg JE, de Jong PE, van der Hem GK, de Zeeuw D. Efficacy and variability of the antiproteinuric effect of ACE inhibition by lisinopril. *Kidney Int* 1989; 36: 272–279.

Hodsman GP, Brown JJ, Cumming AMM, et al. Enalapril in the treatment of hypertension with renal artery stenosis. *Br Med J* 1983; 287: 1413–1417.

Hollenberg NK, Swartz SL, Passan DR, Williams GH. Increased glomerular filtration rate after converting enzyme inhibition in essential hypertension. *N Engl J Med* 1979; 301: 9–12.

Hollenberg NK, Meggs LG, Williams GH, et al. Sodium intake and renal responses to captopril in normal man and in essential hypertension. *Kidney Int* 1981; 20: 240–245.

Hollenberg NK, Williams GH. ACE inhibition, the kidney and non-modulation. *ACE Report* 1990; 67: 1–5.

Hricik DE, Browning PJ, Kopelman R, et al. Captopril-induced functional renal insufficiency in patients with bilateral renal artery stenoses or renal artery stenosis in a solitary kidney. *N Engl J Med* 1983; 308: 373–376.

Ingelfinger JR, Pratt RE, Ellison K, Dzau VJ. Sodium regulation of angiotensinogen mRNA expression in rat kidney cortex and medulla. *J Clin Invest* 1986; 78: 1311–1315.

Kloke HJ, Wetzels JFM, van Hamersvelt HW, et al. Effects of nitrendipine and cilazapril on renal hemodynamics and albuminuria in hypertensive patients with chronic renal failure. *J Cardiovasc Pharmacol* 1990; 16: 924–930.

Lang CC, Rahman AR, Balfour DJK, Struthers AD. Prazosin blunts the antinatriuretic effect of circulating angiotensin-II in man. *J Hypertens* 1992; 10: 1387–1395.

Mann JFE, Reisch C, Ritz E. Use of angiotensin-converting enzyme inhibitors for the preservation of kidney function: a retrospective study. *Nephron* 1990; 55: S38–S42.

Murphy BF, Whitworth JA, Kincaid-Smith P. Renal insufficiency with combinations of angiotensin converting enzyme inhibitors and diuretics. *Br Med J* 1984; 288: 844–845.

Navar LG, Champion WJ, Thomas CE. Effects of calcium channel blockade on renal vascular resistance responses to changes in perfusion pressure and angiotensin-converting enzyme inhibition in dogs. *Circ Res* 1986; 58: 874–881.

Opsahl JA, Abraham PA, Keane WF. Renal effects of angiotensin converting enzyme inhibitors: nondiabetic chronic renal disease. *Cardiovasc Drugs Ther* 1990; 4: 221–228.

Pessina AC, Semplicini A, Rossi G, et al. Effects of captopril on renal function in hypertensive patients. *Am J Cardiol* 1982; 49: 1572–1573.

Raij L, Chiou X-C, Owens R, Wrigley B. Therapeutic implications of hypertension-induced glomerular injury. Comparison of enalapril and a combination of hydralazine, reserpine, and hydrochlorothiazide in an experimental model. *Am J Med* 1985; 79 (Suppl 3C): 37–41.

Reams GP, Bauer JH. Acute and chronic effects of angiotensin converting enzyme inhibitors on the essential hypertensive kidney. *Cardiovasc Drugs Ther* 1990; 4: 207–219.

Robertson JIS. Intrarenal actions of angiotensin converting enzyme inhibitors: their relevance to renal artery stenosis. *ACE Report* 1985; 16: 1–5.

Silas JH, Klenka Z, Solomon SA, Bone JM. Captopril induced reversible renal failure: a marker of renal artery stenosis affecting a solitary kidney. *Br Med J* 1983; 286: 1702–1703.

Staessen J, Bulpitt C, Fagard R, et al. Long-term converting-enzyme inhibition as a guide to surgical curability of hypertension associated with renovascular disease. *Am J Cardiol* 1983; 51: 1317–1322.

Stumpe KO, Overlack A on behalf of the Perindopril Therapeutic Safety Study Group (PUTS). A new trial of the efficacy, tolerability, and safety of angiotensin-converting enzyme inhibition in mild systemic hypertension with concomitant diseases and therapies. *Am J Cardiol* 1993; 71: 32E–37E.

Tolins JP, Raij L. Comparison of converting enzyme inhibitor and calcium channel blocker in hypertensive glomerular injury. *Hypertension* 1990; 16: 452–461.

Wald H, Scherzer P, Popovtzer MM. Na,K-ATPase in isolated nephron segments in rats with experimental heart failure. *Circ Res* 1991; 68: 1051–1058.

Watson ML, Bell GM, Muir AL, et al. Captopril/diuretic combinations in severe renovascular disease: a cautionary note. *Lancet* 1983; 2: 404–405.

CHAPTER 4

ACE Inhibitors
and the Heart

*"Angiotensin-II is clearly emerging as one of the most important
mediators of cardiac hypertrophy in vivo"* (Sadoshima and
Izumo, 1993).

Initially it was thought that ACE inhibitors had only an indirect effect on the heart, for example by decreasing blood
pressure, thereby unloading the heart, and thereby having
an indirect effect in decreasing left ventricular mass in hypertension. More recently, evidence has mounted that
there are angiotensin receptors in the myocardium, that
stimulation of such receptors can alter myocardial contractile function, and that, furthermore, at least some of the
angiotensin involved might be manufactured in cardiac
cells. This chapter will start by analyzing the effects of angiotensin receptor stimulation and ACE inhibitors on the
myocardium, and then examine the possible role of ACE
inhibition in coronary artery disease including angina pectoris, acute myocardial infarction, reperfusion, and postinfarct remodeling. The ultimate question of the cardioprotective effect of ACE inhibitors is examined in Chapter 11.

THE MYOCARDIUM

Myocardial angiotensin-II receptors
and subtypes

Myocardial angiotensin-II receptors, now identified in isolated cardiac myocytes, have high affinity for angiotensin-
II with reversible binding and interact with very low external concentrations of angiotensin-II; in technical terms, the
K_d for angiotensin-II is only about 1 nM (Baker et al., 1984;
Rogers, 1984). There are two receptor subtypes, AT_1 and
AT_2. It is the AT_1 receptor that is linked to the phosphatidylinositol system, whereas the AT_2 is not and has no
known biological role (Dostal and Baker, 1993). There is
controversy about the dominant receptor type in cardiac tis-

sue with one recent study suggesting that it is the AT_1 receptor that is dominant (Meggs et al., 1993).

After occupation of the angiotensin-II receptor, the next step is transmission of the signal to within the cell towards the ultimate effector site. The messenger system stimulated appears to be that involving inositol triphosphate (IP_3) and protein kinase C, with intracellular mobilization of calcium ions (Fig. 4–1). In addition, there also seems to be stimulation of the L-type calcium channel at least in cultured rat myocytes (Dosemeci et al., 1988), thereby enhancing the calcium effect. These observations explain why angiotensin-II, in the nanomolar range, increases contractile frequency in spontaneously beating cultured cells (Allen et al., 1988).

Although angiotensin-II is commonly thought of as possessing positive inotropic properties, as also found in human myocytes (Moravec et al., 1990), in the guinea-pig this effect is not found for unknown reasons. Ultimately, angiotensin-II receptor stimulation is likely to modulate calcium-related physiological events, such as the inotropic and chronotropic state. The physiological role of this system is not clear, and it probably plays a relatively minor modulatory role in the overall regulation of cardiac contraction, especially compared with the effects of sympathetic nervous system control.

Regulation of growth

Besides the mild inotropic effect of angiotensin-II, there is another more intriguing proposed role for the cardiac renin-angiotensin system, namely as a growth regulator (Katz, 1990; Schelling et al., 1991). The idea that angiotensin-II could help to regulate myocardial protein synthesis goes back to at least 1983 (Khairallah and Kanabus, 1983). At least part of the stimulation results from the induction of a variety of complex growth regulating genes called *proto-oncogenes* (Dostal and Baker, 1993) that play an impor-

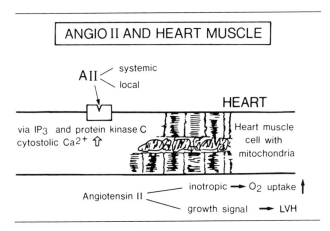

Figure 4–1. Proposed role of myocardial angiotensin-II (AII) receptors in regulating cytosolic calcium in heart muscle cells, with consequences for the inotropic state and for myocardial growth. Fig. © LH Opie.

TABLE 4–1 EVIDENCE FOR CARDIAC AND MYOCARDIAL RENIN-ANGIOTENSIN ACTIVITY

1. Recognition of cardiac components of renin-angiotensin system

a. *Angiotensinogen*

    i. Angiotensinogen synthesis in isolated atria and in ventricles after pressure-loading

    ii. Angiotensinogen release from perfused heart

    iii. Increased mRNA for angiotensinogen in non-infarcted left ventricle in rat (Lindpainter et al, 1993) and in left ventricle of aortic-banded rats (Baker et al, 1990).

    iv. Immunoreactive angiotensinogen in human heart especially in atria, conducting system and subendocardial ventricle (Sawa et al, 1992)

b. *Renin**

    i. Renin gene expression in ventricles more than in atria

    ii. Cyclic AMP-responsive elements in 5′-flanking region of renin gene

    iii. Increased synthesis of renin in response to beta-agonist stimulation.

c. *Activity of angiotensin-converting enzyme (ACE)*

    i. Evidence of occurrence in coronary vasculature and in neonatal myocytes (Dostal et al, 1992)

    ii. Increased ACE activity in pressure-overloaded ventricle (Shunkert et al, 1993)

    iii. Increased mRNA for ACE in right ventricle of rat hearts with post-infarct heart failure (Hirsch et al, 1991)

    iv. Note ACE-insensitive pathways for angiotensin generation in volume-loaded ventricle (Ruzicka et al, 1993). Heart chymase cloned in human heart (Urata et al, 1991)

d. *Angiotensin-II*

    i. Can be formed in perfused rat hearts

    ii. Found in monkey ventricles

    iii. In nephrectomized rabbits with no renal source of renin, ACE inhibition can decrease atrial content of angiotensin-II

2. Myocardial angiotensin-II receptors

a. In sarcolemmal vesicle preparations, receptors are found which meet kinetic requirements for receptor identification.

b. In isolated rat neonatal myocytes, there are about 45,000 receptors per cell.

c. In surviving ventricular myocytes from infarct hearts, AII-receptor density increased (Meggs et al, 1993).

d. Autoradiographic identification in man shows receptors present in myocardial cells, coronary vessels, and in nerves (Urata et al, 1989).

e. Pathways for signal transduction are present chiefly involving phosphotidylinositol pathway, inositol triphosphate and protein kinase C (Meggs et al, 1993).

*Controversial. See von Lutterotti et al. (1994) and Dzau and Re (1994).

TABLE 4–2 ANGIOTENSIN-II AND GROWTH FACTORS

1. Angiotensin-II induces turnover of DNA and RNA, increases RNA content, and induces protein synthesis in chick heart cells.

2. Angiotensin-II activates proto-oncogenes, including c-fos via protein kinase C and cell calcium.

3. Angiotensin-II invokes release of growth factors from vascular smooth muscle cells (Dostal and Baker, 1993).

tant part in regulating the early processes leading to increased cell growth. In addition, angiotensin-II appears to up-regulate the cardiac hypertrophic response by inducing the angiotensinogen gene and the gene for transforming growth factor-β_1 (Sadoshima and Izumo, 1993). (Sadoshima and Izumo, 1993). The proposal that very low doses of an ACE inhibitor, too low to reduce the blood pressure, can regress left ventricular hypertrophy is controversial (Lindpaintner and Ganten, 1991; Scicli, 1994).

Significance of the resident myocardial renin-angiotensin system

That there is a myocardial renin-angiotensin system is now generally accepted (Fig. 4–2). That it has pathophysiological significance is much more difficult to prove. Even more difficult to know is whether the system resides in the cardiac myocytes or in the fibroblasts or in combinations of both or even in other cells, except when the specific cell types have been cultured (Dostal et al., 1992). Furthermore, there may be important species differences between the exact enzyme converting angiotensin-I to angiotensin-II between humans and the common laboratory animal, the rat. Evidence for recognition of the cardiac components of the renin-angiotensin system is summarized in Table 4–1 as are the data showing that there are myocardial angiotensin receptors. The physiological effects of such receptor stimulation could include inotropic and chronotropic changes, but it is difficult to be sure that it is the myocardial renin-angiotensin system that is involved and not circulating components, or components that are located on cardiac cells but have direct access to the extracellular space. Evidence suggesting that the system acts to stimulate growth factors is also good but not conclusive (Table 4–2).

Modification of the renin-angiotensin system has obvious importance in relation to the heart (Table 4–3). However, there is no proof that it is the myocardial myocyte renin-angiotensin system that is the target of ACE inhibitor drug action, as opposed to other systems, for example those in the vascular endothelium, or the circulating renin-angiotensin system. It still remains true that: "To date, no experiments have been reported that provide unequivocal evidence for direct physiological significance of intracardially synthesized angiotensin" (Lindpaintner and Ganten, 1991).

TABLE 4–3 POTENTIAL CARDIOVASCULAR SIGNIFICANCE OF THERAPEUTIC MODIFICATION OF RENIN-ANGIOTENSIN SYSTEM

1. Cardiac hypertrophy in hypertension

a. Therapy with small doses of ACE inhibitor not decreasing blood pressure can reduce left ventricular hypertrophy in aortic banded rats (Baker et al., 1990).

b. However, in spontaneously hypertensive rats, blood pressure reduction rather than ACE inhibition is mechanism for regression of left ventricular hypertrophy with perindopril (Harrap et al., 1993)

c. ACE inhibition normalizes isomyosin profile in rats (Dussaule et al., 1986).

d. Chronic ACE inhibitor therapy completely prevents interstitial fibrosis in genetic hypertension in rats (Brilla et al., 1991).

2. Sympathetic modulation

a. Less effect of sympathetic stimulation on heart rate and contractile activity after ACE inhibitor (Remme et al., 1994).

3. Chronic congestive heart failure

a. ACE inhibitors may have effects above and beyond those of other vasodilators (see Table 5–6).

b. Specific activation of cardiac mRNA for ACE and local synthesis of angiotensin-II in experimental heart failure (Hirsch et al., 1991).

4. Myocardial ischemia

a. Transient ischemia and fewer metabolic defects after addition of ramipril to isolated hearts.

b. Bradykinin inhibition appears to abolish effects.

c. In isolated rat hearts with left ventricular hypertrophy, enalaprilat lessens ischemia-induced diastolic dysfunction (Schunkert et al., 1993).

5. Myocyte necrosis

a. Low-dose infusion of angiotensin-II causes myocytolysis and subsequent fibrosis (Tan et al., 1991). Captopril effective in preventing myocyte injury in renovascular hypertension.

6. Reperfusion arrhythmias in isolated hearts

a. Inhibitory effects of ACE inhibitors abolished by addition of angiotensin-II and by bradykinin inhibition.

b. ACE inhibitor pretreatment lessens reperfusion ventricular fibrillation in pigs (Muller et al., 1993).

7. Postinfarct arrhythmias

a. Complete prevention of inducible ventricular tachycardia in pigs after acute administration of intravenous captopril.

8. Stunned myocardium

a. Enalapril better than hydralazine in preventing stunning in dogs, mechanism unknown.

TABLE 4–3 POTENTIAL CARDIOVASCULAR
SIGNIFICANCE OF THERAPEUTIC MODIFICATION OF
RENIN-ANGIOTENSIN SYSTEM (*Continued*)

9. Ventricular remodeling

   a. Improved experimental and clinical remodeling by use of
ACE inhibitors (Konstam et al., 1993).

10. Increased capillary density in LVH

   a. Subhypertensive doses of ramipril (Unger et al., 1992).

For other references, see Lindpaintner and Ganten (1991).

In the above situations, there is no proof that it is the cardiac myocyte
renin-angiotensin system that is the target of drug action, as opposed to
other cardiac systems such as the fibroblasts or vascular tissue, or circulating renin-angiotensin. See footnote to Table 4–1.

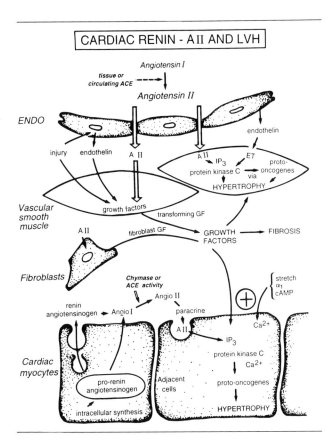

*Figure 4–2. Some proposals for a multicellular interactive renin-
angiotensin system involving cardiac myocytes, fibroblasts, vascular
smooth muscle, and endothelium (for detailed evidence, see Dostal and
Baker, 1993). Although these systems are postulated to have an
important function in regulating vascular and myocardial
hypertrophy, proof of this significance is still awaited. Fig. © LH
Opie.*

Vascular tissue and fibroblasts

Perhaps it is a mistake to expect myocardial cells to have their own active renin-angiotensin system of documented physiological and pathological significance. Rather, the myocardial cells may participate and interact with a variety of other cells, including fibroblasts, vascular smooth muscle cells, and endothelial cells in a multiple cellular interactive manner. Thus, current evidence strongly suggests the existence of a cardiac multicellular renin-angiotensin system, probably helping to regulate cardiac growth, including fibrogenesis (Weber et al., 1994).

Growth factors in vascular cells

Besides stimulation of the phosphatidylinositol signaling system, angiotensin-II may induce the release of a number of growth factors from vascular smooth muscle cells. For example, the platelet-derived growth factor (PDGF) may arise not only from platelets but from smooth muscle cells and be released from them by angiotensin-II. Likewise, the transforming growth factor-$\beta 1$ (TGF-$\beta 1$) can thus be released. The latter growth factor may play a special role in promoting the growth of extracellular matrix, including collagen (Dostal and Baker, 1993).

ACE Inhibitors and Left Ventricular Hypertrophy

Left ventricular hypertrophy (LVH) is currently regarded as one of the serious complications of hypertension, being an independent risk factor for coronary events according to the Framingham data (Levy et al., 1990). ACE inhibitor therapy can reduce blood pressure, left ventricular mass, and early diastolic filling, the agents used include captopril (Muiesan et al., 1988), perindopril (Asmar et al., 1988; Grandi et al., 1991), enalapril (Grandi et al., 1989; Gosse et al., 1990), and ramipril (Eischstadt et al., 1987). The mechanism involved may include, first, the reduction in blood pressure and thereby the reduction in intraluminal pressure; second, a specific effect in modification of the growth-stimulating properties of angiotensin-II (Brilla et al., 1991; Kromer et al., 1991); and, third, a reduction of angiotensin-mediated adrenergic outflow. Which of these is predominantly involved may depend on the model used (compare Harrap et al., 1993 with Baker et al., 1990).

Collagen phenotypes

In experimental LVH, not only is there more myocardial collagen, but its phenotype changes so that there is a relative increase in collagen type I, which is thought to help increase myocardial stiffness. In rats, although both captopril and hydralazine could equally reduce blood pressure, only chronic captopril therapy could lessen the change in collagen phenotypes (Mukherjee and Sen, 1993).

Reduced coronary vascular reserve

Just as increased myocardial collagen impairs mechanical properties of the heart, so does vascular remodeling impair vasodilation (Brilla et al., 1991). This is the proposed explanation for the impaired coronary vasodilator reserve often observed in patients with LVH.

Fibrosis and pathological hypertrophy

In an interesting series of experiments, Weber and Brilla (1991) suggest that not all agents that cause regression of left ventricular hypertrophy also cause regression of fibrosis. For example, verapamil reduced LVH in the spontaneously hypertensive rat without decreasing collagen content (Ruskoaho and Savolainen, 1985), whereas minoxidil actually increased collagen concentration. The ACE inhibitors decreased collagen provided that therapy was sufficiently prolonged. Thus, prolonged therapy with captopril (Jalil et al., 1991) or lisinopril (Brilla et al., 1991) or perindopril (Michel, 1990) or enalapril (Pahor et al., 1991) reduced myocardial fibrosis in the spontaneously hypertensive rat. In some studies, diastolic stiffness decreased, whereas in others chiefly systolic function improved (Gosse et al., 1990).

The exact way in which angiotensin-II activity is related to collagen formation is not clear, but indirect evidence suggests that it works at least in part by stimulation of secretion of aldosterone (Weber and Brilla, 1991; Weber et al., 1994). Ultimately, intracellular calcium may be an important signal (Motz and Strauer, 1989), as shown in Fig. 4–2. The application of these studies to patients is an intriguing challenge that depends on the evolution of techniques to estimate collagen and fibrosis in situ.

Left ventricular hypertrophy and diastolic dysfunction

Commonly, patients with hypertension and left ventricular failure present with exertional dyspnea, and such patients are regarded as having heart failure to be treated by digitalis and diuretics. It is now becoming increasingly apparent, however, that many such patients have normal systolic function as assessed by the ejection fraction (Dougherty et al., 1984; Cuocolo et al., 1990), yet have diastolic dysfunction that is common in concentric left ventricular hypertrophy (Fig. 4–3). In 37 hypertensive patients with radiological cardiomegaly, with none in clinical congestive heart failure, 28 had a normal or high ejection fraction (Jennings et al., 1986). For such patients, digitalis is inappropriate therapy. Rather, it may be supposed on first principles that treatment should be aimed at the regression of left ventricular hypertrophy by beta-blockers, calcium antagonists, or ACE inhibitors (Fig. 4–3). Of note are experimental data that infusion of angiotensin-I to hypertrophied rat hearts impaired diastolic relaxation (Schunkert et al., 1990). Diuretics are often inappropriate because in diastolic dysfunction the

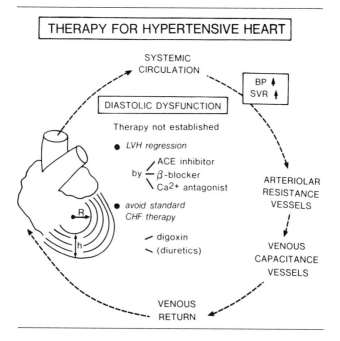

THERAPY FOR HYPERTENSIVE HEART

Figure 4–3. In early left ventricular hypertrophy (LVH), diastolic dysfunction requires different therapy from established systolic failure. Regression of LVH is basic but not yet proven to be the best therapy for diastolic dysfunction. There are arguments to avoid the standard therapy of congestive heart failure (CHF), such as digoxin and possibly diuretics. Digoxin and other digitalis compounds should be avoided because left ventricular systolic function is well maintained or above normal. Fig. © LH Opie.

atrial filling pressure needs to be maintained to achieve maximal left ventricular filling rates despite the diastolic dysfunction.

Although theoretically it should be possible to show improvement in diastolic dysfunction as regression of left ventricular hypertrophy is achieved by ACE inhibition, this aim has not been easy to achieve.

Mitral inflow pattern. In the study by Shahi et al. (1990), captopril (mean daily dose 93 mg, usually with added diuretic) caused regression of left ventricular hypertrophy over 9 months of therapy but did not improve diastolic function as judged by echocardiographic patterns of mitral inflow. Enalapril also did not change the mitral inflow velocity ratios despite decreasing left ventricular mass (Gosse et al., 1990). The mitral inflow pattern may not be a reliable index of diastolic dysfunction since it may remain unchanged when other indices respond to ACE inhibition (Modena et al., 1992).

Enalapril and diastolic dysfunction. Using a different index of diastolic dysfunction, namely the peak lengthening rate in diastole, Grandi et al. (1991) were able to show that enalapril 20 to 40 mg daily given for 4 months was able to increase the mean rate of lengthening (p < 0.01). Of the 12 subjects, 6 had abnormally low lengthening rates at the start, and in each the rate increased, reaching the normal range in the majority. In that study, enalapril also decreased left ventricular mass.

Experimental ischemia-induced diastolic dysfunction in LVH. When hypertrophic rat hearts are subject to acute ischemia, diastolic dysfunction develops (Eberli et al., 1992). Activation of the cardiac renin-angiotensin system is involved in the mechanism, because infusion of enalaprilat attenuated the diastolic abnormality in hypertrophic hearts but not in control hearts.

Lisinopril and diastolic dysfunction. In 35 patients lisinopril 10 to 20 mg daily reduced left ventricular mass over 6 months, but 12 months of therapy was needed to improve some echocardiographic indices of diastolic function (Modena et al., 1992). Even then, the isovolumic relaxation time was still prolonged.

Left ventricular systolic failure in hypertension

With continued left ventricular hypertrophy, eventual left ventricular dilation sets in. Once the radius of the left ventricle is unduly enlarged, wall stress augments, the ventricle stretches, and systolic power production is reduced. The result is diminished left ventricular ejection and a decreased systolic blood pressure (Fig. 4–4). As will be considered in greater detail in Chapter 5, the resultant compensatory increase of adrenergic outflow leads to renin-angiotensin activation, an increased systemic vascular resistance, and a rise in the afterload. At this stage, ACE inhibition should be ideal therapy for the hypertensive patient, able to decrease blood pressure and to lessen the afterload. ACE inhibition should in these circumstances be accompanied by diuretic therapy to correct the volume and sodium retention characteristic of congestive heart failure.

Regression of LVH in patients

Because an increased left ventricular mass is an independent risk factor for cardiovascular events, beyond the risk posed by the level of the blood pressure itself (Levy et al., 1990), lessening the degree of LVH has become a major therapeutic aim. Indirect evidence suggests that ACE inhibitors may be the best drug to achieve most regression of LVH (Dahlof and Hansson, 1992). Direct comparisons show that ACE inhibition is better than diuretic therapy (Dahlof and Hansson, 1992). ACE inhibition is also better than minoxidil as part of triple therapy (Julien et al., 1990). The predicted difference between ACE inhibitors and calcium antagonists on left ventricular regression is small (Dahlof et al., 1992) and it came as no surprise that perindopril and nifedipine were equi-effective in reducing both blood pressure and left ventricular mass (Schulte et al., 1992).

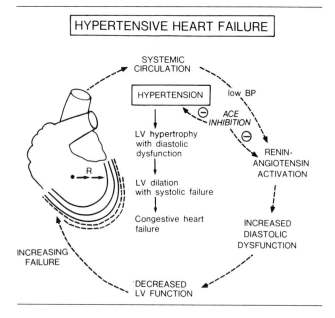

Figure 4–4. In established congestive heart failure due to hypertension, ACE inhibition may have two beneficial effects: first, reduction of the hypertension and, therefore, of the load on the heart and, second, inhibition of renin-angiotensin activation with relief of that component of the increased arteriolar resistance. Note in this figure, compared with the previous one, the increased radius (R) associated with left ventricular dilation and poor left ventricular systolic function. Fig. © LH Opie.

RENIN-SODIUM PROFILE, ANGIOTENSIN AND RISK OF MYOCARDIAL INFARCTION

If angiotensin-II has adverse effects on the myocardium and possibly on the coronary arteries by causing excess growth and fibrosis, then a reasonable hypothesis would be that patients with high circulating renin activities could be more prone to heart attacks than others. Laragh's group has tested their hypothesis that high-renin patients may be at increased cardiovascular risk (Alderman et al., 1991). In 1,717 patients with mild to moderate hypertension, *renin profiles* were obtained by plotting plasma renin activity against urinary excretion of sodium (Fig. 4–5). Their data showed that the ratio rate for high-renin status was about five times that of the low profile group, even when allowing for other cardiovascular risk factors. Of great interest is that black men were twice as likely as white men to have a low-renin profile, which may well explain the clinical findings that (1) this ethnic group is relatively protected from myocardial infarction, and (2) there is a poor response to ACE inhibitor therapy for hypertension (see Chapter 2). The combination of a high-renin profile with other risk factors, such as smoking, a high cholesterol level, or a high fasting blood glucose, increase the risk ratio considerably. For example, patients with the combination of a low-renin profile and a low fasting blood glucose had a risk factor

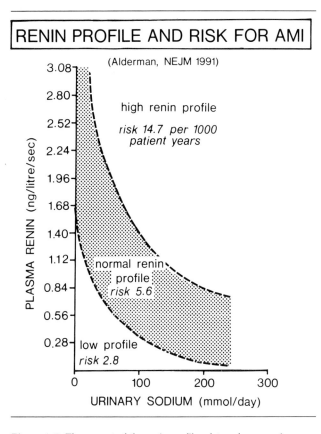

Figure 4–5. *The concept of the renin profile relates plasma renin activity to simultaneously measured urinary sodium excretion. These data taken from Alderman et al. (1991) with permission are modified from Figure 1 and Table 3 in the paper. The zone between the dotted lines show the normal renin profile with the renin rising in relation to the fall in urinary sodium—on a low sodium diet plasma renin is high. In the high-renin profile group, in which the patient had renin values about 2 to 3 times higher for the same urinary sodium excretion, the risk of acute myocardial infarction (AMI) was considerably higher. Low-renin profile patients, on the other hand, appear to be relatively protected. For further details, see Alderman et al. (1991).*

for myocardial infarction of 2.1 per 1,000 patient years, whereas a high-renin profile and a high fasting blood glucose had a risk factor of 48.5 per 1,000 patient years, i.e., 23 times higher. The blood pressure itself was, however, not a direct risk factor for myocardial infarction. These data may explain the promising effects of ACE inhibitor therapy in lessening the incidence of myocardial reinfarction in selected patients (Pfeffer et al., 1992).

ACE INHIBITORS AND CORONARY ARTERY DISEASE

Variable effects on coronary blood flow

In experimental myocardial ischemia, there is activation of the renin-angiotensin system, which appears to exert a coronary constrictive role. Angiotensin-II appears to have different effects on small distal vessels and large conductance vessels (Cohen and Kirk, 1973). With sustained administration, the effect on the small distal vessels becomes blunted, whereas the effect on the large vessels is sustained. These observations would explain why ACE inhibitors could potentially act as coronary vasodilators (Ertl, 1987; Holtz et al., 1987). In patients with mild essential hypertension and no evidence of ischemic heart disease, diuretic administration (furosemide 50 mg daily for 1 week) reduced coronary blood flow, again compatible with the idea of a renin-mediated coronary constriction, whereas a single dose of captopril 25 mg given to the diuretic-treated patients increased blood flow despite reducing the mean arterial pressure (Magrini et al., 1987).

Besides inhibition of coronary vasoconstriction mediated by angiotensin-II (Perondi et al., 1992) and involving the AT_1-receptors (Sudhir et al., 1993), there are two possible additional vasodilatory mechanisms of ACE inhibitors. First, an increase of vasodilatory prostaglandins, such as PGI_2, follows increased formation of bradykinin breakdown, as shown after the administration of ramipril to isolated hearts (van Gilst et al., 1987a). Second, especially in the case of captopril, there may be another mechanism promoting formation of PGI_2, apparently dependent on the SH-groups present in captopril (van Gilst et al., 1987a).

Inconstant antianginal effects of ACE inhibitors in humans

The decrease in myocardial oxygen consumption associated with a decreased blood pressure in the absence of any tachycardia, together with potential coronary vasodilation, should mean that ACE inhibitors have a potential antianginal effect. In some studies (Strozzi et al., 1987; Lai et al., 1987), a modest antianginal effect has been found. Bartels et al. (1993) and Remme et al. (1994) paced 25 untreated normotensive patients with angina but not in heart failure. During pacing there was neurohumoral activation. After the intravenous injection of perindoprilat (0.5 mg), the ACE inhibitor clearly reduced myocardial ischemia by preventing a catecholamine-mediated rise in total peripheral resistance.

On the other hand, in the presence of coronary stenosis, ACE inhibitors might potentially worsen myocardial ischemia because of dilation of the resistance vessels with risk of passive narrowing or even collapse of the coronary stenoses (Schwartz and Bache, 1987). In 11 patients with coronary artery stenosis demonstrated by coronary angiography, the ACE inhibitor benazepril had no overall antianginal effect, although a benefit was noted in 6 of the patients (Thurmann et al., 1991).

Thus, on the whole, ACE inhibitors are not regarded as particularly efficacious antianginal agents. There might be variable results depending on the overall balance between the adverse effects of hypertension, the potential lessening of blood flow across coronary stenoses, the indirect beneficial antiadrenergic effect, and long-term vascular protection.

Hypertension and angina. As expected, in patients with this combination, ACE inhibitor monotherapy could both reduce blood pressure and anginal attacks (Akhras and Jackson, 1991; Stumpe et al., 1993).

Severe heart failure and angina pectoris

It might be anticipated in patients with heart failure that the ACE inhibitors would be particularly effective as antianginal agents because of their capacity to reduce the load on the ventricle and hence to lessen left ventricular dilation. In severe heart failure and angina, however, ACE inhibitor therapy may not be successful (Cleland et al., 1991). The presumed mechanism of this adverse effect is a decreased blood pressure with impaired coronary perfusion. Concurrent therapy with nifedipine was especially harmful.

Unstable angina

In the SOLVD study (1991), patients with low ejection fractions treated by enalapril had a lower incidence of unstable angina and myocardial infarction than those treated by placebo (Yusuf et al., 1992).

Nitrate tolerance during the treatment of angina pectoris

Although ACE inhibitors may not directly have prominent antianginal effects, nonetheless there is increasing evidence that they might benefit patients with angina by facilitating the effects of nitrates (Fig. 4–6). Captopril added to isosorbide dinitrate improved antianginal effects, especially in patients not responding well to nitrates alone (Metelitsa et al., 1992). Depletion of sulfhydryl groups and activation of the renin-angiotensin system are thought to play a role in the production of nitrate tolerance (Katz, 1990). Hence, it might be anticipated that therapy by ACE inhibitors, particularly those containing SH-groups such as captopril, might help to prevent nitrate tolerance. Experimentally, captopril with SH-groups but not ramipril (without SH-groups) is able to potentiate coronary vasodilation in the isolated rat heart in response to isosorbide dinitrate (van Gilst et al., 1987b). Similar data have been obtained on rat aortic rings (Lawson et al., 1991). In patients, however, the venodilator effects of nitrate patches have been tested during therapy by enalapril (10 mg twice daily) and captopril (25 mg three times daily); maintenance of the nitrate effect and lessening of nitrate tolerance was equally well demonstrated during therapy with either captopril or enalapril (Katz et al., 1991) arguing against a specific effect of SH-groups in this situation. Rather, it seems as if nitrate tolerance is prevented by vasodilation, whether by ACE inhibition or by hydralazine (Bauer and Fung, 1991).

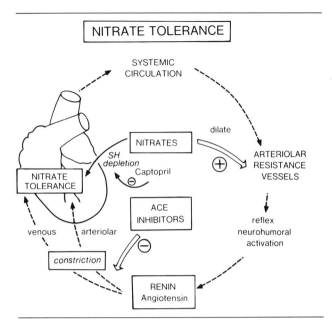

Figure 4–6. There are two major theories for nitrate intolerance. First, there may be a deficiency of vascular SH-groups, and for this, captopril containing SH-groups, would seem logical therapy. Second, the nitrate-induced vasodilation could cause reflex neurohumoral activation with increased renin-angiotensin activity. The result would be arteriolar and venous constriction, thereby diminishing the effects of nitrates on those two systems. For the second mechanism, any type of ACE inhibitor whether or not it contains an SH-group should in practice be appropriate therapy. Although some experimental data support the concept that captopril might be better, clinical data suggest that different ACE inhibitors are almost equieffective for nitrate tolerance. Fig. © LH Opie.

ACE Inhibitors and Early Phase Acute Myocardial Infarction

Initial experimental studies suggested that ACE inhibitors had no effect on myocardial ischemic injury following coronary artery occlusion (Berdeaux et al., 1987) except in the presence of congestive heart failure caused by large myocardial infarction (Drexler et al., 1987). Because of marked neurohumoral activation in patients with acute myocardial infarction, with angiotensin-II levels increasing approximately eightfold (Dargie et al., 1987), it became logical to treat patients with left ventricular failure complicating myocardial infarction by ACE inhibitors (Brivet et al., 1981; Bounhoure et al., 1982; McAlpine et al., 1987). Thus, these agents achieve afterload reduction in patients with acute myocardial infarction (Fig. 4–7). The study by Brivet et al. (1981) is of particular interest because it antedates by some years many of the other studies.

As reduction of the myocardial oxygen demand is known to be a factor decreasing ultimate infarct size, it was not surprising that continuous administration of captopril decreased estimated infarct size over 30 minutes to 6 hours of coronary occlusion in an open-chest dog model (Ertl et

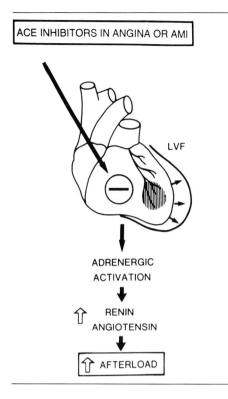

ACE INHIBITORS IN ANGINA OR AMI

LVF

ADRENERGIC
ACTIVATION

⇑   RENIN
ANGIOTENSIN

⇑ AFTERLOAD

Figure 4–7. In acute myocardial infarction (AMI), left ventricular failure (LVF) may develop with adrenergic activation and an increase in afterload mediated by renin-angiotensin. Oral ACE inhibition is logical therapy and is still being tested in a large-scale trial. For use in angina, see Bartels et al. (1993). Fig. © LH Opie.

al., 1982). Regional myocardial blood flow improved and arterial pressure decreased, as did left atrial pressure. This study differs from that of Berdeaux et al. (1987) who used intermittent coronary artery occlusion. In rats with coronary artery ligation, perindopril improved left ventricular performance and decreased myocardial depletion of norepinephrine (Ribuot et al., 1990).

Acute phase infarction: ISIS-IV, GISSI-3 and CONSENSUS-II studies

ACE inhibitors are now freely used and well documented for patients with acute myocardial infarction with overt left ventricular failure (AIRE study, see Chapter 5). The hypothesis that the early administration of an ACE inhibitor to all patients with acute myocardial infarction could be beneficial, has been tested in two massive studies, also considered in Chapter 5 (see Table 5–8). In ISIS-IV, nearly 54,000 patients were randomized to captopril or to placebo within 24 hours of the onset of symptoms. The initial dose of captopril was 6.25 mg, titrated upward to 50 mg twice daily for 4 weeks. In the first 35 days, there were 4.6 fewer deaths per 1,000 patients in the captopril-treated groups with an absolute reduction in mortality of 0.46% (2p = 0.04). Put differently, there was a 6% risk reduction in mortality. In the GISSI-3 study on a total of nearly 19,000 patients, lisinopril was given as an initial dose of 2.5 mg or 5 mg orally, increasing up to 10 mg once daily for 6 weeks. The mortality at 6 weeks was reduced from 7.1% in controls to 6.3% in the lisinopril group, i.e., a reduction of 0.8% (2p = 0.03). Put differently, there was an 11% reduction in the relative risk of mortality when combined with nitrates (intravenous followed by intermittent transdermal nitroglycerin), there was an impressive risk reduction of 17% in mortality.

These modest benefits, to some extent offset by an increased incidence of hypotension (nearly 20% of the captopril-treated patients versus 10% in placebo patients), are probably not sufficient to warrant consideration of the routine use of oral captopril or lisinopril in acute infarction. Furthermore, as shown by the CONSENSUS-II study (1992), an intravenous ACE inhibitor, enalaprilat, does not work because of the frequent occurrence of excess hypotension which, in turn, predisposes to increased mortality. Nevertheless, the data from ISIS-IV and GISSI-3 enlarge the time frame in which ACE inhibitors can safely and beneficially be used in acute myocardial infarction. Whereas ACE inhibitors were started several days after the onset of myocardial infarction in the SAVE and AIRE studies, in the ISIS-IV and GISSI-3 studies they were used as early as possible. To other observers, the benefits in acute phase myocardial infarction are too modest to recommend general use. Rather these agents should be reserved for patients with clinical features of heart failure, or those with large anterior or prior infarcts. Therapy of choice would be an oral ACE inhibitor plus nitrates (GISSI-3, 1994). At present, definite recommendations cannot be made, but clearly these trials will bias more and more cardiologists to use ACE inhibitors when in doubt.

Also of interest is that ACE inhibitors have been tested in three patients with cardiogenic shock in whom there was hemodynamic improvement and short-term survival (Lipkin et al., 1987). In general, however, hypotension is a contraindication to the use of an ACE inhibitor.

ACE INHIBITORS AND REPERFUSION INJURY

Taking the broader concept of reperfusion injury which includes not only arrhythmias but also stunning as well as metabolic damage (Opie, 1989), ACE inhibitors have been reported to decrease early metabolic damage such as noradrenaline overflow and creatine kinase release in a closed-chest pig model (de Graeff et al., 1988). Reperfusion arrhythmias, although decreased in isolated rat heart models (van Gilst et al., 1986; Rochette et al., 1987), were not decreased in the closed-chest pig model (de Graeff et al., 1987; de Langen et al., 1989). Nonetheless, our data (Muller et al., 1994) show that pretreatment of pigs by trandolapril lessens both ischemic and reperfusion arrhythmias. One hypothesis is that ACE inhibitors containing SH-groups are better able to scavenge free radicals during reperfusion. Yet a comparison of the various agents studied by van Gilst et al. (1986) and Elfellah and Ogilvie (1985) strongly suggests that the antiarrhythmic effect, when found, is a class effect (Fig. 4–8).

The mechanism of the antiarrhythmic benefit may include bradykinin formation. In the isolated rat heart, a low concentration of ramiprilat (3×10^{-8} mM) reduces reperfusion arrhythmias, an effect mimicked by bradykinin at a concentration of 10^{-10} mM (Linz et al., 1990). Arrhythmias that had been inhibited by ramiprilat (10^{-7} mM) were precipitated by addition of a bradykinin antagonist (10^{-5} mM).

Late reperfusion arrhythmias

Late arrhythmias, occurring days after ischemic reperfusion in closed-chest pigs, can be prevented by captopril treatment, but in those experiments an effect on the extent of left ventricular dilation seems a probable explanation (Pfeffer and Pfeffer, 1987). An interesting study is that by Tio et al. (1990) who gave oral pretreatment to pigs with zofenopril, a captopril analog, and 2 weeks after reperfusion (following 45 minutes of left anterior descending coronary occlusion) subjected the animals to programmed electrical stimulation. During this test the authors found that the oxygen demand of the heart increased by over 40% and there was an increased efflux of adrenaline, noradrenaline and inosine, as well as hypoxanthine into the coronary venous effluent (Tio et al., 1990). Zofenopril-treated pigs had a reduction of inducibility of sustained ventricular tachyarrhythmias (5 of 9 inducible in untreated animals, 1 of 10 inducible in treated animals, $p < 0.05$).

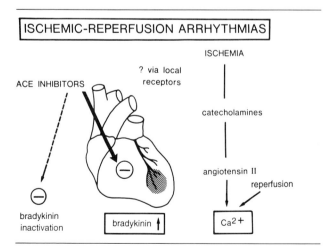

Figure 4–8. The mechanism whereby ACE inhibitors may be effective in ischemic or reperfusion arrhythmias may be because of the capacity of these agents to modulate the increased adrenergic activity associated with acute myocardial infarction. In the reperfusion period, one concept is that enhanced cytosolic calcium helps to promote excess intracellular cycling which predisposes to reperfusion arrhythmias and stunning. Fig. © LH Opie.

Do ACE inhibitors attenuate reperfusion-induced stunning?

In dogs, either high-dose captopril or the isomer with poor ACE activity but equipotent in scavenging superoxide anions, both improve reperfusion-induced stunning (Westlin and Mullane, 1988) and in this system enalaprilat was inactive. However, in another experiment (Przyklenk and Kloner, 1987), treatment by enalapril started 45 minutes after reperfusion in the dog was effective in reducing stunning, and better than the nonspecific vasodilator, nitroprusside. The proposed mechanism of benefit of late enalapril was by coronary vasodilation, but no data on coronary flow were reported.

Thus, as in the case of arrhythmias, there is suggestive evidence that ACE inhibitors can improve stunning without any implication that there is a specific requirement for SH-groups in the structure.

ACE Inhibitors and Postinfarct Ventricular Dilation, Remodeling and Failure

After myocardial infarction some patients undergo a progressive increase in left ventricular size manifest by a long-term increase in the end-diastolic and end-systolic volumes (Gadsboll et al., 1989). The increase in left ventricular volume is particularly found in patients with clinical manifestations of heart failure. This process whereby the left ventricle progressively enlarges is called remodeling. This process stimulates the cardiac renin-angiotensin system (Yamagishi et al., 1993). Evidence both from captopril-treated rats (Pfeffer et al., 1985) and from patient studies (Pfeffer et al., 1988) suggests that ventricular unloading by means of ACE inhibition can beneficially improve the remodeling process, particularly in moderate size rat infarcts (Fig. 4–9). In left ventricular dilation after large myocardial infarctions in rats, captopril but not hydralazine was able to induce hemodynamic benefit which suggests that both preload and afterload reduction is required rather than only afterload reduction as with the use of hydralazine (Raya et al., 1989). Based on the rat heart data, improved postinfarct survival is a potential benefit with the use of ACE inhibitors following acute myocardial infarction (Pfeffer et al., 1988).

Patient studies

In patients with a poor left ventricular ejection fraction ($<45\%$) but without clinical evidence of heart failure, captopril 25 mg three times daily compared with furosemide 40 mg daily prevents progressive left ventricular enlargement (Sharpe et al., 1988). Patients in this study were started 1 week after the onset of acute myocardial infarction or later. In a second study, administration of the ACE inhibitor was started 24 to 48 hours after the onset of symptoms. One hundred patients were given either placebo or

POST−INFARCT REMODELING

WALL STRESS = $\dfrac{\text{Pressure x Radius}}{\text{2 x (wall thickness)}}$

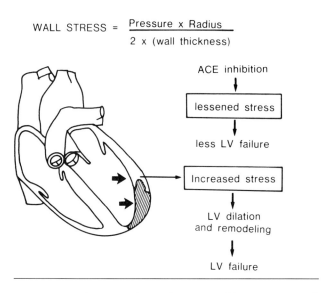

Figure 4–9. In the process of postinfarction remodeling, increased wall stress may promote adverse remodeling and left ventricular (LV) failure. The proposal based on animal data and human studies is that ACE inhibition will attenuate postinfarct left ventricular enlargement and promote beneficial remodeling with better LV mechanical function (Sutton et al., 1994). Fig. © LH Opie.

captopril 50 mg twice daily and followed for 3 months (Sharpe et al., 1991). The captopril group had a decrease in left ventricular end-systolic volume and an increase in the ejection fraction, changes not found in the placebo group. Similar data were obtained with enalapril in patients with more evident heart failure (Konstam et al., 1992).

These studies in relatively small numbers of patients have now been extended to show hard benefits in terms of improved morbidity and mortality in two massive studies, the one specifically on postinfarct patients and using captopril (Pfeffer et al., 1992) and the other on enalapril, showing the prevention of myocardial infarction (Yusuf et al., 1992). Whether such studies will lead to ACE inhibitors being given as routine postinfarction treatment remains to be seen. Strictly speaking, there should be proof of left ventricular dysfunction to benefit from ACE inhibitors given prophylactically to postinfarct patients (Sutton et al., 1994).

As ACE inhibitors are specifically effective in patients with left ventricular failure and as one of the possible adverse effects of beta-blockade is the precipitation of left ventricular failure, the combination of beta-blocker with ACE inhibitor warrants clinical appraisal in postinfarct patients. In the SAVE study (Pfeffer et al., 1992), captopril was beneficial even for patients given concurrent beta-blockers or thrombolytic therapy or aspirin.

Postinfarct ischemic dysfunction

In postinfarct patients with a mean ejection fraction of 40%, captopril (titrated to a dose of 25 mg twice daily for 180 days) improved exercise tolerance, decreased ambulatory ST-segment changes, and lessened the heart volume (Sogaard et al., 1993). Similar functional changes were found in another study wherein captopril compared favorably with digoxin (Bonaduce et al., 1992); ischemia was not an end-point in that study.

Postinfarct failure

The AIRE study (see Chapter 5) has convincingly shown that ramipril (2.5 to 5 mg twice daily), when given to patients with postinfarct failure that is clinically manifest, can improve all-cause mortality. Only a minority of these patients were also receiving digoxin, although the majority had diuretic therapy.

ACE Inhibitors in
Other Cardiac Conditions

In *chronic cor pulmonale*, captopril appears not to decrease pulmonary vascular resistance (hypoxic pulmonary hypertension), and any decrease in pulmonary wedge pressure reflects an effect on the left ventricle not on the pulmonary circulation (Zielinski et al., 1986). In *chronic aortic regurgitation*, acute administration of captopril 25 mg gave benefit by reducing the regurgitant fraction in the absence of any fall in the blood pressure (Reske et al., 1985). The mechanism of this benefit is speculative and may include (1) effects of the ACE inhibitor on aortic compliance (discussed in Chapter 10), and (2) reduction of the preload and thereby an improvement of myocardial wall stress with a consequent increase in myocardial contractile activity. Further studies with much longer follow-up are required before ACE inhibition can be used for this indication. In *murine Coxsackie myocarditis* produced experimentally, captopril whether started early or late in the disease process reduced heart weight and when given early it reduced the extent of necrosis (Rezhalla et al., 1990). In patients with *idiopathic dilated cardiomyopathy*, captopril is better able to reduce wall stress than is nifedipine (Agostini et al., 1986).

In *pediatric cardiomyopathy*, a retrospective study suggested that captopril could improve survival (Lewis and Chabot, 1993).

Summary

Angiotensin-II helps regulate the cardiac inotropic state and acts as a growth signal for the myocardium. There is molecular evidence that the cardiac renin-angiotensin system participates in growth regulation during left ventricular hypertrophy. Nonetheless, the role of angiotensin-converting enzyme in the production of cardiac angiotensin-II in humans is controversial. It is proposed that there is a multicellular interactive renin-angiotensin system involving cardiac myocytes, fibroblasts, vascular smooth muscle, and endothelium. In left ventricular hypertrophy associated with hypertension, ACE inhibition helps to reduce the hypertrophy, acting in part by load reduction and possibly in part by inhibition of the effects of angiotensin-II on collagen formation by fibroblasts. Theoretical grounds suggest that ACE inhibition may play a role in the control of myocardial ischemia, postreperfusion arrhythmias, and, possibly, postreperfusion stunning. Nonetheless, firm data supporting the use of ACE inhibitors to lessen the severity of myocardial ischemia or to decrease reperfusion damage are still lacking. In the case of postinfarct left ventricular dysfunction, both experimental and clinical data available are concordant in supporting the use of ACE inhibition even without additional diuretic therapy and, in fact, in preference to diuretic therapy. The result of recent large-scale postinfarct trials on patients with impaired left ventricular function or failure supports the use of ACE inhibitors in this situation.

Isolated reports suggest that ACE inhibitors containing SH-groups, such as captopril, might have certain specific antiarrhythmic and anti-ischemic effects, and protect from the development of nitrate tolerance. Nonetheless, similar effects have also been found with other ACE inhibitors not containing SH-groups, including enalapril, ramipril, and perindopril. Thus, these proposed benefits of ACE inhibitors are highly likely to be class effects. At least some of the benefit of these drugs may be mediated by increased local formation of bradykinin. Present evidence suggests that nitrate tolerance can be lessened by concurrent therapy by ACE inhibitors or by hydralazine.

Apart from the reduction of left ventricular hypertrophy, the most important cardiac indication for ACE inhibition is likely to be in postinfarct patients with either (1) left ventricular dysfunction in whom ACE inhibitors improve function and prognosis, and help lessen the incidence of reinfarction and unstable angina; or (2) postinfarct clinical heart failure in whom mortality is reduced. In acute phase infarction, ACE inhibition plus nitrates may be appropriate for patients at risk of LV dysfunction, e.g., large anterior infarcts.

REFERENCES

Agostoni PG, De Cesare N, Doria E, et al. Afterload reduction: a comparison of captopril and nifedipine in dilated cardiomyopathy. *Br Heart J* 1986; 55: 391–399.

Akhras F, Jackson G. The role of captopril as single therapy in hypertension and angina pectoris. *Int J Cardiol* 1991; 33: 259–266.

Alderman MH, Madhavan S, Ooi WL, et al. Association of the renin sodium profile with the risk of myocardial infarction in patients with hypertension. *N Engl J Med* 1991; 324: 1098–1104.

Allen IS, Cohen NM, Dhallan RS, et al. Angiotensin-II increases spontaneous contractile frequency and stimulates calcium current in cultured neonatal rat heart myocytes: insights into the underlying biochemical mechanisms. *Circ Res* 1988; 62: 524–534.

Asmar RG, Pannier B, Santoni JPh, et al. Reversion of cardiac hypertrophy and reduced arterial compliance after converting enzyme inhibition in essential hypertension. *Circulation* 1988; 78: 941–950.

Baker KM, Campanile CP, Trachte GJ, Peach MJ. Identification and characterization of the rabbit angiotensin-II myocardial receptor. *Circ Res* 1984; 54: 286–293.

Baker KM, Cherin MI, Wixon SK, Aceto JF. Renin angiotensin system involvement in pressure-overload cardiac hypertrophy in rats. *Am J Physiol* 1990; 259: H324–H332.

Bartels L, Remme WJ, van der Ent M, Kruijssen D. ACE inhibitors reduce myocardial ischemia through modulation of ischemia-induced catecholamine activation, experience with perindoprilat. *J Am Coll Cardiol* 1993; 21: 19A.

Bauer JA, Fung H-L. Concurrent hydralazine administration prevents nitroglycerin-induced hemodynamic tolerance in experimental heart failure. *Circulation* 1991; 84: 35–39.

Berdeaux A, Bonhenry C, Giudicelli JF. Effects of four angiotensin-I converting enzyme inhibitors on regional myocardial blood flow and ischemia injury during coronary artery occlusion in dogs. *Fundam Clin Pharmacol* 1987; 1: 201–212.

Bonaduce D, Petretta M, Arrichiello P, et al. Effects of captopril treatment on left ventricular remodeling and function after anterior myocardial infarction: comparison with digitalis. *J Am Coll Cardiol* 1992; 19: 858–863.

Bounhoure JP, Kayanakis JG, Fauvel JM, Puel J. Beneficial effects of captopril in left ventricular failure in patients with myocardial infarction. *Br J Clin Pharmacol* 1982; 14: 187S–191S.

Brilla CG, Janicki JS, Weber KT. Cardioreparative effects of lisinopril in rats with genetic hypertension and left ventricular hypertrophy. *Circulation* 1991; 83: 1771–1779.

Brivet F, Delfraissy J-F, Giudicelli J-F, et al. Immediate effects of captopril in acute left ventricular failure secondary to myocardial infarction. *Eur J Clin Invest* 1981; 11: 369–373.

Cleland JGF, Henderson E, McLenachan J, et al. Effect of captopril, an angiotensin-converting enzyme inhibitor, in patients with angina pectoris and heart failure. *J Am Coll Cardiol* 1991; 17: 733–739.

Cohen MV, Kirk ES. Differential response of large and small coronary arteries to nitroglycerin and angiotensin. Autoregulation and tachyphylaxis. *Circ Res* 1973; 33: 445–453.

Cuocolo A, Sax FL, Brush JE, et al. Left ventricular hypertrophy and impaired diastolic filling in essential hypertension. Diastolic mechanisms for systolic dysfunction during exercise. *Circulation* 1990; 81: 978–986.

Dahlof B, Hansson L. Regression of left ventricular hypertrophy in previously untreated essential hypertension: different effects of enalapril and hydrochlorothiazide. *J Hypertens* 1992; 10: 1513–1524.

Dahlof B, Pennert K, Hansson L. Reversal of left ventricular hypertrophy in hypertensive patients. A meta-analysis of 109 treatment studies. *Am J Hypertens* 1992; 5: 95–110.

Dargie HJ, McAlpine HM, Morton JJ. Neuroendocrine activation in acute myocardial infarction. *J Cardiovasc Pharmacol* 1987; 9 (Suppl 2): S21–S24.

de Graeff PA, van Gilst WK, Bel K, et al. Concentration-dependent protection by captopril against myocardial damage during ischemia and reperfusion in a closed chest pig model. *J Cardiovasc Pharmacol* 1987; 9 (Suppl 2): S37–S42.

de Graeff PA, de Langen CDJ, van Gilst WH, et al. Protective effects of captopril against ischemia/reperfusion-induced ventricular arrhythmias in vitro and in vivo. *Am J Med* 1988; 84 (Suppl 3A): 67–74.

de Langen CDJ, de Graeff PA, van Wilst WH, et al. Effects of angiotensin-II and captopril on inducible sustained ventricular tachycardia two weeks after myocardial infarction in the pig. *J Cardiovasc Pharmacol* 1989; 13: 186–191.

Dosemeci A, Dhallan RS, Cohen NM, et al. Phorbol ester increases calcium current and simulates the effects of angiotensin-II on cultured neonatal rat heart myocytes. *Circ Res* 1988; 62: 347–357.

Dostal DE, Baker KM. Evidence for a role of an intracardiac renin-angiotensin system in normal and failing hearts. *Trends Cardiovasc Med* 1993; 3: 67–74.

Dostal DE, Rothblum KN, Conrad KM, et al. Detection of angiotensin-I and II in cultured rat cardiac myocytes and fibroblasts. *Am J Physiol* 1992; 263: C851–C863.

Dougherty AH, Naccarelli GV, Gray EL, et al. Congestive heart failure with normal systolic function. *Am J Cardiol* 1984; 54: 778–782.

Drexler H, Depenbusch JW, Truog AG, et al. Acute regional vascular effects of intravenous captopril in a rat model of myocardial infarction and failure. *J Pharmacol Exp Ther* 1987; 241: 13–19.

Dussaule J-C, Michel J-B, Auzan C, et al. Effect of antihypertensive treatment on the left ventricular isomyosin profile in one-clip, two-kidney hypertensive rats. *J Pharmacol Exp Ther* 1986; 236: 512–518.

Dzau VJ, Re R. Tissue angiotensin system in cardiovascular medicine. A paradigm shift? *Circulation* 1994; 89: 493–498.

Eberli FR, Apstein CS, Ngoy S, Lorell BH. Exacerbation of left ventricular ischemic diastolic dysfunction by pressure-overload hypertrophy. Modification by specific inhibition of cardiac angiotensin converting enzyme. *Circ Res* 1992; 70: 931–943.

Eischstadt HW, Felix R, Langer M, et al. Use of nuclear magnetic resonance imaging to show regression of hypertrophy with ramipril treatment. *Am J Cardiol* 1987; 59: 98D–103D.

Elfellah MS, Ogilvie RI. Effect of vasodilator drugs on coronary occlusion and reperfusion arrhythmias in anesthetized dogs. *J Cardiovasc Pharmacol* 1985; 7: 826–832.

Ertl G. Coronary vasoconstriction in experimental myocardial ischemia. *J Cardiovasc Pharmacol* 1987; 9 (Suppl 2): S9–S17.

Ertl G, Kloner RA, Alexander W, Braunwald E. Limitation of experimental infarct size by an angiotensin-converting enzyme inhibitor. *Circulation* 1982; 65: 40–48.

Gadsboll N, Hoilund-Carlsen P-F, Badsberg JS, et al. Late ventricular dilatation in survivors of acute myocardial infarction. *Am J Cardiol* 1989; 64: 961–966.

GISSI-3 (Gruppo Italiano per lo Studio della Sopravvivenza Nell' Infarto Miocardico). GISSI-3: effects of lisinopril and transdermal glyceryl trinitrate singly and together on 6-week mortality and ventricular function after acute myocardial infarction. *Lancet* 1994; 343: 1115–1122.

Gosse P, Roudaut R, Herrero G, Dallocchio M. Beta-blockers vs angiotensin-converting enzyme inhibitors in hypertension: effects on left ventricular hypertrophy. *J Cardiovasc Pharmacol* 1990; 16 (Suppl 5): S145–S150.

Grandi AM, Venco A, Barzizza F, et al. Effect of enalapril on left ventricular mass and performance in essential hypertension. *Am J Cardiol* 1989; 63: 1093–1097.

Grandi AM, Venco A, Barzizza F, et al. Double-blind comparison of perindopril and captopril in hypertension. Effects on left ventricular morphology and function. *Am J Hypertens* 1991; 4: 516–520.

Harrap SB, Mitchell GA, Casley DJ, et al. Angiotensin-II, sodium, and cardiovascular hypertrophy in spontaneously hypertensive rats. *Hypertension* 1993; 21: 50–55.

Hirsch AT, Talsness CE, Schunkert H, et al. Tissue-specific activation of cardiac angiotensin converting enzyme in experimental heart failure. *Circ Res* 1991; 69: 475–482.

Holtz J, Busse R, Sommer O, Bassenge E. Dilation of epicardial arteries in conscious dogs induced by angiotensin-converting enzyme inhibition with enalaprilat. *J Cardiovasc Pharmacol* 1987; 9: 348–355.

ISIS-IV study (1994)(Fourth International Study of Infarct Survival). Preliminary results presented at the American Heart Association meeting, November 1993. *Circulation* 1994; 89: 545–547.

Jalil JE, Janicki JS, Weber KT. Coronary vascular remodeling and myocardial fibrosis in the rat with renovascular hypertension. Response to captopril. *Am J Hypertens* 1991; 4: 51–55.

Jennings AA, Jee LD, Smith JA, et al. Acute effect of nifedipine on blood pressure and left ventricular ejection fraction in severely hypertensive outpatients. Predictive effects of acute therapy and prolonged efficacy. *Am Heart J* 1986; 111: 557–563.

Julien J, Dufluoux M-A, Prasquier R, et al. Effects of captopril and minoxidil on left ventricular hypertrophy in resistant hypertensive patients: A 6-month double-blind comparison. *J Am Coll Cardiol* 1990; 16: 137–142.

Katz RJ. Mechanisms of nitrate tolerance. A Review. *Cardiovasc Drugs Ther* 1990; 4: 247–252.

Katz RJ, Levy WS, Buff L, Wasserman AG. Prevention of nitrate tolerance with angiotensin converting enzyme inhibitors. *Circulation* 1991; 83: 1271–1277.

Khairallah PA, Kanabus J. Angiotensin and myocardial protein synthesis. In: Tarazi RC, Dunbar JB (eds), *Perspectives in Cardiovascular Research*, Vol 8. Raven Press, New York, 1983, 337–347.

Konstam MA, Rousseau MF, Kronenberg MW, et al. Effects of the angiotensin-converting enzyme inhibitor enalapril on the long-term progression of left ventricular dysfunction in patients with heart failure. *Circulation* 1992; 86: 431–438.

Kromer EP, Elsner D, Riegger GAJ. Role of neurohumoral systems for pressure induced left ventricular hypertrophy in experimental supravalvular aortic stenosis in rats. *Am J Hypertens* 1991; 4: 521–524.

Lai C, Onnis E, Orani E, et al. Antiischaemic activity of ACE inhibitor enalapril in normotensive patients with stable effort angina (abstr). *J Am Coll Cardiol* 1987; 9: 192A.

Lawson DL, Nichols WW, Mehta P, Mehta JL. Captopril-induced reversal of nitroglycerin tolerance: role of sulfhydryl group vs ACE inhibitory activity. *J Cardiovasc Pharmacol* 1991; 17: 411–418.

Levy D, Garrison RJ, Savage DD, et al. Prognostic implications of echocardiographically determined left ventricular mass in the Framingham heart study. *N Engl J Med* 1990; 322: 1561–1566.

Lewis AB, Chabot M. The effect of treatment with angiotensin-converting enzyme inhibitors on survival of pediatric patients with dilated cardiomyopathy. *Pediatr Cardiol* 1993; 14: 9–12.

Lindpaintner K, Ganten D. The cardiac renin-angiotensin system. An appraisal of present experimental and clinical evidence. *Circ Res* 1991; 68: 905–921.

Lindpaintner K, Lu W, Niedermajer N, et al. Distribution and functional significance of cardiac angiotensin converting enzyme in hypertrophied rat hearts. *J Mol Cell Cardiol* 1993; 25: 133–143.

Linz W, Martorana PA, Grotsch H, et al. Antagonizing bradykinin (BK) obliterates the cardioprotective effects of bradykinin and angiotensin-converting enzyme (ACE) inhibitors in ischemic hearts. *Drug Development Research* 1990; 19: 393–408.

Lipkin DP, Frenneaux M, Maseri A. Beneficial effect of captopril in cardiogenic shock (Letter). *Lancet* 1987; 2: 327.

McAlpine HM, Morton JJ, Leckie B, Dargie HJ. Haemodynamic effects of captopril in acute left ventricular failure complicating myocardial infarction. *J Cardiovasc Pharmacol* 1987; 9 (Suppl 2): S25–S30.

Magrini F, Shimizu M, Roberts N, et al. Converting enzyme inhibition and coronary blood flow. *Circulation* 1987; 75 (Suppl I): I-168-I-174.

Meggs LG, Coupet J, Huang H, et al. Regulation of angiotensin-II receptors on ventricular myocytes after myocardial infarction in rats. *Circ Res* 1993; 72: 1149–1162.

Metelitsa WI, Martsevich SY, Kozyreva MP, Slastnikova ID. Enhancement of the efficacy of isosorbide dinitrate by captopril in stable angina pectoris. *Am J Cardiol* 1992; 69: 291–296.

Michel J-B. Relationship between decrease in afterload and beneficial effects of ACE inhibitors in experimental cardiac hypertrophy and congestive heart failure. *Eur Heart J* 1990; 11 (Suppl D): 17–26.

Modena MG, Mattioli AV, Parato VM, Mattioli G. Effectiveness of the antihypertensive action of lisinopril on left ventricular mass and diastolic filling. *Eur Heart J* 1992; 13: 1540–1544.

Moravec C, Schuluchter MD, Paranandi L, et al. Inotropic effects of angiotensin-II on human cardiac muscle in vitro. *Circulation* 1990; 82: 1973–1984.

Motz W, Strauer BE. Left ventricular function and collagen content after regression of hypertensive hypertrophy. *Hypertension* 1989; 13: 43–50.

Muiesan ML, Agabiti-Rosei E, Romanelli G, et al. Beneficial effects of one year's treatment with captopril on left ventricular anatomy and function in hypertensive patients with left ventricular hypertrophy. *Am J Med* 1988; 84 (Suppl 3A): 129.

Mukherjee D, Sen S. Alteration of cardiac collagen phenotypes in hypertensive hypertrophy: role of blood pressure. *J Mol Cell Cardiol* 1993; 25: 185–196.

Muller CA, Opie LH, Peisach M, Pineda CA. Chronic oral pretreatment with angiotensin converting enzyme inhibitor trandolapril decreases ventricular fibrillation and cardiac converting enzyme activity in a pig model of acute ischemia and reperfusion. *Eur Heart J* 1994, in press.

Opie LH. Reperfusion injury and its pharmacological modification. *Circulation* 1989; 80: 1049–1062.

Pahor M, Bernabei R, Sgadari A, et al. Enalapril prevents cardiac fibrosis and arrhythmias in hypertensive rats. *Hypertension* 1991; 18: 148–157.

Perondi R, Saino A, Tio RA, et al. ACE inhibition attenuates sympathetic coronary vasoconstriction in patients with coronary artery disease. *Circulation* 1992; 85: 2004–2013.

Pfeffer MA, Pfeffer JM. Ventricular enlargement and reduced survival after myocardial infarction. *Circulation* 1987; 75 (Suppl IV): IV-93–IV-97.

Pfeffer MA, Pfeffer JM, Steinberg C, Finn P. Survival after an experimental myocardial infarction: beneficial effects of long-term therapy with captopril. *Circulation* 1985; 72: 406–412.

Pfeffer MA, Lamas GA, Vaughan DE, et al. Effect of captopril on progressive ventricular dilatation after anterior myocardial infarction. *N Engl J Med* 1988; 319: 80–86.

Pfeffer MA, Braunwald E, Moye LA, et al. Effect of captopril on mortality and morbidity in patients with left ventricular dysfunction after myocardial infarction. Results of the Survival and Ventricular Enlargement Trial. *N Engl J Med* 1992; 327: 669–677.

Przyklenk K, Kloner RA. Acute effects of hydralazine and enalapril on contractile function of postischemic "stunned" myocardium. *Am J Cardiol* 1987; 60: 934–936.

Raya TE, Gay RG, Aguirre M, Goldman S. Importance of venodilation in prevention of left ventricular dilatation after chronic large myocardial infarction in rats: A comparison of captopril and hydralazine. *Circ Res* 1989; 64: 330–337.

Remme WJ, Kruyssen DACM, Look MP, et al. Systemic and cardiac neuroendocrine activation and severity of myocardial ischemia in humans. *J Am Coll Cardiol* 1994; 23: 82–91.

Reske SN, Heck I, Kropp J, et al. Captopril mediated decrease of aortic regurgitation. *Br Heart J* 1985; 54: 415–419.

Rezhalla S, Kloner RA, Khatib G, Khatib R. Beneficial effects of captopril in acute Coxsackie virus B$_3$ murine myocarditis. *Circulation* 1990; 81: 1039–1046.

Ribuot C, Mossiat C, Devissaguet M, Rochette L. Beneficial effect of perindopril, an angiotensin-converting enzyme inhibitor, on left ventricular performance and noradrenaline myocardial content during cardiac failure development in the rat. *Can J Physiol Pharmacol* 1990; 68: 1548–1551.

Rochette L, Ribout C, Belichard P, et al. Protective effect of angiotensin converting enzyme inhibitors (CEI): captopril and perindopril on vulnerability to ventricular fibrillation during myocardial ischemia and reperfusion in rat. *Clin Exp Theory Pract* 1987; A9: 365–368.

Rogers TB. High affinity angiotensin-II receptors in myocardial sarcolemmal membranes. Characterization of receptors and covalent linkage of ^{125}I-angiotensin-II to a membrane component of 116,000 daltons. *J Biol Chem* 1984; 259: 8106–8114.

Ruskoaho HJ, Savolainen E-R. Effects of long-term verapamil treatment on blood pressure, cardiac hypertrophy and collagen metabolism in spontaneously hypertensive rats. *Cardiovasc Res* 1985; 19: 355–362.

Ruzicka M, Yuan B, Harmsen E, Leenen FHH. The renin-angiotensin system and volume overload-induced cardiac hypertrophy in rats. Effects of angiotensin-converting enzyme inhibitor versus angiotensin-II receptor blocker. *Circulation* 1993; 87: 921–930.

Sadoshima J, Izumo S. Molecular characterization of angiotensin-II-induced hypertrophy of cardiac myocytes and hyperplasia of cardiac fibroblasts. Critical role of the AT$_1$ receptor subtype. *Circ Res* 1993; 73: 413–423.

Sawa H, Tokuchi F, Mochizuki N, et al. Expression of the angiotensinogen gene and localization of its protein in the human heart. *Circulation* 1992; 86: 138–146.

Schelling P, Fischer H, Ganten D. Angiotensin and cell growth: a link to cardiovascular hypertrophy? *J Hypertens* 1991; 9: 3–15.

Schulte K-L, Meyer-Sabellek W, Liederwald K, et al. Relation of regression of left ventricular hypertrophy to changes in ambulatory blood pressure after long-term therapy with perindopril versus nifedipine. *Am J Cardiol* 1992; 70: 468–473.

Schunkert H, Dzau VJ, Tang SS, et al. Increased rat cardiac angiotensin-converting enzyme activity and mRNA expression in pressure overload left ventricular hypertrophy. *J Clin Invest* 1990; 86: 1913–1920.

Schunkert H, Jackson B, Tang S, et al. Distribution and functional significance of cardiac angiotensin converting enzyme in hypertrophied rat hearts. *Circulation* 1993; 87: 1328–1339.

Schwartz JS, Bache RJ. Pharmacologic vasodilators in the coronary circulation. *Circulation* 1987; 75 (Suppl I): I-162–I-167.

Scicli AG. Increases in cardiac kinins as a new mechanism to protect the heart. *Hypertension* 1994; 23: 419–421.

Shahi M, Thom S, Poulter N, et al. Regression of hypertensive left ventricular hypertrophy and left ventricular diastolic function. *Lancet* 1990; 336: 458–461.

Sharpe N, Murphy J, Smith H, Hannan S. Treatment of patients with symptomless left ventricular dysfunction after myocardial infarction. *Lancet* 1988; 1: 255–259.

Sharpe N, Smith H, Murphy J, et al. Early prevention of left ventricular dysfunction after myocardial infarction with angiotensin-converting enzyme inhibition. *Lancet* 1991; 337: 872–876.

Sogaard P, Gotzsche C-O, Ravkilde J, Thygesen K. Effects of captopril on ischemia and dysfunction of the left ventricle after myocardial infarction. *Circulation* 1993; 87: 1093–1099.

SOLVD Investigators. Effect of enalapril on survival in patients with reduced left ventricular ejection fractions and congestive heart failure. *N Engl J Med* 1991; 325: 293–302.

Strozzi C, Cocco G, Portaluppi F, et al. Effects of captopril on the physical work capacity of normotensive patients with stable effort angina pectoris. *Cardiology* 1987; 74: 226–228.

Stumpe KO, Overlack A on behalf of the Perindopril Therapeutic Safety Study Groups (PUTS). A new trial of the efficacy, tolerability, and safety of angiotensin-converting enzyme inhibition in mild systemic hypertension with concomitant diseases and therapies. *Am J Cardiol* 1993; 71: 32E–37E.

Sudhir K, MacGregor JS, Gupta M, et al. Effect of selective angiotensin-II receptor antagonism and angiotensin-converting enzyme inhibition on the coronary vasculature in vivo. Intravascular two-dimensional and Doppler ultrasound studies. *Circulation* 1993; 87: 931–938.

Sutton MStJ, Pfeffer MA, Plappert T, et al. Quantitative two-dimensional echocardiographic measurements are major predictors of adverse cardiovascular events after acute myocardial infarction. The protective effects of captopril. *Circulation* 1994; 89: 68–75.

Swedberg K, Held P, Kjekshus J, et al on behalf of the CONSENSUS II Study Group. Effects of the early administration of enalapril on mortality in patients with acute myocardial infarction. Results of the Cooperative New Scandinavian Enalapril Survival Study II (CONSENSUS II). *N Engl J Med* 1992; 327: 678–684.

Tan L-B, Jalil JE, Pick R, et al. Cardiac myocyte necrosis induced by angiotensin-II. *Circ Res* 1991; 69: 1185–1195.

Thurmann P, Odenthal HJ, Rietbrock N. Converting enzyme inhibition in coronary artery disease: a randomized, placebo-controlled trial with benazepril. *J Cardiovasc Pharmacol* 1991; 17: 718–723.

Tio RA, de Langen CDJ, de Graeff PA, et al. The effects of oral pretreatment with zofenopril, an angiotensin-converting enzyme inhibitor, on early reperfusion and subsequent electrophysiologic stability in the pig. *Cardiovasc Drugs Ther* 1990; 4: 695–704.

Unger T, Mattfeldt T, Lamberty V, et al. Effect of early onset angiotensin-converting enzyme inhibition on myocardial capillaries. *Hypertension* 1992; 20: 478–482.

Urata H, Healy B, Stewart RW, et al. Angiotensin-II receptors in normal and failing human hearts. *J Clin Endocrinol Metab* 1989; 69: 54–66.

van Gilst WH, de Graeff PA, Wesseling H, de Langen CDJ. Reduction of reperfusion arrhythmias in the ischemic isolated rat heart by angiotensin converting enzyme inhibitors: a comparison of captopril, enalapril and HOE 498. *J Cardiovasc Pharmacol* 1986; 8: 722–728.

van Gilst WH, van Wijngaarden J, Scholtens E, et al. Captopril-induced increase in coronary flow: An SH-dependent effect on arachidonic acid metabolism *J Cardiovasc Pharmacol* 1987a; 9 (Suppl II): S31–S36.

van Gilst WH, de Graeff PA, Scholtens E, et al. Potentiation of isosorbide dinitrate-induced coronary dilatation by captopril. *J Cardiovasc Pharmacol* 1987b; 9: 254–255.

Weber KT, Brilla CG. Pathological hypertrophy and cardiac interstitium. Fibrosis and renin-angiotensin-aldosterone system. *Circulation* 1991; 83: 1849–1865.

Westlin W, Mullane K. Does captopril attenuate reperfusion-induced myocardial dysfunction by scavenging free radicals? *Circulation* 1988; 77 (Suppl I): I-30–I-39.

Yamagishi H, Kim S, Nishikimi T, et al. Contribution of cardiac renin-angiotensin system to ventricular remodelling in myocardial-infarcted rats. *J Mol Cell Cardiol* 1993; 25: 1369–1380.

Yusuf S, Pepine CJ, Garces C, et al. Effect of enalapril on myocardial infarction and unstable angina in patients with low ejection fractions. *Lancet* 1992; 340: 1173–1178.

Zielinski J, Hawrylkiewicz I, Gorecka D, et al. Captopril effects on pulmonary and systemic hemodynamics in chronic cor pulmonale. *Chest* 1986; 90: 562–565.

CHAPTER 5

ACE Inhibitors for Congestive Heart Failure

"ACE inhibitors—a cornerstone of the treatment of heart failure"
(Braunwald, 1991).

"ACE inhibitors are now part of established therapeutic practice for congestive heart failure" (Braunwald, 1991). There is a tendency to use ACE inhibitors earlier and earlier including now for the milder degrees of congestive heart failure. Extensive hemodynamic studies have shown acute and chronic benefit with these agents, generally without the development of tolerance. Three major outcome studies in congestive heart failure, in patients mostly already treated by diuretics and digoxin, have shown improved mortality (CONSENSUS Trial Study Group, 1987; SOLVD Investigators, 1991; Cohn et al., 1991). Two major outcome trials in patients with left ventricular systolic dysfunction but without advanced heart failure attest to the preventative benefits of these agents (SAVE study–Pfeffer et al., 1992; SOLVD Investigators, 1992). Despite these persuasive trials, which justify the widespread and increasing use of ACE inhibitors, many aspects of their role in the therapy of congestive heart failure remain unanswered, particularly because the typical patient enrolled in these trials has been white, male, about 60, and with a previous myocardial infarction. Data on females, blacks, and valvular heart disease are strikingly absent. This chapter will first briefly review the presumed stages of development of heart failure. The possible use of ACE inhibitors at each stage will be considered, with particular reference to the information made available by each of the therapeutic trials. Emphasis will be laid on factors that govern the success of addition of ACE inhibitors to existing therapy, as well as factors that may predict their likely failure.

Rationale for ACE Inhibitors at Each Stage of Development of Myocardial Failure

Meerson (1969) has proposed that excess mechanical load-ing of the left ventricle leads to myocardial failure through three phases (Fig. 5–1): (1) an acute adaptation to the hemo-dynamic load, which leads to (2) compensatory ventricular hypertrophy, and eventually to (3) myocardial failure. In the phase of left ventricular failure, the well known neu-rohumoral adaptation is thought to be a reaction to sys-temic hypotension, according to the proposals of Harris (1987): "In these ways the syndrome of congestive heart failure may be regarded as one which arises when the heart becomes chronically unable to maintain an appropriate ar-terial pressure without support". This basic role of hypo-tension in the vicious circle that exists in severe congestive heart failure is shown in Fig. 5–2. Compensatory vasocon-strictive and volume-retaining mechanisms having their origin in baroreceptor control overwhelm opposing vaso-dilatory mechanisms mediated through atrial natriuretic peptide and having their origin in atrial distension (Harris, 1989), as shown in Fig. 5–3.

In the early stages of the Meerson progression, ACE inhibitors should act both on the early first loading stage of myocardial hypertrophy as well as during the phase of left ventricular hypertrophy. ACE inhibitors reduce the load on the myocardium (Table 5–1) by acting both as arteriolar and venous dilators, by reducing the blood pressure and de-creasing ventricular dimensions.

By similar logic, ACE inhibitors decrease left ventricu-lar hypertrophy, which in itself is the cause of diastolic dys-function and predisposes to the third phase of the failing left ventricle. Whereas the second phase is characterized by

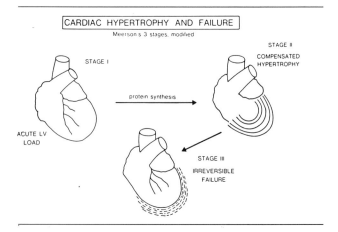

Figure 5–1. Meerson's three stages, as modified for clinical application. The acute hemodynamic load (Stage 1) calls forth protein synthesis and compensated hypertrophy (Stage II) before failure develops (Stage III). Fig. © LH Opie.

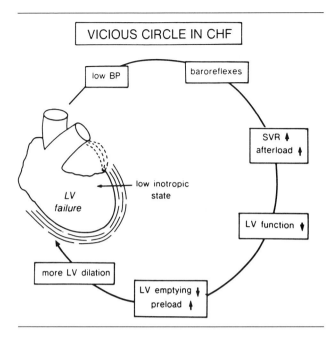

VICIOUS CIRCLE IN CHF

Figure 5–2. Potential vicious circle in congestive heart failure (CHF) in which a low inotropic state of the left ventricle (LV) causes a low arterial blood pressure (BP), which activates the baroreflexes to increase the systemic vascular resistance (SVR) and the afterload. Consequently, the failing left ventricle must work against a greater resistance so that left ventricular function falls, left ventricular emptying is depressed, left ventricular preload is increased, and there is more left ventricular dilation. Fig. © LH Opie.

normal indices of systolic function but abnormal diastolic function, the third phase is characterized by abnormalities both of systolic and diastolic function and is symptomatically divided by the severity of dyspnea according to the New York Heart Association (NYHA) classification.

Effects on neurohumoral activation

ACE inhibitors are commonly used in advanced failure, in which a neurohumoral syndrome is elicited that includes enhanced renin secretion by the kidney. It may be supposed that circulating renin and angiotensin-II levels should therefore be elevated in all patients with congestive heart failure and that the degree of elevation should bear relation to the severity of the congestive heart failure. However, in untreated early congestive heart failure, in patients with NYHA Disability Class I or Class II, plasma renin activity is not raised, although atrial natriuretic peptide values and plasma adrenaline are increased (Remes et al., 1991). Likewise, in untreated patients with slightly more severe congestive heart failure (NYHA Classes II and III), plasma renin and aldosterone levels were normal, although plasma norepinephrine levels were high (Bayliss et al., 1987). In patients with even more severe congestive heart failure, almost all in NYHA Class III or IV, the major con-

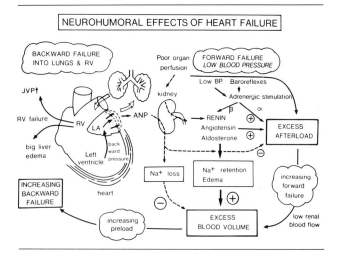

Figure 5–3. *The failing heart can elicit two types of neurohumoral signals to the circulation. First, as the left ventricle (LV) fails and left atrial (LA) pressure increases, distension of the atrial walls releases atrial natriuretic peptide (ANP), which acts on the kidneys to cause sodium loss and hence to inhibit the excess blood volume found in congestive heart failure. It is also vasodilatory. Further aspects of backward failure are the increase in the jugular venous pressure (JVP) and other features of right ventricular (RV) heart failure, such as an enlarged liver and edema. Another aspect of the failing left ventricle is a low cardiac output (forward failure). Hypotension (low blood pressure) elicits an adrenergic reflex response that increases the afterload. The low cardiac output as well as the adrenergic stimulation cause release of renin from the kidneys, which activates angiotensin-II, thus increasing the afterload. In addition, secretion of the hormone aldosterone from the adrenal cortex is increased, thereby causing sodium retention and edema. Excess blood volume contributes to the excess preload. The disadvantageous responses induced by forward failure outweigh the advantageous release of ANP induced by backward failure. The heart is, therefore, caught in an increasing vicious circle, leading to further deterioration of ventricular function. Fig. © LH Opie.*

sistent finding was water and sodium retention as well as an increased plasma norepinephrine (Anand et al., 1989). Plasma renin activity was increased in only 5 of the 8 patients. On the other hand, in diuretic-treated patients, plasma renin activity is consistently elevated (Bayliss et al., 1987). The findings of Remes et al (1991) suggest that an elevation in plasma renin activity only follows other stages of the neurohumoral adaptation such as an increase in plasma catecholamines (Fig. 5–4). Thus, logically, whereas it could be expected that ACE inhibitors should be effective therapy in patients with heart failure treated by diuretics (which would increase renin activity) and in the majority of patients with severe congestive heart failure in whom plasma renin activity is increased, nonetheless there should be reservations about their use in early congestive heart failure when plasma renin activity is not elevated in the absence of treatment.

TABLE 5–1 STAGES OF DEVELOPMENT OF CONGESTIVE HEART FAILURE WITH POSSIBLE ROLE OF ACE INHIBITION

Meerson stage	Clinical modification of Meerson classification	Rationale for ACE inhibition
1. Acute load	Initial loading stage, normal left ventricle (early post-AMI, early valve disease, early hypertension)	Load reduction prevents left ventricular hypertrophy (hypothetical)
2. Compensatory hypertrophy	Left ventricular hypertrophy often with diastolic failure	Load reduction improves left ventricular hypertrophy and diastolic function
3. Failure	Left ventricular hypertrophy and dilation with systolic and diastolic failure. Neurohumoral adaptation	Load reduction lessens dilation. Decrease of angiotensin-II and plasma norepinephrine. Sometimes aldosterone levels fall.

AMI, acute myocardial infarction

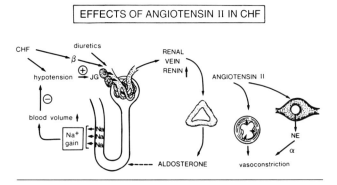

EFFECTS OF ANGIOTENSIN II IN CHF

Figure 5–4. Congestive heart failure (CHF) increases renin secretion from the juxtaglomerular (JG) cells in the kidney by two mechanisms: hypotension and increased beta-adrenergic stimulation. Circulating renin then stimulates a plasma substrate to convert circulating angiotensinogen to angiotensin-I, which is converted to angiotensin-II in the tissue to cause vasoconstriction. Angiotensin-II also increases release of norepinephrine (NE) further to promote vasoconstriction. Angiotensin-II releases aldosterone from the adrenal glands, thereby causing sodium retention. As a result of aldosterone secretion, there is sodium and water retention, which helps to maintain blood pressure and renal perfusion, thereby acting as a feedback loop on the kidney to diminish renin secretion. Note, in addition, the role of diuretic therapy in promoting renin release. Fig. © LH Opie.

Additional mechanisms of benefit

In early heart failure, even when patients have normal renin values, there are abnormalities in response to acute salt and water loading (Volpe et al., 1992). The response is favorably changed by the ACE inhibitor, quinapril.

Cardiac parasympathetic activity may be increased by ACE inhibition, which may also benefit heart failure (Flapan et al., 1992).

ACE Inhibitors as Preventative Therapy for Early Myocardial Failure

Preventative role in the postinfarct phase: SAVE study

In patients with recent acute myocardial infarction, ACE inhibitor therapy given to those with low ejection fractions but without symptoms improved the depressed left ventricular function better than did furosemide (Sharpe et al., 1988). Presumably load reduction was helping to prevent adverse left ventricular remodeling. In the large SAVE · study (Pfeffer et al., 1992) on over 2,000 patients, captopril achieved some striking benefits. It was given to patients 3 to 16 days postinfarct who had ejection fractions of below 40% but were not in overt heart failure, at an initial dose of 6.25 mg and titrated up to 50 mg three times daily. The benefits over an average of 42 months were several (Fig.

5–5). Most importantly, mortality from all causes was reduced by 19%, the development of severe heart failure was down by 37%, and (a surprise) recurrent myocardial infarction was reduced by 25%.

Does ACE inhibition act in some specific way or as a nonspecific load reducer? Judgutt et al. (1990) compared prophylactic ACE inhibition with prophylactic nitrate administration early after acute myocardial infarction and followed the effects on left ventricular dimensions and function. Both agents had a similar prophylactic benefit on remodeling. Therefore, it seems as if, in this early stage, ACE inhibitors act as nonspecific unloaders.

ACE inhibitors do not appear to act beneficially in postinfarct remodeling by only arteriolar dilation—it seems as if the added venous dilation is crucial, both shown by the study of Jugdutt et al. (1990) in patients and by the failure of hydralazine beneficially to improve postinfarct remodeling in rats (Raya et al., 1989).

Other etiologies for early myocardial failure

Does the benefit extend to other clinical conditions that predispose to eventual left ventricular failure? Two such conditions would be early valvular heart disease and early hypertension. Logically, patients with aortic stenosis or mitral

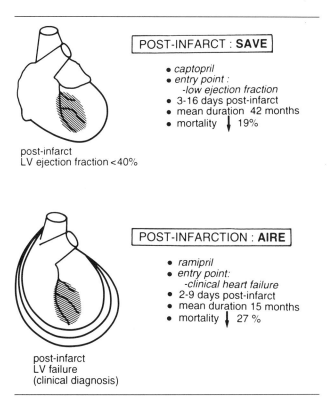

Figure 5–5. Summary of benfits of ACE inhibition by captopril in the SAVE study (Pfeffer et al., 1992), or by ramipril in the AIRE study (1993). LVEF, left ventricular ejection fraction; CHF, congestive heart failure. Fig. © LH Opie.

stenosis should be excluded from any such therapeutic therapy with ACE inhibitors, but equally logically, ACE inhibition that improves the hemodynamics of mitral and aortic regurgitation (see Chapter 4) could be given at an early stage as part of prophylactic therapy to prevent eventual left ventricular hypertrophy and dilation. This particular use is, as yet, completely unexplored.

Likewise, in early hypertension, before the development of left ventricular hypertrophy, prophylactic use of ACE inhibitors would also be logical. Nonetheless, there are no outcome trials nor data to support this proposed use.

In none of these situations can it be expected that plasma renin activity would be elevated, so that the logical basis for the use of ACE inhibitors postinfarct would be the mechanical unloading effect, or an effect on LV growth.

Early symptomatic left ventricular hypertrophy with diastolic dysfunction

Because the mechanism of the symptomatology, chiefly dyspnea, is thought to be by diastolic dysfunction, which is a consequence of left ventricular hypertrophy, and because ACE inhibition by itself can improve left ventricular hypertrophy, such therapy is likely to improve symptoms. Again, this seemingly logical sequence of events has not been established. Although some studies (Shahi et al., 1990) have shown that ACE inhibitor therapy by captopril did not improve echocardiographic indices of diastolic dysfunction (Shahi et al., 1990), much depends on the technique and parameters used (see Chapter 4).

POSSIBLE USE OF ACE INHIBITORS AS FIRST-LINE THERAPY IN HEART FAILURE

Strictly speaking, there have been only three studies on the possible use of ACE inhibitors as *sole therapy* (i.e., no diuretics, no digoxin) in clinical heart failure. First, Richardson et al. (1987) studied 14 patients who were previously stable on diuretic therapy. Patients were randomly assigned to either captopril 25 mg three times daily or a loop diuretic once daily (furosemide 40 mg, amiloride 5 mg). After 8 weeks patients were crossed over without washout to the other therapy. Captopril by itself was as effective as prior diuretic therapy in 10 of 14 patients in that this group remained stable, whereas in the other 4 patients who had had a history of pulmonary edema, captopril was not sufficient as monotherapy.

Second, Riegger (1991) studied the effects of quinapril given as monotherapy to 26 patients with heart failure (NYHA Class II and III). The increase of exercise time in patients receiving quinapril monotherapy was greater than in those receiving placebo. However, the data are not given in detail, so this report must be regarded as provisional.

Third, in 5 patients with untreated but severe heart failure, Anand et al. (1990) gave an acute dose of enalapril and found surprisingly few hemodynamic changes; systemic vascular resistance fell and cardiac index rose, but pulmonary wedge and pulmonary artery pressures did not fall. Thereafter, 3 of the 5 patients responded to 1 month of enalapril therapy by weight loss. The authors felt unable to recommend a longer formal trial for ACE inhibition as monotherapy in patients with severe congestive heart failure.

SOLVD preventative study

In the huge SOLVD study (1992) on over 4,000 patients, only 17% were taking diuretics and 66% were in NYHA Class I—so that the question was whether enalapril could prevent overt heart failure. Not surprisingly, the most striking benefits were found in patients with the lowest initial ejection fractions, below 28%, with only borderline results in those with values of 33% to 35%. Enalapril in a mean daily dose of 17 mg was associated with less hospitalization and less development of symptomatic heart failure. Of note is that 80% of these patients were postinfarct, so that the prophylactic benefit of an ACE inhibitor in other types of asymptomatic early heart failure is not established.

ACE INHIBITORS AS SECOND-LINE THERAPY WITH DIURETICS FOR CONGESTIVE HEART FAILURE

Diuretic therapy is universally accepted as first-step and first-line therapy in left ventricular failure and congestive heart failure. Whereas in congestive heart failure, it is logical to be rid of the fluid retention that is causing the symptoms, in left ventricular failure, where the problem may be chiefly diastolic dysfunction, diuretic therapy could theoretically decrease the left atrial filling pressure and the capacity of the left ventricle to fill. Nonetheless, there are no trials available in which diuretic therapy and placebo have been compared with left ventricular function as end-point. This section, therefore, details studies where patients already treated with diuretics were given additionally an ACE inhibitor or digoxin.

ACE inhibition versus digoxin versus combination in early left ventricular failure

This important question has been studied by Kromer et al. (1990) in 19 patients, all treated with hydrochlorothiazide 25 mg and all categorized as having mild congestive heart failure with NYHA Class II symptoms. In a randomized single-blind cross-over study, patients first were given placebo therapy for 4 weeks, then 6 weeks of treatment with either digoxin or the ACE inhibitor quinapril, then a 4 week placebo washout period and a cross-over to the other agent for a final 6 weeks of combination therapy. The digoxin dose in 17 patients was 0.25 mg daily and in 2 patients the dose was 0.375 mg daily. The quinapril dose was 5 to 10 mg twice daily to achieve a systolic blood pressure below 120 mmHg.

In these patients, ACE inhibitor therapy was markedly more effective than digoxin as it increased exercise tolerance, decreased heart size, and decreased circulating norepinephrine and aldosterone levels. All of these were left unchanged by digoxin therapy. Combination therapy gave virtually identical results to ACE inhibition except that, in addition, fractional shortening increased significantly.

This important study clearly shows that relatively short-term therapy with an ACE inhibitor is preferable to digoxin in early heart failure already treated by diuretics. Digoxin exerted no benefit of note. While these data cannot be extrapolated to longer periods and need further follow-up and supportive studies, nonetheless the data support a widespread clinical impression that ACE inhibitor therapy combined with a mild diuretic is highly effective in early heart failure.

When should an ACE inhibitor be added to the diuretic?

Whereas the Kromer et al. (1990) study clearly showed the benefits of addition of an ACE inhibitor to low-dose thiazide therapy, apparently contradictory results were obtained by Cowley et al. (1986). They claimed that in patients treated with a low-dose diuretic, it was preferable to increase the diuretic dose rather than add the ACE inhibitor captopril. Using exercise testing and visual analogue scores as indices of the severity of heart failure, Cowley et al (1986) showed that in their patients better results could be obtained by increasing the furosemide from 40 mg daily up to 120 mg daily rather than adding captopril 25 to 50 mg three times daily. Although the addition of captopril increased the exercise tolerance significantly, higher doses of furosemide did likewise and, furthermore, were better on the analogue score. Both drugs caused a similar reduction in the perceived exertion score in an exercise protocol, and both drugs improved the scores for fatigue and wellbeing. Surprisingly, captopril did not alter the visual analog score for breathlessness over the period of therapy.

Thus, Cowley et al. (1986) clearly showed that, from the short-term symptomatic point of view, an increase of diuretic dose may achieve at least as much as ACE inhibition in selected patients. Their study did not go on to show that there are long-term benefits of the increase of diuretic dose and, on first principles, it could be supposed that there would be many adverse effects including activation of the renin-angiotensin axis. Of interest is the finding that in postinfarct patients with modestly depressed left ventricular function, the ACE inhibitor captopril was better able to maintain left ventricular function and size than the diuretic furosemide (Sharpe et al., 1988).

Clearly, longer term observations are required to settle the comparable benefits of addition of ACE inhibition and increased diuretic therapy in heart failure. Many clinicians will be impressed by the Kromer et al. (1990) study and, in addition, by the Captopril-Digoxin Multicenter Research Group (1988) study that compared captopril with digoxin in mild to moderate heart failure (next section). Furthermore, the general protective effects of ACE inhibition in

TABLE 5–2 COMPARATIVE EFFECTS OF CAPTOPRIL VERSUS DIGOXIN VERSUS PLACEBO IN MILD TO MODERATE CONGESTIVE HEART FAILURE IN A MULTICENTER STUDY

	Pretreatment	Captopril	Digoxin	Placebo
Effort tolerance	563 sec	+17%*	+11%	+9%
Ejection fraction	26%	+1/8%	+4.4%**	+0.9%
VPB score	67/hr	−15/hr	+61/hr	+33/hr
NYHA class	2.3	+41%***	+31%	+22%

Difference *from P (p < 0.05), **from P (p < 0.005) and C (p < 0.05), ***from P (p < 0.01).

NYHA class, New York Heart Association functional class, mean values.

VPB, ventricular premature beats

For further details, see Captopril–Digoxin Multicenter Study (1988).

early heart failure are now evident so that these drugs are being added earlier and earlier.

Dose of ACE inhibitor added to furosemide

In a fascinating report (Motwani et al., 1992), the addition of a minute dose of captopril (1 mg) was able to facilitate a diuresis when added to furosemide (median dose 80 mg/day). In contrast, 25 mg captopril decreased blood pressure and glomerular filtration and slightly decreased the diuretic response to furosemide in the same study. Possibly the higher dose of captopril had a negative pharmacokinetic interaction with furosemide (see Chapter 7).

Captopril-Digoxin Multicenter study in mild to moderate heart failure

Three hundred patients with mild to moderate heart failure and an average functional classification (NYHA) of 2.3 were allocated randomly in a double-blind manner to captopril, digoxin, or placebo. Most were maintained on furosemide. Captopril was better than digoxin in increasing the effort tolerance and the functional classification as well as decreasing ventricular premature beats (Table 5–2). However, only digoxin increased the ejection fraction. The improvement in the effort tolerance with captopril and in mechanical performance with digoxin correspond well to the data of Kromer et al. (1990).

ACE Inhibitors as Third Component Therapy in Combination with Diuretics and Digoxin

Can ACE inhibition reduce diuretic requirements in congestive heart failure? Because angiotensin-II affects the release of aldosterone and, in several studies, use of ACE inhibitors has been associated with decreased aldosterone levels, it is logical to suppose that the introduction of ACE inhibitor therapy to patients already on optimal diuretic doses may lead to a lessened requirement for diuretics. In patients with severe congestive heart failure (NYHA Class IV), captopril did not reduce diuretic requirements (Odemuyiwa et al., 1989). In patients with NYHA Class III heart failure, about half of a small series required a lower diuretic dose (Odemuyiwa et al., 1989). Likewise, the addition of enalapril to patients already treated by digoxin and a diuretic required reduction of diuretic dose in about half but eventually the diuretic dose was increased in the other half (Sharpe et al., 1984).

The fundamental logic for triple therapy (diuretic–ACE inhibitor–inotropic agent) lies in the self-evident different mode of action of these three types of agents (Smith and Pfeffer, 1989). From the hemodynamic point of view, the combination ACE inhibitor–inotropic agent gives better results than either therapy alone both in mild heart failure (Kromer et al., 1990) and in severe heart failure (Gheorghiade et al., 1989). Withdrawal of digoxin from triple therapy results in deterioration (Packer et al., 1992). When, however, comparing the effects of an ACE inhibitor with an inhibitor of phosphodiesterase-III, such as enoximone, there are few differences (Scriven et al., 1988).

ACE inhibition versus nonspecific vasodilation

A question only recently answered is whether ACE inhibition confers any specific advantages over nonspecific vasodilators in advanced heart failure. It is possible to hazard a guess that ACE inhibition is going to be better in the long run, because captopril inhibited the release of norepinephrine from the failing heart compared with hydralazine-nitrate (Daly et al., 1986), and this reduction in myocardial sympathetic tone should logically have long-term benefits. A retrospective analysis of the CONSENSUS Study proposed that enalapril was most effective in patients with neuroendocrine and renin-angiotensin activation (Swedberg et al., 1990). In fact, the Veterans Administration Heart Failure Trial (V-HeFT-II) shows the expected advantage for ACE inhibition over hydralazine-nitrate therapy (Cohn et al., 1991).

Acute hemodynamic effects of ACE inhibitors

In many acute studies, various ACE inhibitors given to patients with heart failure have reduced the pulmonary wedge pressure (= left ventricular filling pressure), the systemic vascular resistance, the blood pressure, and the right atrial pressure. Heart rate has generally been unaffected. The stroke volume (stroke volume index) and, therefore, the cardiac index (cardiac output) correspondingly increased. The study of Nishimura et al. (1989) with captopril is of particular interest because they also measured venous distensibility and showed an increase in venous volume (i.e., venous pooling) resulting from acute ACE inhibition. All the other hemodynamic changes can readily be explained by acute afterload reduction. Furthermore, renal blood flow is specifically increased (Thuillez et al., 1990).

An important point is that, when measured, right atrial pressure falls as does pulmonary vascular resistance (Chatterjee et al., 1985). Therefore both sides of the heart are unloaded.

Chronic hemodynamic and echocardiographic studies with ACE inhibitors

In a series of studies reviewed in Table 5–3, it can be seen that nearly consistent effects of captopril or enalapril are in the increase in exercise time, in reduction of the preload and afterload, in decreased echocardiographic size, and in increased indices of function such as fractional shortening, as well as an increased ejection fraction measured by radionuclide techniques.

Several cautionary aspects must, however, be emphasized. First, one study did not show a chronic increase in exercise time (Timmis et al., 1984), and in the study by

TABLE 5–3 CHRONIC EFFECTS OF ACE INHIBITORS ON EXERCISE TIME, INVASIVE HEMODYNAMICS, AND ECHOCARDIOGRAPHIC INDICES AS WELL AS RADIONUCLIDE EJECTION FRACTION IN PATIENTS WITH CONGESTIVE HEART FAILURE ALREADY TREATED BY DIGOXIN AND/OR DIURETICS

Author	Patient number	Trial design	Dose	Exercise time	Invasive hemodynamics		Echocardiographic parameters			Radionuclide ejection fraction or cardiac index
					Preload	Afterload	EDD	ESD	FS	
Captopril										
Chatterjee et al. (1985)	124	Open, up to 20 mths	Mean daily dose 250 mg	+	ND	ND	ND	ND	ND	ND
Cleland et al. (1984)	14	DB, PI, CO, 6 wks	Mean daily dose 94 mg	+	ND	ND	–	–	↑	ND
Packer et al. (1984a)	14	Open 2–8 wks (hyperreninemia)*	75–450 mg daily	ND	–	–	ND	ND	ND	+
Packer et al. (1984a)	12	Open 2–8 wks (nonresponders)	75–450 mg daily	ND	↑	↑	ND	ND	ND	↑
Powers et al. (1987)	65	DB, CO no PI, vs lisinopril	dose titration 12.5–50 mg tds Mean daily dose 98 mg	+	ND	ND	ND	ND	ND	↑

	n	Design	Dose							
Riegger and Kochsiek (1986)	10	Open	50 mg 3×	ND	+	ND	↑	ND	ND	ND
Timmis et al. (1987)	10	4 weeks	25 mg 3×	↑	ND	ND	ND	↑	↑	↑
Enalapril										
Brilla et al. (1989)	38	SB 12 wks	5 mg 1×	ND	+	ND	—	ND	ND	ND
Cleland et al. (1985)	20	Open 8 wks	5–40 mg daily mean 37 mg	ND	↑	—	—	ND	ND	+
Creager et al. (1985)	11	PI 12 wks	Mean daily dose 24 mg	↑	ND	ND	ND	ND	ND	+
DiCarlo et al. (1983)	7	Open 4 wks	10 mg 2×	+	ND	ND	ND	—	—	ND
Sharpe et al. (1984)	16	DB, PI, R, 12 wks	5 mg 2×	+	+	—	—	—	—	+

TABLE 5–3 Chronic Effects of ACE Inhibitors on Exercise Time, Invasive Hemodynamics, and Echocardiographic Indices as Well as Radionuclide Ejection Fraction in Patients with Congestive Heart Failure Already Treated by Digoxin and/or Diuretics (Continued)

Author	Patient number	Trial design	Dose	Exercise time	Invasive hemodynamics		Echocardiographic parameters			Radionuclide ejection fraction or cardiac index
					Preload	Afterload	EDD	ESD	FS	
Lisinopril										
Chalmers et al. (1987)	87	DB, Prl, Pl; 12 wks	5–40 mg 1×	+	ND	ND	ND	ND	ND	+
Powers et al. (1987)	64	DB, CO vs captopril, 12 wks	Titrated to mean daily dose of 12 mg	+	ND	ND	ND	ND	ND	+
Perindopril										
Bounhoure et al. (1988)	103	DB, Pl, R, Prl, 12 wks	2–4 mg 1×	+	ND	ND	ND	ND	ND	ND
Desche et al. (1993)	208	Open label 24 wks	2–4 mg 1×	+	ND	ND	ND	ND	ND	ND
Flammang et al. (1993)	11	Open label, 12 wks	2–4 mg 1×	ND	−	−	ND	ND	ND	+

	n	Design	Dose						
Quinapril**									
Riegger (1991)	225	DB, Pl, R, Prl, 12 wks	10–20 mg 2×	+	ND	ND	ND	ND	ND
Northridge et al. (1993)	32	DB, Pl, R, Prl, 8 wks	5–20 mg in 2 doses	+	ND	ND	ND	ND	↑
Ramipril									
de Graeff et al. (1989)	4	Open 12 wks	5 mg acute	ND	—	—	ND	ND	↑

For 11 earlier studies with captopril, see Heel et al. (1980) and Turini et al. (1983).

For 7 earlier studies with enalapril, see Todd and Heel (1986).

SB, single-blinded; DB, double-blinded; Pl, placebo-controlled; R, randomized; CO, cross-over; Prl, parallel EDD, left ventricular end-diastolic diameter; EDS, left ventricular end-systolic diameter; FS, fractional shortening; ND, no data; +, increase; −, decrease; →, no significant change

1×, once daily; 2×, twice daily; 3×, three times daily.

Preload = pulmonary wedge pressure or pulmonary artery pressure measured invasively; afterload = systemic vascular resistance measured invasively, except for ramipril study where blood pressure is taken.

*Low-renin patients with rise in renin <4 ng/ml/hr during therapy.

**Some patients reveived quinapril monotherapy; details not given.

TABLE 5–4 EFFECT OF CHRONIC ACE INHIBITION ON NEUROHUMORAL PARAMETERS IN CONGESTIVE HEART FAILURE IN PATIENTS TREATED BY DIGOXIN AND/OR DIURETICS

Author	Drug and dose	Plasma renin	Plasma angiotensin-II	Plasma aldosterone	Plasma norepinephrine	Plasma epinephrine	Plasma vasopressin
Bayliss et al (1986)	Captopril 25–50 mg 3× daily for 1 month after 1 week of placebo; DB comparison with prazosin, 15 patients	+	ND	–	→*	ND	ND
Brilla et al (1989)	Enalapril 5 mg daily 38 patients, 3 months SB, controlled	+	ND	–	ND	ND	ND
Cleland et al (1984)	Captopril mean dose 94 mg daily, 6 wks, PI, 14 patients	+	–	↑	–	↑	ND

Study					
Cleland et al (1985)	Enalapril 5–40 mg daily, 20 patients, 8 wks Mean daily dose 37 mg	+	—	—	↑	—
Mettauer et al (1986)	Captopril, 6.25–25 mg 4×, 1 month, 26 patients, open	+	ND	—	↑	→ or —
Riegger and Kochsiek (1986)	Captopril, 50 mg 3×, 4 weeks, 10 patients, Open	+	ND	ND	ND	ND
Swedberg et al (CONSENSUS) (1990)	Enalapril mean dose 19 mg daily, 6 weeks, DB vs placebo, 127 patients	No	—	—	↑	ND

ND, no data; +, increased; −, decreased; →, unchanged; pl, placebo
*mean plasma norepinephrine decreased by 15%, not significant.

Packer et al. (1984a) only about half of the patients chronically responded to captopril. Those who responded could not be predicted in advance by the circulating renin level but rather by an increase of renin during captopril therapy (reactive hyperreninemia). Second, only a few studies have been double-blinded, placebo-controlled, and randomized. The study by Sharpe et al. (1984) is an outstanding example of a thorough study in which the exercise time increased, hemodynamic loading decreased, echocardiographic size decreased, and functional shortening increased.

The problem of the poor response of certain patients to long-term ACE inhibitor therapy is evaluated later in this chapter, but the incidence of poor response can vary from 100% (Timmis et al., 1984) to a much lower percentage as appears to hold in most of the other studies, with the Packer study (Packer et al., 1984a) showing response in just over 50%.

Neurohumoral effects of ACE inhibitors added to digoxin and diuretics

As shown in Table 5–4, administration of ACE inhibitors has, on the whole, a consistent effect in increasing plasma renin (by virtue of the inhibition of the converting enzyme), decreasing angiotensin-II (the consequence of the enzyme inhibition), with also a decrease in aldosterone (which is stimulated by angiotensin-II), and a fall in norepinephrine and vasopressin, the elevation of which are among consequences of severe congestive heart failure. Parasympathetic activity, reduced in heart failure, is improved by ACE inhibition. Although there are some exceptions to the patterns noted, most of the results are reasonably consistent. From these data it can be concluded that chronic ACE inhibition ameliorates the neurohumoral changes found in congestive heart failure. Generally, such changes are thought to be adverse because of increased vasoconstriction following enhanced levels of angiotensin-II and norepinephrine, because of fluid and sodium retention associated with increased aldosterone levels, and a dilutional hyponatremia associated with increased vasopressin levels.

ACE INHIBITION AS PART OF QUADRUPLE THERAPY INCLUDING DIURETICS, DIGOXIN, AND VASODILATORS

Logically, there should be scope for added vasodilator therapy to the now standard triple therapy in congestive heart failure, the latter consisting of diuretics–digoxin–ACE inhibition. Although pulmonary vascular dilation and a decrease in right atrial pressure is part of the hemodynamic response to acute ACE inhibition in patients already treated by digoxin and digitalis (see Table 5–3), nonetheless *nitrates* are better able to decrease pulmonary arteriolar resistance and right atrial pressure than captopril (Packer et al., 1985a). The greater functional obstruction in the pulmonary circuit during ACE inhibition limits the degree to which the right ventricular output can increase, and this is proposed as a cause of more hypotensive effects during ACE inhibitor therapy by captopril than with isosorbide dinitrate (Packer et al., 1985a).

The acute administration of *isosorbide dinitrate* 40 mg every 6 hours for 24 hours relieved pulmonary hypertension and improved left ventricular filling in 10 of 14 patients with chronic heart failure already treated with captopril (Mehra et al., 1992).

An additional and indirect argument for concomitant vasodilator therapy is that in the well known CONSENSUS study (1987) 47% of patients were already receiving nitrates, while in the treatment arm of SOLVD (1991) 40% were on nitrates. In the Hy-C trial (Fonarow et al., 1992), 84% of the patients were on nitrate therapy. Thus, in nitrate-treated patients, ACE inhibition can produce further clinical benefit.

In these trials, very few patients were receiving hydralazine. There is a specific disadvantage of hydralazine in that active arteriolar dilation increases reflex sympathetic output. This aspect has not been specifically tested in congestive heart failure, although the combination of nitrate and hydralazine increased release of norepinephrine from the failing human myocardium, whereas captopril left the release unchanged (Daly et al, 1986). Furthermore, when either captopril or hydralazine was added to the therapy of patients mostly already receiving digitalis, furosemide, and nitrates, mortality was worse in the hydralazine group (Fonarow et al., 1992).

Therefore, there appear to be good arguments for *adding* nitrates to conventional triple therapy, even though the extra combination has not been formally tested in prospective trials. First principles and currently available data suggest that nitrates would most benefit patients in severe heart failure as part of quadruple therapy.

DIASTOLIC DYSFUNCTION

The preceding discussion has concentrated on the role of ACE inhibition in systolic heart failure and the indices of improvement in systolic function. Currently, however, the emphasis is shifting to diastolic heart failure, thought to be an early event particularly in left ventricular hypertrophy. There are relatively few studies with ACE inhibitor therapy in diastolic heart failure, and results depend on the technique used to assess diastolic dysfunction (see Chapter 4). Results are controversial. More data are required on the effects of ACE inhibitors on diastolic dysfunction.

SKELETAL MUSCLE METABOLISM IN HEART FAILURE

Poor blood flow to working skeletal muscle may be one cause of fatigue and exercise intolerance in congestive heart failure and, furthermore, there may be chronic metabolic abnormalities in such muscle (Wilson et al., 1989).

It is, therefore, logical to ask whether ACE inhibitor therapy can improve blood flow and metabolism in the leg muscle of patients with congestive heart failure. Wilson and Ferraro (1985) studied 12 patients already treated by digitalis and diuretics and added captopril at a mean oral dose of 20 mg daily, while studying conventional hemodynamics at rest and exercise and also in particular measuring indices of skeletal muscle metabolism. Whereas there was the expected improvement in pulmonary wedge pressure and systemic vascular resistance both at rest and during exercise, the oxygen uptake of the leg muscle was not increased by the addition of captopril, nor did leg blood flow rise, nor was lactate release altered, even though the vascular resistance in the leg muscle fell. In other words, there was no acute benefit on leg muscle metabolism. Likewise, Timmis et al. (1987) found that neither acute nor chronic captopril therapy improved the oxygen uptake of exercising leg muscle.

COMPARATIVE STUDIES OF ACE INHIBITORS

Enalapril versus captopril

The study by Packer et al. (1986a) could be cited as evidence favoring the view that enalapril in high dose is more likely to cause hemodynamic tolerance than captopril, also in high dose, which would correspond to the concept of receptor downgrading by prolonged blood levels of a therapeutic drug, as in the case of nitrates. Further evidence for this point of view could be that no tolerance was found over a period of 18 months when captopril was used in patients with congestive heart failure (Chatterjee et al., 1985). This subject needs considerable further study. The fact that enalapril was able to save lives in the CONSENSUS study (1987) and in SOLVD (1991) could actually constitute an argument favoring the view that the ideal drug evokes no hemodynamic changes when chronically administered but does achieve neurohormonal changes.

An important retrospective analysis of patients treated by either captopril or enalapril, and serving as controls for a xamoterol study, showed an excess of mortality in the captopril group (Pouleur et al., 1991). By their nature, retrospective analyses cannot be firm in their conclusions, yet the authors believe that captopril was often given in doses too low or too infrequently. They recommend captopril 25 mg three times daily as the usual dose.

Lisinopril versus captopril

In a short-term 12-week comparison, in patients already treated by digitalis and diuretics, lisinopril at a mean daily dose of 12 mg was more effective in prolonging exercise time than was captopril at a mean daily dose of 98 mg (Powers et al., 1987). Only lisinopril increased left ventricular ejection fraction. There are two important reservations to the apparent conclusion that lisinopril is better than captopril for congestive heart failure. First, hypotension induced by lisinopril was later in onset and more prolonged as well as more frequent than with captopril. Second, blood urea nitrogen and plasma potassium increased more frequently during lisinopril than during captopril therapy.

Ramipril versus captopril

In patients with severe congestive heart failure (NYHA Classes III and IV), an acute dose of ramipril 5 mg decreased pulmonary wedge pressure more than did captopril 12.5 mg and for a longer time, with correspondingly more severe first dose hypotensive effects (de Graeff et al., 1989). After 3 months of open treatment, the same dose of ramipril reduced pulmonary wedge pressure less and more transiently (at that stage there were no comparisons with captopril). The hypotensive effect of ramipril was also less at 3 months.

Enalapril versus xamoterol

In a short-term cross-over study, enalapril titrated to a mean dose of about 14 mg twice daily was compared with xamoterol in a fixed dose of 200 mg twice daily (Jamieson et al., 1991). Each agent was given for 3 weeks followed by 2 weeks of placebo washout before cross-over. Background therapy was with diuretics and digoxin (details not given). Enalapril was marginally better ($p < 0.04$) on Doppler indices of cardiac output, yet at the cost of a daytime fall of blood pressure that was not found in the xamoterol group. Neither agent altered indices of renal function.

In another large-scale study in which xamoterol or placebo was compared with enalapril/captopril plus diuretic, the mortality in the xamoterol group was greater (Xamoterol Study Group, 1990).

Captopril versus hydralazine

Captopril and hydralazine were compared in a randomized short-term (12 weeks) study, partially blinded, on a total of 50 consecutive patients (Schofield et al., 1991). All patients were receiving diuretics, and some were receiving nitrates and/or digoxin as well. Captopril was titrated to a mean total dose of about 50 mg daily and hydralazine to about 200 mg daily, each drug given in divided doses every 8 hours. Captopril was better at improving dyspnea, decreasing tiredness, and increasing treadmill exercise time more than hydralazine. Only captopril improved the ejection fraction.

ACE Inhibitor Therapy for Congestive Heart Failure Success, Tolerance, and Failure

The response to ACE inhibitor therapy in congestive heart failure, depending on how measured, varies from a very high positive response, such as 85% positive (Packer, 1986), to a very high rate of failure, such as 100% failing (Timmis et al., 1987). When large numbers of patients are studied as in SAVE, SOLVD, and CONSENSUS, then the overall benefits are obvious. For the individual patient, ACE inhibitor therapy may achieve more or less than expected. In addition, there may be a variable response according to the drug used, as proposed by Packer et al. (1986a), although most clinicians appear to feel that if one ACE inhibitor does not work then there is little point in switching to another in the treatment of congestive heart failure.

One of the fundamental questions is whether patient response to an ACE inhibitor can be predicted in advance.

Predictors of response to ACE inhibitor therapy

Because activation of the renin-angiotensin-aldosterone axis is often supposed to have adverse effects in congestive heart failure, it might be supposed that the higher the initial renin value, the better the response to ACE inhibitor therapy. That expectation has not been met in at least four studies (Davis et al., 1979; Packer et al., 1984a; Packer et al., 1985b; Mettauer et al., 1986). Packer et al. (1984a) did claim that an initial low renin was not relevant, but rather that there should be a reactive hyperreninemia during treatment in responders. This does not seem to be a practical test as the only way of detecting such a renin increase is actually to treat the patient and to remeasure the renin, by which time it is as simple to see whether or not the patient responds clinically.

A group of nonresponders appear to be those in whom the mean right atrial pressure exceeds 12 mmHg and the serum creatinine exceeds 1.5 mg/dl (Packer et al., 1986a). In that case, up to 65% of patients failed to respond, in contrast to the usual situation in which a somewhat similar percentage of patients usually do respond to ACE inhibitor therapy.

Hyponatremia, if present, first indicates that the congestive heart failure is sufficiently severe to call forth a vasopressin response. Second, there may be an excessive or brisk response to ACE inhibitor therapy. Third, initial loop diuretic therapy is required to correct the hyponatremia, which may not respond to ACE inhibitor therapy of its own (Dzau and Hollenberg, 1984). Finally, hyponatremia is associated with an excess incidence of hypotension (Packer et al., 1984b). Packer's proposal is that the hyponatremia may in some way be linked to the relatively inadequate pulmonary vasodilator capacities of ACE inhibitors (Packer et al., 1985c). In the SOLVD study (1991), hyponatremia (sodium <140 mmol/liter) was not associated with any special adverse effect during the use of enalapril at a mean dose of 17 mg daily.

Tolerance to ACE inhibitor therapy has been found in the studies of Packer et al. (1986a) with high-dose enalapril (40 mg daily) and with captopril (25 mg three times daily) in the absence of digoxin therapy (Timmis et al., 1987).

The *sodium status* may be an important factor determining the response to ACE inhibitor therapy. According to Laragh (1986), a relatively modest intake of salt (100 mmol daily) could markedly suppress renin and aldosterone values in congestive heart failure without changing peripheral resistance. Thus, a non-renin but sodium-related mechanism must be able to regulate arterial constriction. A captopril challenge with an acute dose evoked no response during a normal sodium intake but a large response after sodium depletion in patients with congestive heart failure (Laragh, 1986). As in many studies in congestive heart failure, the exact sodium intake is not stipulated. Variations in the sodium status could help determine the response to ACE inhibitor therapy. Thus, *dietary sodium depletion appears highly desirable.*

Atrial natriuretic peptide (ANP) is released in response to angiotensin-II stimulation and therefore would act as a natural vasodilator to counter vasoconstriction induced by angiotensin-II (Ferrari and Anand, 1989; Harris, 1989). ANP is not, however, equally effective in experimental models with or without heart failure, and the suggestion is that ANP receptors might become downgraded to explain the lack of response to ANP. Thus, one reason why a patient might not respond to ACE inhibitor therapy is that, with a decrease in circulating angiotensin-II (Table 5–4), there could follow a fall in ANP, of consequence only in patients without ANP receptor downgrading. These complex interrelations between ANP and angiotensin-II point to a balancing role of the ANP system and the vasoconstrictor system in congestive heart failure (Ferrari and Anand, 1989).

ACE INHIBITORS FOR CONGESTIVE HEART FAILURE: CONTRAINDICATIONS AND CAUTIONS

Renal function in congestive heart failure

Whereas hemodynamic and hormonal effects of ACE inhibition are uniformly favorable, some of the renal effects can be construed as being unfavorable. Packer et al. (1986b) have argued that renin-angiotensin activation serves to preserve glomerular function in heart failure, in keeping with the known hemodynamic effects of angiotensin-II on efferent renal arteriolar tone. Thus, it is not surprising that there may be a tendency for urea and creatinine to rise, with a fall in the glomerular filtration rate and creatinine clearance. These occur despite an increase in the effective plasma flow and presumably reflect a fall in efferent arteriolar tone, thereby decreasing intraglomerular filtration pressure (see Chapter 3). Among the benefits of chronic ACE inhibition, there is a sodium diuresis and improved handling of a water load (Table 5–5). The apparent lessening of sodium diuresis in the study of Crozier et al. (1987) probably reflects excess hypotension with the acute high dose of the ACE inhibitor used.

Enalapril versus captopril and renal function

Packer et al. (1986a) have claimed that enalapril, by virtue of prolonged blood pressure reduction, is more likely to cause renal impairment than is captopril with its shorter

TABLE 5–5 Effect of Chronic ACE Inhibition Added to Digoxin and Diuretic Therapy in Patients with Congestive Heart Failure on Parameters of Renal Function

| Author | Drug and dose | Type of study | Serum/plasma | | | | | Urine | | | GFR or CCl | Filtration fraction | Effective plasma flow | Renal vascular resistance |
			Na+	K+	Mg++	Urea	Creat	Vol	Na+	K+				
Cleland et al. (1984)	Captopril Mean dose 94 mg	14 pts, Pl, R, DB	↑	+	ND	+	+	ND	→*	ND	↑	ND	+	ND
Cleland et al. (1985)	Enalapril 5–40 mg daily; mean dose 37 mg	20 pts, Pl, DB, 8 weeks	↑	+	+	+	+	ND	→*	ND	−	ND	+	ND
Crozier et al. (1987)	Ramipril 10 and 20 mg on two consecutive days	9 pts, Open	−	+	ND	+	+	ND	−	−	ND	ND	ND	ND
Kubo et al. (1985)	Captopril 75 mg 3 ×, 1 week	10 pts, Open 1 week	ND	ND	ND	ND	ND	+	+	↑	↑	−	+	−
Mettauer et al. (1986)	Captopril 25–50 mg 4 × mean daily dose 46 mg	26 pts, Open 1 month	↑	ND	ND	↑	−	+**	+	ND	+	ND	ND	ND

Creat, creatinine; GFR, glomerular filtration rate; CCl, creatinine clearance
*Total body sodium unchanged; **Over 5 hours in response to water load

lived action. They have raised an important point in that blood pressure reduction with captopril is episodic, whereas with enalapril it is sustained. It is difficult to know whether or not this difference between the two agents is an advantage for either. During prolonged captopril therapy, the addition of further captopril as an acute dose produced acute hemodynamic changes, such as a further fall in the wedge pressure, right atrial pressure, and a rise in the cardiac index and stroke work index. These changes were not seen with the further addition of enalapril which could be interpreted to mean that the prolonged effect of enalapril had given rise to a certain amount of hemodynamic tolerance so that the acute dose had no specific effect. The greater renal impairment achieved with enalapril could be the result of the more prolonged hypotension or, otherwise, more prolonged intrarenal hemodynamic change. Despite these supposed disadvantages of enalapril, it is the drug that was used in the CONSENSUS and SOLVD studies to show improved mortality. It should be noted that the doses of drugs used by Packer et al. (1986a), captopril 50 mg three times daily and enalapril 20 mg twice daily, could be regarded as high by current standards and that no initial test dose was given to eliminate patients more likely to develop hypotension.

Practical policies: renal function in heart failure

Because temporary renal failure is most likely to develop in patients with excess diuretic therapy and volume depletion, in whom there is a greater hypotensive response to ACE inhibitor therapy (Packer et al., 1987a), it is logical to start ACE inhibitors with low initial doses, such as captopril 6.25 mg or enalapril 2.5 mg. A low initial dose of perindopril (2 mg) is less likely to cause initial hypotension than a low first dose of either enalapril (2.5 mg) or captopril (6.25 mg) for unknown reasons (MacFadyen et al., 1991). The temporary renal failure caused by excess hypotension resulting from high-dose ACE inhibitor therapy is well documented in a single patient reported by Crozier et al. (1987). Urine volume and sodium fell during the hypotensive episode only to recover as the blood pressure rose. Second, special caution is required in diabetics in whom renal failure is a particular hazard (Packer et al., 1987b) doubtlessly because diabetes predisposes to renal disease.

Patients with severe hyponatremia are 30 times more likely to develop hypotension in response to ACE inhibitor therapy and require special care. The cause of the hyponatremia is at least in part renin-angiotensin activation (Dzau et al., 1984) as can result from intense diuretic therapy.

Thus, it may seem contradictory that the combination of furosemide and ACE inhibitor therapy is advised for patients with hyponatremia (Dzau and Hollenberg, 1984). However, it is essential to avoid excess diuresis and volume depletion before using the furosemide–ACE inhibitor combination. A very low starting dose of the ACE inhibitor is advisable (Motwani et al., 1992).

In patients who are not volume-depleted, restriction of water intake is important in view of the delayed water diuresis that may occur in severe congestive heart failure and thereby contribute to hyponatremia.

Risk of hyperkalemia: combination with spironolactone

In patients treated by diuretics and ACE inhibitors, a potassium-retaining diuretic should not routinely be used nor should potassium supplements be added because of the risk of hyperkalemia. This risk is greatest in patients with pre-existing renal failure. In other patients with severe heart failure already stabilized on captopril, furosemide, and digitalis, the addition of spironolactone to low-dose captopril can improve the clinical status without excess hyperkalemia (Dahlstrom and Karlsson, 1993).

Nonsteroidal anti-inflammatory drugs (NSAIDs)

Also contributing to the risk of hyperkalemia is associated therapy by NSAIDs, because NSAIDs inhibit the formation of vasodilatory prostaglandins that help to maintain renal blood flow in severe heart failure (Orme, 1986). NSAIDs in their own right sometimes precipitate renal failure and are known to cause sodium retention. For these reasons, they should not be prescribed in patients with congestive heart failure.

CARDIAC COMPLICATIONS OF ACE INHIBITOR THERAPY

Angina pectoris and severe congestive heart failure

In the SOLVD studies, treatment with enalapril reduced the rate of hospital admission for unstable angina (Yusuf et al., 1992). Sometimes ACE inhibitors are not ideal therapy in patients with angina pectoris and severe congestive heart failure at risk of hypotension. In a small series of patients (18 in total; mean age 63 years), captopril actually worsened the symptoms of angina and increased consumption of nitrates. Possibly the drop in mean blood pressure values from 127/81 mmHg to 105/67 mmHg in the erect position might have exaggerated the angina. Four patients who did particularly badly were also receiving nifedipine. "The combination of captopril with nifedipine in patients with severe ventricular dysfunction, especially if blood pressure is already low, seems unwise" (Cleland et al., 1991).

First-dose hypotension

A test dose of captopril (6.25 mg as in the SAVE study) is often used at the initiation of therapy for heart failure. Although there is little difference between the hypotensive effects of 6.25 mg and 25 mg as first dose (McLay et al., 1992), logically the lower dose should be preferred in case a severe reaction occurs. A new finding is that some ACE inhibitors are more likely than others to avoid first-dose hypotension (see Fig. 8–2). It would seem a commonsense procedure to initiate therapy with those ACE inhibitors that decrease the blood pressure less acutely in the setting of heart failure. Possibly, perindopril could be the drug to use in this situation (MacFadyen et al., 1991). A preliminary report (Squire et al., 1994) shows that a second dose of enalapril (2.5 mg) is again more likely to reduce the blood pressure than a second dose of perindopril (2 mg) despite equivalent degrees of inhibition of plasma ACE.

RECENT LARGE-SCALE TRIALS
SOLVD, SAVE, AIRE, AND OTHERS

SOLVD (Studies of Left Ventricular Dysfunction)

In the CONSENSUS trial (1987) that showed that enalapril decreased mortality, this ACE inhibitor was added to treatment by digitalis and diuretics in severely ill patients (NYHA Class IV). The question of whether ACE inhibitor therapy improves mortality or morbidity in lesser degrees of heart failure has now been settled. Recently several large-scale studies, involving several thousands of treated patients and a comparable number of controls, have been published (Table 5–6). The SOLVD treatment trial (Studies Of Left Ventricular Dysfunction) has shown that ACE inhibition by enalapril in a recommended dose of 10 mg twice daily can beneficially alter mortality (decreased by 16%) in patients with depressed left ventricular function (ejection fraction equal to or less than 35%) and mostly in NYHA Class II or III.

In the treatment arm of the SOLVD trial, a history of overt congestive heart failure was required for entry (SOLVD Investigators, 1991). In the prevention arm of the trial, no such history was required. The trial lasted three years with further follow-up for two years. The treatment arm showed that enalapril reduced mortality in patients with congestive heart failure and reduced the risk of heart failure worsening (SOLVD Investigators, 1991). *In the prevention arm of the trial,* enalapril was given to patients mostly postinfarct and in NYHA Class I, not receiving digoxin or diuretics (Table 5–6). Hospitalization for congestive heart failure and development of overt heart failure were both lessened (SOLVD Investigators, 1992).

Because the majority of the patients in the prevention arm of the trial were receiving monotherapy with enalapril alone, this trial is a powerful argument for the role of ACE inhibition per se in postinfarct patients with asymptomatic LV dysfunction.

SAVE (Survival and left Ventricular Enlargement)

This trial in early postinfarct patients provides the most spectacular example of the prophylactic power of ACE inhibition in that all-cause mortality was reduced (Fig. 5–5)

TABLE 5–6 THREE TREATMENT TRIALS WITH ACE INHIBITORS IN PATIENTS WITH OVERT CHRONIC HEART FAILURE, THE MAJORITY RECEIVING DIURETIC THERAPY; COMPARISON WITH ONE PREVENTION TRIAL

	CONSENSUS-I (treatment)	SOLVD-I (treatment)	V-Heft-II (treatment)	SOLVD-II (prevention)
Total number treated	127	1,285	403	2,111
Drug and dose (daily)	Enalapril[+] 18.4 mg	Enalapril[+] 16.6 mg	Enalapril 5–20 mg	Enalapril mean dose 16.7 mg
Mean duration (months)	6	41	24	37
Patient population	Severe heart failure	Chronic heart failure	Chronic heart failure	"Asymptomatic"; EF 35% or less, no antifailure drugs
Age (years), mean	71	61	61	60
Gender, male (%)	70	81	100	89
Race, white (%)	100	79	70	86
NYHA (%) I	0	11	6	66
II	0	57	52	33
III	0	30	42	0
IV	100	2	0.5	0

Postinfarct (%)	47	66	46	81
Hypertension (%)	24	43	50	37
Diuretics (%)	100	86	100	16
Digitalis (%)	92	66	100	12
Ejection fraction (%), mean	?	25	29	28
Mortality reduction (%)	40	16	28	8 (NS)
Worsening of or development of new heart failure (%) (reduction in risk)	13*	26	None	37
Sudden death (reduction)	None	NS	38**	Not stated

NS, not significant
EF, LV ejection fraction
+ mean daily dose
*improvement in mean NYHA classification, calculated from Table 4 of the study.
**calculated from Table 2 of the study.

when captopril was given to patients with an ejection fraction of 40% or less. Furthermore, the effect was additive to that of beta-blockade and aspirin. The reason for the benefit of captopril was probably that widespread neurohumoral activation occurred in these patients (Rouleau et al., 1993).

AIRE (Acute Infarction Ramipril Efficacy)

This recently published trial shows a striking benefit for ramipril given to early postinfarct patients with clinically diagnosed heart failure (Fig. 5–5). The drug was given 3 to 10 days after the onset of acute myocardial infarction in an initial dose of 2.5 mg and titrated upwards to 5 mg twice daily. All-cause mortality and a variety of softer end-points were all reduced (Table 5–7).

V-HeFT-II (Veterans Administration Cooperative Vasodilator-Heart Failure Trial)

The first Veterans Administration vasodilator heart failure trial (V-HeFT-I) established the beneficial effects of vasodilation by nitrate-hydralazine therapy in patients with congestive heart failure (Cohn et al., 1986). In that trial, the two year mortality rate was reduced by 34%. In the V-HeFT-II trial, enalapril was more effective than nitrate-hydralazine therapy in reducing mortality (Cohn et al., 1991) and of interest was the reduction in sudden death, in line with the experimental antiarrhythmic effect (Chapter 11). In black patients, in contrast, vasodilator therapy seemed more effective than ACE inhibition (Carson et al., 1994).

Which ACE inhibitor?

Are the data obtained from the large-scale studies (Tables 5–6 and 5–7) only applicable to the actual ACE inhibitor used? This possibility seems highly unlikely for several reasons. First, both captopril and enalapril have been used, and these two agents belong to two different pharmacokinetic categories of ACE inhibitors (see Chapter 7). There are clear structural differences between them, with captopril possessing an SH-group and enalapril not. Second, in the Hy-C trial, captopril was able to reduce mortality in advanced heart failure, when compared with hydralazine (Fonarow et al., 1992). Third, enalapril is representative of a large group of ACE inhibitors that become activated by liver metabolism (see Chapter 7). At least one of these agents, quinapril, is able to improve exercise time over one year, albeit in an open-label study (Riegger, 1991). Ramipril, another representative of this group, improves prognosis in postinfarct patients with heart failure (see Table 5–7). Fourth, the benefits found are likely to be those of the specific inhibition of the renin-angiotensin axis, not just the consequences of nonspecific vasodilation, as shown by the V-HeFT-II study (Cohn et al., 1991). All ACE inhibitors are by definition able to interrupt a sequence leading from renin to angiotensin-II. It is this pathway that is activated in the myocardium by either post-infarct remodeling or in heart failure (Chapter 4).

Which doses?

Whereas an extremely low dose (1 mg) of captopril can enhance the diuretic effect of furosemide (Motwani et al., 1992), when the aim is suppression of neurohumoral activation and long-term survival, then the ideal dose of captopril is "high", 75 mg or more per day, rather than low (Pacher et al., 1993). A similar conclusion was based on the retrospective analysis of another study on severe heart failure (Pouleur et al., 1991). Thus, the dose of ACE inhibitors used in severe heart failure should be high rather than low, although hypotension may often be a limiting factor. In that case, the addition of spironolactone may suppress urinary aldosterone excretion and achieve clinical benefit even in the presence of low-dose captopril (Dahlstrom and Karlsson, 1993). When using an ACE inhibitor prophylactically, first principles suggest that lower doses should be effective despite the fact that in the SAVE study the total daily dose of captopril was close to 150 mg per day. Osterziel and Dietz (1993) argue the case for lower doses to achieve postinfarct protection.

Comment

A series of six major trials on nearly 12,000 patients have established the beneficial effects of ACE inhibition in heart failure, both in its treatment and its prevention (see Tables 5–6 and 5–7). The first SOLVD trial and V-HeFT-II have shown a benefit on mortality of patients with congestive heart failure in categories of patients less seriously ill than those already studied in CONSENSUS-I. In the SOLVD prevention trial, ACE inhibitor monotherapy by enalapril helped to prevent the development of heart failure. Similar data were obtained in the SAVE study. The postinfarct trials (SAVE, SOLVD preventative arm, and AIRE) showed that ACE inhibition could help prevent or treat congestive heart failure and also reduce all-cause mortality.

Reservations

At a time when the virtues of ACE inhibitor therapy seem incontrovertible, it must be pointed out that the trials have been predominantly on middle-aged or elderly white males, by far the majority suffering from ischemic heart disease. In the therapy of hypertension, it is well accepted that ACE inhibitor therapy is less efficacious in blacks than in whites. There may be a similar situation in heart failure. Where are the data on females? What about noninfarct patients? Why are nonischemic patients not well studied? Although a sizeable percentage of the population in the V-HeFT studies consisted of patients with dilated cardiomyopathy, there appear to be no data in heart failure associated with valvular heart disease.

Cost-effectiveness of ACE inhibitors in treatment of heart failure

While all calculations of cost-effectiveness must be based on extrapolations, an interesting calculation was recently undertaken (Hart and McMurray, 1993). They worked out

TABLE 5–7 Treatment Trials with ACE Inhibitors in Early Postinfarct Patients with Left Ventricular Dysfunction or Overt Heart Failure

	SAVE	AIRE
Total number treated	1,115	1,986
Drug and dose (daily)	Captopril 50 mg 3× in 79%	Ramipril 2.5–5 mg 2×
Mean duration (months)	42	15
Patient population	3–16 days postinfarct	2–9 days postinfarct
Entry criteria	Ejection fraction 40% or less	Clinical heart failure
Age (years), mean	59	65
Gener, male (%)	83	74

Clinical classification	60% Killip Class I	Severe heart failure excluded (all received ACE inhibitors)
Hypertension (%)	43	28
Diuretics (%)	32 at end	60
Digitalis (%)	?	12
Ejection fraction (%), mean	31	?
Mortality reduction (%)	19	27
Worsening heart failure (%) (reduction in risk)	37	29
Sudden death (reduction)	? none	Reduced

that the cost per life year gained varied from $300 to $1,000 according to the dose and according to whether the treatment was initiated in hospital or outside hospital by a general practitioner. These calculations were based on the SOLVD treatment arm studies. It is likely that if similar calculations had been carried out for the AIRE study, an even more impressive result would have been obtained.

It is therefore apparent that the use of ACE inhibitors in the treatment of heart failure, whether caused by the type of diseases covered by the SOLVD study or whether caused by acute infarction (AIRE study), is highly cost-effective. At a time when governments are examining their policy in relation to drugs that might often be considered relatively expensive, such as the ACE inhibitors, this high cost-effectiveness needs to be considered as a further argument in favor of the use of these agents.

EARLY PHASE INFARCT STUDIES WITH ACE INHIBITORS

Now that the results of three large studies with patients treated in the acute phase of myocardial infarction by ACE inhibitors have become available, it is reasonable to ask how much benefit has been achieved. Of a total of nearly 40,000 patients so treated, the majority were entered into the ISIS-IV study (see Table 5–8). In that study, captopril was started at a low oral dose of 6.25 mg and increased to 50 mg twice daily for 28 days. Mortality in control patients at 35 days was already low at 7.3%, possibly because the majority had received fibrinolytic therapy and almost all had received antiplatelet therapy. Captopril reduced mortality to 6.9%, an absolute change of only 0.46% or 4.6 lives saved per 1,000 treated. Although this decrease was significant ($p = 0.04$), the benefit must be weighed against the risk of hypotension—20% in captopril patients versus 10% in controls, the difference being highly significant.

The fear of hypotension in the acute stage is real. In response to intravenous enalaprilat in the CONSENSUS-II study (Swedberg et al., 1992), the incidence of first-dose hypotension increased from 12% in controls to 17% and was linked to an increased mortality. The incidence of hypotension at any time was 25% in the enalapril group and 10% in controls ($p < 0.001$). The cause of this increased harmful hypotension could have been the fixed high intravenous dose of enalaprilat given at the start of the study.

In GISSI-3 (1994), lisinopril, started as a low dose within 24 hours of the onset of symptoms and increased to 10 mg daily, reduced mortality at 6 weeks with a risk reduction of 12% ($p = 0.03$). Mortality fell by 17% when lisinopril was combined with nitroglycerin, given intravenously for the first 24 hours and then as an intermittent patch for the rest of the 6 weeks. Hypotension was found in 36% of controls and 20% of lisinopril-treated patients. In studies on patients with heart failure, both captopril and enalapril caused more first-dose hypotension than did another ACE inhibitor, perindopril (MacFadyen et al., 1991), raising the possibility that not all ACE inhibitors are equal when it comes to this side-effect.

Hypothetically, the increased hypotension induced by captopril, with a mean fall of 10% in blood pressure after a

TABLE 5–8 TRIALS OF ACE INHIBITORS GIVEN AT THE START OF TREATMENT OF ACUTE MYOCARDIAL INFARCTION

	Consensus-II	ISIS-IV	GISSI-3
Total number treated	3,044	27,442	9,435
Drug and daily dose	Enalaprilat IV 1 mg over 2h; then enalapril up to 20 mg 2 × daily	Captopril 6.25 mg initially, increased to 50 mg 2 × daily	Lisinopril 2.5–5 mg initially, increased to 10 mg 1 × daily
Duration	41 to 180 days	28 days	42 days
Patient population	AMI within 24h of onset	AMI within 24h of onset	AMI within 24h of onset
Age, years	66 mean	72% below 70	70 or below in 73%
Gender male (%)	73	74	78
BP exclusion levels	100/60	100 systolic	100 systolic
Hypotension as side-effect (%)	25 (control 10)	21 (control 10)	20 (control 36)
Mortality change, (absolute %)	0.8 increase	0.46 decrease*	0.88 decrease[+]
Mortality change as risk reduction	10% increase	9% decrease* (p = 0.04)	12% decrease (p = 0.03)[+]

*35 days, + 6 weeks.

dose of only 6.25 mg in a subgroup of patients with an initial blood pressure of 129/81 mmHg (Pipilis et al., 1993), could have detracted from other benefits of captopril.

SUMMARY

ACE inhibitor therapy has now become firmly ensconced in the modern therapeutic approach to congestive heart failure. While its benefit is abundantly proven as add-on therapy after digitalis and diuretics, smaller and shorter studies have shown that as second-line therapy it may be preferable to digoxin. ACE inhibition given prophylactically to postinfarct patients may help to prevent the onset of heart failure as shown in the SAVE and SOLVD studies. These data suggest a role for ACE inhibitors as effective first-line monotherapy in early heart failure and an undoubted benefit in postinfarct failure (AIRE Study, 1993). When there is diastolic dysfunction on the basis of left ventricular hypertrophy, then the arguments favoring early ACE inhibitor therapy are strong, because both diuretics and digitalis are theoretically contraindicated.

The benefits of ACE inhibitor therapy can also be shown by acute hemodynamic changes with reduction of preload and afterload and increased left ventricular performance, as monitored both by classic invasive hemodynamic techniques and by echocardiography, the latter showing decreased left ventricular dimensions. In a few studies, ejection fractions have been measured and have increased. The neurohumoral changes associated with chronic ACE inhibitor therapy include increased plasma renin, decreased angiotensin-II, decreased aldosterone, decreased plasma norepinephrine, a tendency to decreased epinephrine, and decreased vasopressin. These changes are thought to be beneficial in the therapy of congestive heart failure. Many workers now believe that these neurohumoral changes are essential in explaining the benefits of ACE inhibitor therapy and provide an argument for the benefits of ACE inhibitor therapy over conventional vasodilators. Evidence favoring this point of view is provided by the VeHeFT-II trial.

There are some contraindications or cautions for the use of ACE inhibitors in congestive heart failure, such as pre-existing hypotension, high-renin states such as bilateral renal artery stenosis with hypertensive heart failure, aortic stenosis combined with congestive heart failure, and the combination of severe angina pectoris and advanced congestive heart failure. Overdiuresis predisposes to hypotension.

ACE inhibitor therapy may have deleterious effects on renal function in heart failure, for example by decreasing the glomerular filtration rate. There is some evidence that longer acting agents are more likely to result in renal impairment than short-acting agents, such as captopril, but this point is by no means fully studied. In general, it is likely that serum urea and creatinine will rise slightly and the glomerular filtration rate fall slightly during ACE inhibitor therapy, whereas it might have been supposed that improved renal blood flow, together with an effective increase in renal plasma flow, would improve the glomerular filtration rate.

A final mystery about ACE inhibitor therapy is that a relatively large number of patients may not respond. An analogy could be made with hypertension in which mean values of blood pressure in a group of patients are consistently reduced by, for example, thiazide therapy, but when the individual patient response is considered, there may be only about a 60% response. Thus, in considering the individual patients, there may be failures with ACE inhibitor therapy. Such failure of therapy may occur especially in patients with a very high right atrial pressure, with a high serum creatinine, with hyponatremia if not also treated by loop diuretics, and, speculatively, in patients with a brisk response of the ANP system to angiotensin (so that reduction of angiotensin decreases ANP levels). The question of the one-third of patients who do not respond well to ACE inhibitor therapy merits much more intense study. At least some of these patients might be black, in whom standard vasodilators might work better. In others, severe hepatic dysfunction might reduce the rate of conversion of enalapril-like compounds to the active form (Oberg et al., 1994).

REFERENCES

AIRE (Acute Infarction Ramipril Efficacy) Study Investigators. Effect of ramipril on mortality and morbidity of survivors of acute myocardial infarction with clinical evidence of heart failure. *Lancet* 1993; 342: 821–828.

Anand IS, Ferrari R, Kalra GS, et al. Edema of cardiac origin. Studies of body water and sodium, renal function, hemodynamic indexes, and plasma hormones in untreated congestive cardiac failure. *Circulation* 1989; 80: 299–305.

Anand IS, Kalra GS, Ferrari R, et al. Enalapril as initial and sole treatment in severe chronic heart failure with sodium retention. *Int J Cardiol* 1990; 28: 341–346.

Bayliss J, Canepa-Anson R, Norell M, et al. The renal response to neuroendocrine inhibition in chronic heart failure: double-blind comparison of captopril and prazosin. *Eur Heart J* 1986; 7: 877–884.

Bayliss J, Norell M, Canepa-Anson R, et al. Untreated heart failure: clinical and neuroendocrine effects of introducing diuretics. *Br Heart J* 1987; 57: 17–22.

Bounhoure JP, Lechat P, Richard C, et al. Perindopril versus placebo: a double-blind multicenter study in chronic congestive heart failure (abstr). *Circulation* 1988; Suppl 2: II–619.

Braunwald E. ACE inhibitors—a cornerstone of the treatment of heart failure. *N Engl J Med* 1991; 325: 351–353.

Brilla CG, Kramer B, Hoffmeister HM, et al. Low-dose enalapril in severe chronic heart failure. *Cardiovasc Drugs Ther* 1989; 3: 211–218.

Captopril-Digoxin Multicenter Research Group. Comparative effects of therapy with captopril and digoxin in patients with mild to moderate heart failure. *JAMA* 1988; 259: 539–544.

Carson PE, Johnson GR, Singh SN, et al for the VA Cooperative Study Group. Differences in vasodilator response by race in heart failure: VHeFT (abstr). *J Am Coll Cardiol* 1994; 23: 382A.

Chalmers JP, West MJ, Cyran J, et al. Placebo-controlled study of lisinopril in congestive heart failure: a multicentre study. *J Cardiovasc Pharmacol* 1987; 9 (Suppl 3): S89–S97.

Chatterjee K, Parmley WW, Cohn JN, et al. A cooperative multicenter study of captopril in congestive heart failure: hemodynamic effects and long-term response. *Am Heart J* 1985; 110: 439–447.

Cleland JGF, Dargie HJ, Hodsman GP, et al. Captopril in heart failure. A double-blind controlled trial. *Br Heart J* 1984; 52: 530–535.

Cleland JGF, Dargie HJ, Ball SG, et al. Effects of enalapril in heart failure: a double-blind study of effects on exercise performance, renal function, hormones, and metabolic state. *Br Heart J* 1985; 54: 305–312.

Cleland JGF, Henderson E, McLenachan J, et al. Effect of captopril, an angiotensin-converting enzyme inhibitor, in patients with angina pectoris and heart failure. *J Am Coll Cardiol* 1991; 17: 733–739.

Cohn JN, Archibald DG, Ziesche S, et al. Effect of vasodilator therapy on mortality in chronic congestive heart failure. Results of a Veterans Administration Cooperative Study. *N Engl J Med* 1986; 314: 1547–1552.

Cohn JN, Johnson G, Ziesche S, et al. Comparison of enalapril with hydralazine-isosorbide dinitrate in the treatment of chronic congestive heart failure. *N Engl J Med* 1991; 325: 303–310.

CONSENSUS Trial Study Group. Effects of enalapril on mortality in severe congestive heart failure. Results of the Cooperative North Scandinavian Enalapril Survival Study (CONSENSUS). *N Engl J Med* 1987; 316: 1429–1435.

Cowley AJ, Stainer K, Wynne RD, et al. Symptomatic assessment of patients with heart failure: double-blind comparison of increasing doses of diuretics and captopril in moderate heart failure. *Lancet* 1986; 2: 770–772.

Creager MA, Massie BM, Faxon DP, et al. Acute and long-term effects of enalapril on the cardiovascular response to exercise and exercise tolerance in patients with congestive heart failure. *J Am Coll Cardiol* 1985; 6: 163–170.

Crozier IG, Ikram H, Nicholls MG, Jans S. Acute hemodynamic, hormonal and electrolyte effects of ramipril in severe congestive heart failure. *Am J Cardiol* 1987; 59: 155D–163D.

Dahlstrom U, Karlsson E. Captopril and spironolactone therapy for refractory congestive heart failure. *Am J Cardiol* 1993; 71: 29A–33A.

Daly P, Rouleau J-L, Cousineau D, et al. Effects of captopril and a combination of hydralazine and isosorbide dinitrate on myocardial sympathetic tone in patients with severe congestive heart failure. *Br Heart J* 1986; 56: 152–157.

Davis R, Ribner HS, Keung E, et al. Treatment of chronic congestive heart failure with captopril, an oral inhibitor of angiotensin-converting enzyme. *N Engl J Med* 1979; 301: 117–121.

de Graeff PA, Kingma JH, Viersma JW, et al. Acute and chronic effects of ramipril and captopril in congestive heart failure. *Int J Cardiol* 1989; 23: 59–67.

Desche P, Antony I, Lerebours G, et al. Acceptability of perindopril in mild-to-moderate chronic congestive heart failure. Results of a long-term open study in 320 patients. *Am J Cardiol* 1993; 71: 61E–68E.

DiCarlo L, Chatterjee K, Parmley WW, et al. Enalapril: a new angiotensin-converting enzyme inhibitor in chronic heart failure: acute and chronic hemodynamic evaluations. *J Am Coll Cardiol* 1983; 2: 865–871.

Dzau VJ, Hollenberg NK. Renal response to captopril in severe heart failure: role of furosemide in natriuresis and reversal of hyponatremia. *Ann Intern Med* 1984; 100: 777–782.

Dzau VJ, Packer M, Lilly LS, et al. Prostaglandins in severe congestive heart failure. Relation to activation of the renin-angiotensin system and hyponatremia. *N Engl J Med* 1984; 310: 347–352.

Ferrari R, Anand I. Neurohumoral changes in untreated heart failure. *Cardiovasc Drugs Ther* 1989; 3: 979–986.

Flammang D, Waynberger M, Chassing A. Acute and long-term efficacy of perindopril in severe chronic congestive heart failure. *Am J Cardiol* 1993; 71: 48E–56E.

Flapan AD, Nolan J, Neilson JMM, Ewing DJ. Effect of captopril on cardiac parasympathetic activity in chronic cardiac failure secondary to coronary artery disease. *Am J Cardiol* 1992; 69: 532–535.

Fonarow GC, Chelimsky-Fallick C, Stevenson LW, et al. Effect of direct vasodilation with hydralazine versus angiotensin-converting enzyme inhibition with captopril on mortality in advanced heart failure: the Hy-C Trial. *J Am Coll Cardiol* 1992; 19: 842–850.

Gheorghiade M, Hall V, Lakier JB, Goldstein S. Comparative hemodynamic and neurohumoral effects of intravenous captopril and digoxin and their combinations in patients with severe heart failure. *J Am Coll Cardiol* 1989; 13: 134–142.

GISSI-3 (Gruppo Italiano per lo Studio della Sopravvivenza Nell' Infarto Miocardico). GISSI-3: effects of lisinopril and transdermal glyceryl trinitrate singly and together on 6-week mortality and ventricular function after acute myocardial infarction. *Lancet* 1994; 343: 1115–1122.

Harris P. Congestive cardiac failure: central role of the arterial blood pressure. *Br Heart J* 1987; 58: 190–203.

Harris P. Congestive cardiac failure: the syndrome of volume expansion. *Cardiovasc Drugs Ther* 1989; 3: 941–945.

Hart W, McMurray J. The cost-effectiveness of enalapril in the treatment of heart failure (abstr). *Eur Heart J* 1993; 14 (Suppl): 14.

Heel RC, Brogden RN, Speight TM, Avery GS. Captopril: a preliminary review of its pharmacological properties and therapeutic efficacy. *Drugs* 1980; 20: 409–452.

ISIS-IV study (1994)(Fourth International Study of Infarct Survival)—Ferguson JJ. Meeting highlights. *Circulation* 1994; 89: 545–547.

Jamieson MJ, Webster J, Fowler G, et al. A comparison of the chronic effects of oral xamoterol and enalapril on blood pressure and renal function in mild to moderate heart failure. *Br J Clin Pharmacol* 1991; 31: 305–312.

Judgutt B, Tymchak W, Humen D, et al. Prolonged nitroglycerin versus captopril therapy on remodeling after transmural myocardial infarction (abstr). *Circulation* 1990; 82 (Suppl III): III–442.

Kromer EP, Elsner D, Riegger GAJ. Digoxin, converting-enzyme inhibition (quinapril), and the combination in patients with congestive heart failure function class II and sinus rhythm. *J Cardiovasc Pharmacol* 1990; 16: 9–14.

Kubo S, Nishioka A, Nishimura H, et al. Effects of converting-enzyme inhibition on cardiorenal hemodynamics in patients with chronic congestive heart failure. *J Cardiovasc Pharmacol* 1985; 7: 753–759.

Laragh JH. Endocrine mechanisms in congestive cardiac failure: renin, aldosterone and atrial natriuretic hormone. *Drugs* 1986; 32 (Suppl 5): 1–12.

MacFadyen RJ, Lees KR, Reid JL. Differences in first dose response to ACE inhibition in congestive cardiac failure—a placebo controlled study. *Br Heart J* 1991; 66: 206–211.

McLay JS, McMurray J, Bridges A, Struthers AD. Practical issues when initiating captopril therapy in chronic heart failure. What is the appropriate dose and how long should patients be observed? *Eur Heart J* 1992; 13: 1521–1527.

Meerson FZ. The myocardium in hyperfunction, hypertrophy and heart failure. *Circ Res* 1969; 25 (Suppl 2): 1–163.

Mehra A, Ostrzega E, Shotan A, et al. Persistent hemodynamic improvement with short-term nitrate therapy in patients with chronic congestive heart failure already treated with captopril. *Am J Cardiol* 1992; 70: 1310–1314.

Mettauer B, Rouleau J-L, Bichet D, et al. Differential long-term intrarenal and neurohormonal effects of captopril and prazosin in patients with chronic congestive heart failure: importance of initial plasma renin activity. *Circulation* 1986; 73: 492–502.

Motwani JG, Fenwick MK, Morton JJ, Struthers AD. Furosemide-induced natriuresis is augmented by ultra low-dose captopril but not by standard doses of captopril in chronic heart failure. *Circulation* 1992; 86: 439–445.

Moye LA, Pfeffer MA, Braunwald E for the SAVE Investigators. Rationale, design and baseline characteristics of the survival and ventricular enlargement trial. *Am J Cardiol* 1991; 68: 70D–79D.

Nishimura H, Kubo S, Ueyama M, et al. Peripheral hemodynamic effects of captopril in patients with congestive heart failure. *Am Heart J* 1989; 117: 100–105.

Northridge DB, Rose E, Raftery ED, et al. A multicentre, double-blind, placebo-controlled trial of quinapril in mild, chronic heart failure. *Eur Heart J* 1993; 14: 403–409.

Oberg KC, Just VL, Bauman JL, Papp MA. Reduced bioavailability of enalapril in patients with severe heart failure (abstr). *J Am Coll Cardiol* 1994; 23: 381A.

Odemuyiwa O, Gilmartin J, Kenny D, Hall RJC. Captopril and the diuretic requirements in moderate and severe chronic heart failure. *Eur Heart J* 1989; 10: 586–590.

Orme M L'E. Non-steroidal anti-inflammatory drugs and the kidney. *Br Med J* 1986; 292: 1621–1622.

Osterziel KJ, Dietz R. Dosing of ACE inhibitors in post-infarct protection. *Cardiovasc Drugs Ther* 1993; 7: 881–883.

Pacher R, Globits S, Bergler-Klein J, et al. Clinical and neurohumoral response of patients with severe congestive heart failure treated with two different captopril dosages. *Eur Heart J* 1993; 14: 273–278.

Packer M. The role of vasodilator therapy in the treatment of severe chronic heart failure. *Drugs* 1986; 32 (Suppl 5): 13–26.

Packer M, Medina N, Yushak M. Efficacy of captopril in low-renin congestive heart failure: importance of sustained reactive hyperreninemia in distinguishing responders from non-responders. *Am J Cardiol* 1984a; 54: 771–777.

Packer M, Medina N, Yushak M. Relation between serum sodium concentration and the hemodynamic and clinical responses to converting enzyme inhibition with captopril in severe heart failure. *J Am Coll Cardiol* 1984b; 3: 1035–1043.

Packer M, Medina N, Yushak M, Lee WH. Comparative effects of captopril and isosorbide dinitrate on pulmonary arteriolar resistance and right ventricular function in patients with severe left ventricular failure: results of a randomized crossover study. *Am Heart J* 1985a; 109: 1293–1299.

Packer M, Medina N, Yushak M, Lee WH. Usefulness of plasma renin activity in predicting haemodynamic and clinical responses and survival during long term converting enzyme inhibition in severe chronic heart failure. Experience in 100 consecutive patients. *Br Heart J* 1985b; 54: 298–304.

Packer M, Lee WH, Medina N, Yushak M. Hemodynamic and clinical significance of the pulmonary vascular response to long-term captopril therapy in patients with severe chronic heart failure. *J Am Coll Cardiol* 1985c; 6: 635–645.

Packer M, Lee WH, Yushak M, Medina N. Comparison of captopril and enalapril in patients with severe chronic heart failure. *N Engl J Med* 1986a; 315: 847–853.

Packer M, Lee WH, Kessler PD. Preservation of glomerular filtration rate in human heart failure by activation of the renin-angiotensin system. *Circulation* 1986b; 74: 766–774.

Packer M, Lee WH, Medina N, et al. Functional renal insufficiency during long-term therapy with captopril and enalapril in severe chronic heart failure. *Ann Intern Med* 1987a; 106: 346–354.

Packer M, Lee WH, Medina N, et al. Influence of diabetes mellitus on changes in left ventricular performance and renal function produced by converting enzyme inhibition in patients with severe chronic heart failure. *Am J Med* 1987b; 82: 1119–1126.

Packer M, Gheorghiade M, Young JB, et al on behalf of the RADIANCE study. Randomized, double-blind, placebo-controlled, withdrawal study of digoxin in patients with chronic heart failure treated with converting-enzyme inhibitors (abstr). *J Am Coll Cardiol* 1992; 19: 260A.

Pfeffer MA, Braunwald E, Moye LA, et al. Effect of captopril on mortality and morbidity in patients with left ventricular dysfunction after myocardial infarction. Results of the Survival and Ventricular Enlargement Trial. *N Engl J Med* 1992; 327: 669–677.

Pipilis A, Flather M, Collins R, et al. Hemodynamic effects of captopril and isosorbide mononitrate started early in acute myocardial infarction: a randomized placebo-controlled study. *J Am Coll Cardiol* 1993, 21; 73–79.

Pouleur H, Rousseau MF, Oakley C, Ryden L for the Xamoterol in Severe Heart Failure Study Group. Difference in mortality between patients treated with captopril or enalapril in the Xamoterol in Severe Heart Failure Study. *Am J Cardiol* 1991; 68: 71–74.

Powers ER, Chiaramida A, DeMaria AN, et al. A double-blind comparison of lisinopril with captopril in patients with symptomatic congestive heart failure *J Cardiovasc Pharmacol* 1987; 9 (Suppl 3): S82–S88.

Raya TE, Gay RG, Aguirre M, Goldman S. Importance of venodilatation in prevention of left ventricular dilatation after chronic large myocardial infarction in rats: a comparison of captopril and hydralazine. *Circ Res* 1989; 64: 330–337.

Remes J, Tikkanen I, Fyhrquist F, Pyorala K. Neuroendocrine activity in untreated heart failure. *Br Heart J* 1991; 65: 249–255.

Richardson A, Bayliss J, Scriven A, et al. Double-blind comparison of captopril alone against frusemide plus amiloride in mild heart failure. *Lancet* 1987; 2: 709–711.

Riegger GAJ. Effects of quinapril on exercise tolerance in patients with mild to moderate heart failure. *Eur Heart J* 1991; 12: 705–711.

Riegger GAJ, Kochsiek K. Vasopressin, renin and norepinephrine levels before and after captopril administration in patients with congestive heart failure due to idiopathic dilated cardiomyopathy. *Am J Cardiol* 1986; 58: 300–303.

Rouleau JL, de Champlain J, Klein M, et al. Activation of neurohumoral systems in postinfarction left ventricular dysfunction. *J Am Coll Cardiol* 1993; 22: 390–398.

Schofield PM, Brooks NH, Lawrence GP, et al. Which vasodilator drug in patients with chronic heart failure? A randomised comparison of captopril and hydralazine. *Br J Clin Pharmacol* 1991; 31: 25–32.

Scriven AJI, Lipkin DP, Anand IS, et al. Double-blind, randomised, cross-over comparison of oral captopril and enoximone added to diuretic treatment in patients with severe heart failure. *J Cardiovasc Pharmacol* 1988; 11: 45–50.

Shahi M, Thom S, Poulter N, et al. Regression of hypertensive left ventricular hypertrophy and left ventricular diastolic function. *Lancet* 1990; 336: 458–461.

Sharpe N, Murphy J, Coxon R, Hannan SF. Enalapril in patients with chronic heart failure: a placebo-controlled, randomized, double-blind study. *Circulation* 1984; 70: 271–278.

Sharpe N, Murphy J, Smith H, Hannan, S. Treatment of patients with symptomless left ventricular dysfunction after myocardial infarction. *Lancet* 1988; 1: 255–259.

Smith TW, Pfeffer MA. The rationale for combined use of diuretics, digitalis and vasodilators in congestive heart failure. *Cardiovasc Drugs Ther* 1989; 3: 13–17.

SOLVD Investigators. Effect of enalapril on survival in patients with reduced left ventricular ejection fractions and congestive heart failure. *N Engl J Med* 1991; 325: 293–302.

SOLVD Investigators. Effect of enalapril on mortality and the development of heart failure in asymptomatic patients with reduced left ventricular fractions. *N Engl J Med* 1992; 327: 685–691.

Squire IB, MacFadyen RJ, Lees KR, Reid JL. Differing blood pressure and renin angiotensin system responses to ACE inhibition in heart failure (abstr). *J Am Coll Cardiol* 1994; 23: 376A.

Swedberg K, Eneroth P, Kjekshus J, Wilhelmsen L, for the CONSENSUS Trial Study Group. Hormones regulating cardiovascular function in patients with severe congestive heart failure and their relation to mortality. *Circulation* 1990; 82: 1730–1736.

Swedberg K, Held P, Kjekshus J, Rasmussen K, et al on behalf of the CONSENSUS II Study Group. Effects of the early administration of enalapril on mortality in patients with acute myocardial infarction. Results of the Cooperative New Scandinavian Enalapril Survival Study II (CONSENSUS II). *N Engl J Med* 1992; 327: 678–684.

Thuillez C, Richard C, Loueslati H, et al. Systemic and regional hemodynamic effects of perindopril in congestive heart failure. *J Cardiovasc Pharmacol* 1990; 15: 527–535.

Timmis AD, Smyth P, Kenny JF, et al. Effects of vasodilator treatment with felodipine on haemodynamic responses to treadmill exercise in congestive heart failure. *Br Heart J* 1984; 52: 314–320.

Timmis AD, Bojanowski LMR, Najm YC, et al. Captopril versus placebo in congestive heart failure: effects on oxygen delivery to exercising skeletal muscle. *Eur Heart J* 1987; 8: 1295–1304.

Todd PA, Heel RC. Enalapril. A review of its pharmacodynamic and pharmacokinetic properties, and therapeutic use in hypertension and congestive heart failure. *Drugs* 1986; 31: 198–248.

Turini GA, Waeber B, Brunner HR. The renin-angiotensin system in refractory heart failure: clinical, hemodynamic and hormonal effects of captopril and enalapril. *Eur Heart J* 1983; 4 (Suppl A): 189–197.

Volpe M, Tritto C, De Luca N, et al. Angiotensin-converting enzyme inhibition restores cardiac and hormonal responses to volume overload in patients with dilated cardiomyopathy and mild heart failure. *Circulation* 1992; 86: 1800–1809.

Wilson JR, Ferraro N. Effect of the renin-angiotensin system on limb circulation and metabolism during exercise in patients with heart failure. *J Am Coll Cardiol* 1985; 6: 556–563.

Wilson JR, Mancini DM, Chance B. Skeletal muscle metabolism in congestive heart failure. *Cardiovasc Drugs Ther* 1989; 3: 995–1000.

Xamoterol in Severe Heart Failure Study Group. Xamoterol in severe heart failure. *Lancet* 1990; 336: 1–6.

Yusuf S, Pepine CJ, Garces C, et al. Effect of enalapril on myocardial infarction and unstable angina in patients with low ejection fractions. *Lancet* 1992; 340: 1173–1178.

CHAPTER 6

ACE Inhibitors and the Central Nervous System

"Behavioral studies have provided clear evidence that the ACE inhibitors have potential to improve cognitive performance"
(Barnes et al., 1989).

Angiotensinogen is locally made in the brain (Campbell et al., 1984). There are also angiotensin-II receptors in the brain and their activity may be concerned with certain types of hypertension (Nazarali et al., 1990). ACE inhibitors are likely to interact with these receptors and also at several other levels of the central and autonomic nervous systems. First, ACE inhibitors should indirectly modify the release of norepinephrine; second, there may be effects on baroreceptors; third, cerebral blood flow regulation could be altered; and fourth, there could be direct effects on mood and other higher functions.

AUTONOMIC NERVOUS SYSTEM

Modulation of sympathetic activity

Angiotensin-II is thought to have a "permissive" role in the release of norepinephrine from the terminal adrenergic neurons, both by enhancing the release of norepinephrine and by inhibiting the re-uptake of norepinephrine into the terminal neurons. Furthermore, angiotensin-II facilitates ganglionic transmission and also has a role in central adrenergic activation (see Chapter 1). Normally, exercise induces a rise in plasma catecholamine levels. During ACE inhibition therapy, this rise is attenuated probably because less norepinephrine is released from terminal neurons (Morioka et al., 1983). This indirect antiadrenergic effect of ACE inhibition may be important not only in blood pressure reduction but also in helping to explain the antiarrhythmic effects in myocardial ischemia.

Enhanced parasympathetic activity

ACE inhibitor therapy reduces the blood pressure without any reflex tachycardia. Logically, this could result from resetting of baroreflexes (Vidt et al., 1982; Raman et al., 1985) or enhanced activity of the parasympathetic nervous system. A relative increase of the activity of the parasympathetic nervous system compared with that of the sympathetic nervous system has been found after captopril (Campbell et al., 1985), lisinopril (Ajayi et al., 1985), perindopril (Ajayi et al., 1986), enalapril (Boni et al., 1990), and benazepril (West et al., 1991). By enhancing parasympathetic outflow, baroreceptor activity can be reset without any change in the actual sensitivity of the receptors (West et al., 1991). In diabetics with mild vagal impairment, a single dose of 25 mg captopril enhanced the reflex bradycardic response to apneic face immersion in water (Moore et al., 1987).

EFFECTS ON CEREBRAL PERFUSION

Cerebral autoregulation

Cerebral autoregulation is the process whereby the cerebral vascular bed maintains a constant blood flow in the face of variations in the perfusion pressure, the latter for practical purposes corresponding to the blood pressure. Regulation of cerebral blood flow is of dual importance in relation to hypertensive patients, particularly in the elderly in whom autoregulation may be impaired by several possible concurrent disease processes, such as stroke, diabetes, and dementia (Strandgaard, 1990; Paulson and Strandgaard, 1994). First, limits of autoregulation are altered by the hypertensive process and, second, various drugs may have different influences on the patterns of autoregulation. Thus, the lowest tolerated mean blood pressure in normotensives is about 43 mmHg (Strandgaard, 1976). In treated hypertensive patients, this lower limit is about 53 mmHg and, in ineffectively treated severe hypertension, the limit is about 65 mmHg (Strandgaard, 1976).

Effect of angiotensin-II on cerebral circulation

In general, there is a lack of response of cerebral blood flow to intraluminal angiotensin-II (Brown and Brown, 1986). Degradation products of angiotensin-II, such as angiotensin-III, and the combination of angiotensin-II-(3–8) with L-arginine may produce vasodilatory rather than vasoconstrictory responses in cerebral arterioles (Haberl et al., 1991). Local generation of angiotensin-II by the renin-angiotensin system in the vascular wall does, however, occur (Speth and Harik, 1985) and may have different effects. As in the case of other tissues, it is unclear to what extent the circulating renin-angiotensin system and locally synthesized components interact. Nonetheless, it is the luminal ACE activity of large cerebral arteries that probably plays the most important role in determining the effects of ACE inhibitors on cerebral blood flow. Thus, whether or not ACE inhibitors penetrate to deeper sites in the central nervous system is not crucial to the control of the cerebral circulation by these agents (Starr and Whalley, 1994).

ACE inhibitors and autoregulation

ACE inhibitor therapy alters the range over which autoregulation of cerebral blood flow occurs, bringing down the upper and lower limits in hypertensive rats (Barry et al., 1984; Muller et al., 1990; Bray et al., 1991). In humans, ACE inhibitors also reset cerebral autoregulation at lower blood pressures (Paulson et al., 1985), influencing mostly the systolic value. Such resetting of autoregulation has been thought to be protective against sudden decreases of blood pressure, especially during the treatment of congestive heart failure, so that low arterial blood pressure values are not associated with symptoms of cerebral ischemia (Paulson et al., 1986). Conversely, Brown and Brown (1986) propose that the decrease in the upper limit of autoregulation by ACE inhibitor therapy, for example from 200 to 140 mmHg (Barry et al., 1984), could be harmful because it would not protect against any sudden upward surges of the blood pressure.

ACE Inhibitors and Stroke

Angiotensin-II and circulation in cerebral ischemia

Currently, there are two opposing hypotheses on the possible effects of angiotensin-II in cerebral ischemia. These hypotheses are particularly important in the evaluation of cerebral vascular disease. First, it is proposed that the activity of angiotensin-II, by potentially increasing collateral flow to ischemic brain tissue, could protect the brain (Fernandez et al., 1986). In keeping with this hypothesis, Brown and Brown (1986) proposed that angiotensin-II normally plays a protective role in the cerebral circulation, acting by (1) maintenance of the blood pressure during hypotensive episodes, protecting by maintenance of the upper limit of cerebral autoregulation, and by (2) vasodilation of smaller cerebral vessels by release of prostacyclin or other vasodilator prostaglandins (Toda and Miyazaki, 1981).

Conversely, angiotensin-II by virtue of its vasoconstrictive effect can be expected to exaggerate the cerebral vascular spasm associated with stroke and, hence, to make stroke worse. Furthermore, by generally elevating blood pressure, angiotensin is likely to predispose to stroke, and when stroke does occur, to make it worse. Evidence supporting the potential harmful effects of angiotensin-II is summarized by Werner et al. (1991).

Existing data on therapy of hypertension and stroke

There are as yet no outcome data on the effect of ACE inhibitors in the reduction of stroke in hypertensive patients, although one such study is under way (CAPP Group, 1990; Chapter 3). A large prospective study has defined the risks for stroke in middle-aged men: a high systolic blood pressure, smoking, heavy alcohol consumption, and ischemic heart disease with left ventricular hypertrophy (Shaper et al., 1991). Another equally large retrospective survey found that an elevated diastolic blood pressure was an even greater risk (Palmer et al., 1992).

In general, a fall of diastolic blood pressure of 5 to 10 mmHg should reduce the incidence of stroke by 34% to 56% (MacMahon et al., 1990). The blood pressure reduction should be effective however achieved. Currently, this proposal would appear to be the most logical one available and is supported by animal data showing that an ACE inhibitor, perindopril, reduces stroke mortality in renovascular hypertension (Atkinson et al., 1990).

Could there be a special protective effect of ACE inhibitors?

Laragh and his group in New York have proposed that there could basically be two different forms of hypertension with different consequences for stroke: the first being sodium-dependent and related to abnormal membrane function, while the second is renin-dependent and related to vasoconstriction. Simply put, the former is "wet" hypertension and the latter "dry" hypertension. The proposed hypothetical difference between these two types is that vascular sequelae, such as stroke and heart attack, are more likely to occur in the high-renin "dry" type (Laragh, 1987). Although Laragh's concept has been much criticized, support for the proposed relationship has been forthcoming in the case of heart attacks but not stroke (Alderman et al., 1991).

Possible vascular protective role of ACE inhibitors

Nonetheless, the vascular hypothesis lives on. Angiotensin-II is an important regulator of vascular growth (Chapter 10) and, hence, of vascular hypertrophy. Vascular disease may predispose to stroke or cognitive impairment even in the absence of hypertension (Starr and Whalley, 1994). Hypothetically, ACE inhibitors could be protective against stroke even in the absence of any antihypertensive effect.

Stroke-prone spontaneously hypertensive rats

There is a specific strain of spontaneously hypertensive rat, namely the stroke-prone animal (Kim et al., 1991). As the rats mature, there are higher adrenal levels of angiotensin-I and angiotensin-II. In addition, the circulating levels of plasma renin, angiotensin-I, and angiotensin-II, as well as aldosterone, are all high in the adult animal, even after bilateral nephrectomy. Therefore, there must have been a nonrenal source for the renin, which is thought to be contributory to stroke development in this strain of rats.

Comment

Clearly, there are three different situations to consider in relation to the possible harm of angiotensin-II in relation to stroke. First, in relation to the general mechanism of stroke development, increased circulating angiotensin-II activity has a hypertensive effect, in part central, that must promote the risk of stroke. Second, angiotensin-II as a growth factor may promote cerebral vascular disease and predispose to stroke even in the absence of hypertension. Third, in at least some special situations, angiotensin-II may be able to maintain collateral circulation to the ischemic zone of the brain and, thereby, exert a paradoxical protective effect against cerebral ischemia. In humans, it is likely that cerebral vasospasm contributes to the overall symptomatology of cerebrovascular accidents, as shown by the benefits of successful treatment by calcium antagonists, such as nimodipine. Therefore, it may be anticipated that, in general, the therapy of hypertension by ACE inhibitors should be beneficial in the prevention of cerebral vascular disease. However, a firm answer to this important question could only be given when the outcome data on the incidence of stroke from large and reliable clinical trials become available.

EFFECTS OF ACE INHIBITORS ON MOOD AND OTHER HIGHER FUNCTIONS

In contrast to several other antihypertensive agents acting centrally or having central effects such as methyldopa and propranolol, ACE inhibitors are thought to improve mood (Croog et al., 1986). In addition, it has been proposed that ACE inhibitors have unique behavioral and cognitive actions unlike those of other antihypertensive agents (Barnes et al., 1989; Ferrario et al., 1990).

Memory and behavior

When angiotensin is given intraperitoneally to animals or into a brain ventricle, there is facilitation of certain types of motivated behavior (Ferrario et al., 1990) or reversal of the helpless behavior induced by repetitive electrical shocks (Martin et al., 1990). There is some evidence that angiotensin-II may promote memory. In humans, there is less definitive evidence for such central effects (see review by Jern, 1988).

When an ACE inhibitor was given to 23 normal volunteers in an antihypertensive dose, it had no effect on memory performance nor on sleep patterns (Dietrich and Herrmann, 1989). Isolated case reports have suggested that the ACE inhibitor, captopril, has a mood elevating effect in depressed patients (Zubenko and Nixon, 1984), but their patients were suffering from heart failure or from diastolic hypertension, so that it is not certain that the benefits in mood were achieved as a direct result of the ACE inhibitor therapy or indirectly by improving the symptomatology of heart failure or hypertension.

Hypertensive patients with psychological depression

Depression may be an organic syndrome caused by decreased formation of certain biogenic amines. Especially reserpine and methyldopa are therapies for hypertension that may actually cause depression (Beers and Passman,

1990). Patients receiving propranolol are five times more likely to be given concurrent antidepressants, and in the users of beta-blockers aged 20 to 39 years, the relative risk of antidepressant therapy use was 17 times higher (Thiessen et al., 1990). This risk of depression is much less for other beta-blockers (Thiessen et al., 1990). Hence, in patients subject to depression, beta-blockade especially by propranolol should be avoided, and the agents of choice include ACE inhibitors. Although ratings of "well being" improved during ACE inhibitor therapy in hypertensive patients (Croog et al., 1986), it is not clear that the effect is specific (Hjemdahl and Wiklund, 1992).

In a randomized, double-blind parallel group study on 360 hypertensive men, captopril but not enalapril improved the depressed mood when compared with propranolol or atenolol (Steiner et al., 1990). Another tantalizing result was found in 379 hypertensive men: captopril preserved a high quality of life, which worsened with enalapril (Testa et al., 1993). In neither study was there a concurrent placebo group.

CENTRAL ANTIHYPERTENSIVE MECHANISMS OF ACE INHIBITORS

Unger et al. (1981) review evidence for a central mechanism, at least in part, for the antihypertensive effects of ACE inhibitors. Such effects of ACE inhibitors, exerted chiefly at the level of the brain stem, might be more important in blood pressure reduction than the peripheral vasodilation (Starr and Whalley, 1994). A number of peptides besides angiotensin, such as kinins, substance P, and opioid peptides such as beta-endorphin (Handa et al., 1991), all thought to participate in central blood pressure regulation, are substrates for converting enzyme activity or closely related enzymes that are also inhibited by ACE inhibitor therapy. Angiotensin-II acts in part through release of vasopressin which is a major component of the central blood pressure controlling system (Starr and Whalley, 1994). Of great interest is that atrial natriuretic peptide (ANP) in general opposes the effects of angiotensin-II on the brain (Starr and Whalley, 1994). Thus, the proposal is that ACE inhibitors have central effects that may make a major contribution to the antihypertensive action, at least in part by suppression of central peptidergic blood pressure regulation and/or of brain ACE activity (Sakaguchi et al., 1988). Because the centers involved in blood pressure control lie outside the blood brain barrier, there is no particular difference between those ACE inhibitors, such as zofenopril, that penetrate this barrier and those, such as enalapril, that do not.

SUMMARY

ACE inhibitors affect the autonomic nervous system by indirectly diminishing adrenergic activity and by relatively increasing parasympathetic activity. Thereby baroreceptor control may be altered without changing the sensitivity of the receptors.

ACE inhibitors decrease the limits of cerebral autoregulation, clearly beneficial in patients with congestive heart failure and low blood pressure levels. The effects of ACE inhibitors on stroke in hypertensive patients is not yet established. First principles would suggest that a reduction of blood pressure by any means should induce a corresponding fall in the stroke rate. Nonetheless, there are some conflicting experimental data that need to be considered.

ACE inhibitors maintain the quality of life at normal levels. Some claim that ACE inhibitors positively improve the quality of life and that there may be differences between captopril and enalapril (for other reviews, see Chapter 8).

In general, the cerebral effects of angiotensin-II and of ACE inhibitors are still relatively poorly understood.

REFERENCES

Ajayi AA, Campbell BC, Howie CA, Reid JL. Acute and chronic effects of the converting enzyme inhibitors enalapril and lisinopril on reflex control of heart rate in normotensive man. *J Hypertens* 1985; 3: 47–53.

Ajayi AA, Lees KR, Reid JL. Effects of angiotensin-converting enzyme inhibitor, perindopril, on autonomic reflexes. *Eur J Clin Pharmacol* 1986; 30: 177–182.

Alderman MH, Madhavan S, Ooi WL, et al. Association of the renin sodium profile with the risk of myocardial infarction in patients with hypertension. *N Engl J Med* 1991; 324: 1098–1104.

Atkinson J, Bentahila S, Scalbert E, et al. Perindopril and cerebral ischaemia in renovascular hypertension (abstr). *Eur J Pharmacol* 1990; 183: 2066–2067.

Barnes JM, Barnes NM, Costall B, et al. ACE inhibition and cognition. In: MacGregor GA, Sever PS (eds). *Current Advances in ACE Inhibition.* Churchill Livingstone, Edinburgh, 1989, 159–171.

Barry DI, Paulson OB, Jarden JO, et al. Effects of captopril on cerebral blood flow in normotensive and hypertensive rats. *Am J Med* 1984; 76: 79–85.

Beers MH, Passman LJ. Antihypertensive medications and depression. *Drugs* 1990; 40: 792–799.

Boni E, Alicandri C, Fariello R, et al. Effect of enalapril on parasympathetic activity. *Cardiovasc Drugs Ther* 1990; 4: 265–268.

Bray L, Lartaud I, Muller F, et al. Effects of the angiotensin-I converting enzyme inhibitor perindopril on cerebral blood flow in awake hypertensive rats. *Am J Hypertens* 1991; 4: 246S–252S.

Brown MJ, Brown J. Does angiotensin-II protect against strokes? *Lancet* 1986; 2: 427–429.

Campbell BC, Sturani A, Reid JL. Evidence of parasympathetic activity of the angiotensin converting enzyme inhibitor, captopril, in normotensive man. *Clin Sci* 1985; 68: 49–56.

Campbell DJ, Bouhnik J, Menard J, Corvol P. Identity of angiotensinogen precursors of rat brain and liver. *Nature* 1984; 308: 206–208.

CAPP Group. The Captopril Prevention Project: a prospective intervention trial of angiotensin converting enzyme inhibition in the treatment of hypertension. *J Hypertens* 1990; 8: 985–990.

Croog SH, Levine S, Testa MA, et al. The effect of antihypertensive therapy on the quality of life. *N Engl J Med* 1986; 314: 1657–1664.

Dietrich B, Herrmann WM. Influence of cilazapril on memory functions and sleep behaviour in comparison with metoprolol and placebo in healthy subjects. *Br J Clin Pharmacol* 1989; 27: 249S–261S.

Fernandez LA, Spencer DD, Kaczmar T. Angiotensin-II decreases mortality rate in gerbils with unilateral carotid ligation. *Stroke* 1986; 17: 82–85.

Ferrario CM, Block CH, Zelenski SG. Behavioral and cognitive effects of ACE inhibitors. *ACE Report* 1990; 70: 1–7.

Haberl RL, Decker PJ, Einhaupl KM. Angiotensin degradation products mediate endothelium-dependent dilation of rabbit brain arterioles. *Circ Res* 1991; 68: 1621–1627.

Handa K, Sasaki J, Tanaka H, et al. Effects of captopril on opioid peptides during exercise and quality of life in normal subjects. *Am Heart J* 1991; 122: 1389–1394.

Hjemdahl P, Wiklund IK. Quality of life on antihypertensive drug therapy: scientific end-point or marketing exercise? *J Hypertens* 1992; 10: 1437–1446.

Jern S. Evaluation of mood and the effect of angiotensin-converting enzyme inhibitors. *Drugs* 1988; 35 (Suppl 5): 86–88.

Kim S, Hosoi M, Shimamoto K, et al. Increased production of angiotensin-II in the adrenal gland of stroke-prone spontaneously hypertensive rats with malignant hypertension. *Biochem Biophys Res Comm* 1991; 178: 151–157.

Laragh JH. Two forms of vasoconstriction in systemic hypertension. *Am J Cardiol* 1987; 60: 82G–93G.

MacMahon S, Peto R, Cutler J, et al. Blood pressure, stroke, and coronary artery disease. Part 1, prolonged differences in blood pressure: prospective observational studies corrected for the regression dilution bias. *Lancet* 1990; 335: 765–774.

Martin P, Massol J, Scalbert E, Puech AJ. Involvement of angiotensin-converting enzyme inhibition in reversal of helpless behavior evoked by perindopril in rats. *Eur J Pharmacol* 1990; 187: 165–170.

Moore MV, Jeffcoate WJ, MacDonald IA. Apparent improvement in diabetic autonomic neuropathy induced by captopril. *J Human Hypertens* 1987; 1: 161–165.

Morioka S, Simon G, Cohn JN. Cardiac and hormonal effects of enalapril in hypertension. *Clin Pharmacol Ther* 1983; 34: 583–589.

Muller F, Lartaud I, Bray L, et al. Chronic treatment with the angiotensin-I converting enzyme inhibitor, perindopril, restores the lower limit of autoregulation of cerebral blood flow in the awake renovascular hypertensive rat. *J Hypertens* 1990; 8: 1037–1042.

Nazarali AJ, Gutkind JS, Correa FMA, Saavedra JM. Decreased angiotensin-II receptors in subfornical organ of spontaneously hypertensive rats after chronic antihypertensive treatment with enalapril. *Am J Hypertens* 1990; 3: 59–61.

Palmer AJ, Bulpitt CJ, Fletcher AE, et al. Relation between blood pressure and stroke mortality. *Hypertension* 1992; 20: 601–605.

Paulson OB, Strandgaard S. The brain. In: Messerli FH (ed.). *The ABCs of Antihypertensive Therapy.* Authors' Publishing House, 1994, 59–68.

Paulson OB, Vorstrup S, Andersen AR, et al. Converting enzyme inhibition resets cerebral autoregulation at lower blood pressure. *J Hypertens* 1985; 3: S487–S488.

Paulson OB, Jarden JO, Vorstrup A, et al. Effect of captopril on the cerebral circulation in chronic heart failure. *Eur J Clin Invest* 1986; 16: 124–132.

Raman GV, Waller DG, Warren DJ. The effect of captopril on autonomic reflexes in human hypertension. *J Hypertens* 1985; 3 (Suppl 2): S111–S115.

Sakaguchi K, Chai S-Y, Jackson B, et al. Differential angiotensin-converting enzyme inhibition in brain after oral administration of perindopril demonstrated by quantitative in vitro autoradiography. *Neuroendocrinology* 1988; 48: 223–228.

Shaper AG, Phillips AN, Pocock SJ, et al. Risk factors for stroke in middle-aged British men. *Br Med J* 1991; 302: 1111–1115.

Speth RC, Harik SI. Angiotensin-II receptor binding sites in brain microvessels. *Proc Natl Acad Sci* 1985; 82: 6340–6343.

Starr JM, Whalley LJ. *ACE Inhibitors: Central Actions.* Raven Press, New York, 1994, pp 1–254.

Steiner SS, Friedhoff AJ, Wilson BL, et al. Antihypertensive therapy and quality of life: a comparison of atenolol, captopril, enalapril and propranolol. *J Human Hypertens* 1990; 4: 217–225.

Strandgaard S. Autoregulation of cerebral blood flow in hypertensive patients. The modifying influence of prolonged antihypertensive treatment on the tolerance to acute, drug-induced hypotension. *Circulation* 1976; 53: 720–727.

Strandgaard S. Cerebral blood flow in the elderly: impact of hypertension and antihypertensive treatment. *Cardiovasc Drugs Ther* 1990; 4: 1217–1222.

Testa MA, Anderson RB, Nackley JF, Hollenberg NK and the Quality of Life Hypertension Study Group. Quality of life and antihypertensive therapy in men. A comparison of captopril with enalapril. *N Engl J Med* 1993; 328: 907–913.

Thiessen BQ, Wallace SM, Blackburn JL, et al. Increased prescribing of antidepressants subsequent to beta-blocker therapy. *Arch Intern Med* 1990; 150: 2286–2290.

Toda N, Miyazaki M. Angiotensin-induced relaxation in isolated dog renal and cerebral arteries. *Am J Physiol* 1981; 240: H247–H254.

Unger T, Rockhold RW, Kaufmann-Buhler I, et al. Effects of angiotensin converting enzyme inhibitors on the brain. In: Horovitz ZP (ed), *Angiotensin Converting Enzyme Inhibitors.* Urban and Schwarzenberg, Baltimore, 1981, 55–79.

Vidt DG, Bravo EL, Fonad FM. Captopril. *N Engl J Med* 1982; 306: 214–219.

Werner C, Hoffman WE, Kochs E, et al. Captopril improves neurologic outcome from incomplete cerebral ischemia in rats. *Stroke* 1991; 22: 910–914.

West JNW, Champion de Crespigny PC, et al. Effects of the angiotensin converting enzyme inhibitor, benazepril, on the sino-aortic baroreceptor heart rate reflex. *Cardiovasc Drugs Ther* 1991; 5: 747–752.

Zubenko GS, Nixon RA. Mood-elevating effect of captopril in depressed patients. *Am J Psychiatry* 1984; 141: 110–111.

CHAPTER 7

ACE Inhibitors: Specific Agents and Pharmacokinetics

"Trust all but verify everything" (Russian proverb, quoted by
Ronald Reagan to Mikhail Gorbachev)

CLASSIFICATION

Chemical classification

The best known classification is that based on the nature of
the ligand to the zinc ion of the enzyme (Table 7–1). The
three major groups are the sulfhydryl-containing inhibitors, such as captopril; the carboxyl-containing inhibitors,
such as enalapril; and the phosphoryl-containing inhibitors, such as fosinopril. Nonetheless, in current clinical
practice, there seems to be little direct relevance in group-
ings based on these chemical properties. It would seem
more natural to separate the drugs on their marked pharmacokinetic differences.

Pharmacokinetic classification

There are three types of ACE inhibitors from the pharmacokinetic point of view. The first class of compound is
captopril-like (Fig. 7–1), already in the active form, yet
undergoing further metabolism. Such metabolic conversion
produces disulfides with pharmacological activity. Both the
parent compound and the disulfides are eliminated by the
kidney. The second class of compounds are prodrugs (Fig.
7–2). For example, enalapril becomes active only on conversion to enalaprilat, which occurs chiefly in the liver. This
diacid form can then either be eliminated in the kidneys or
may be taken up into the tissues where it is thought inhibition of tissue ACE activity may occur. Examples of such
prodrugs include benazepril, cilazapril, perindopril, quinapril, and ramipril. In the case of very highly lipophilic
compounds, such as fosinopril, there is also biliary excretion following hepatic cellular uptake of the diacid. The
third class of compound is water-soluble and does not
undergo metabolism (Fig. 7–3). Lisinopril is the prototype.

TABLE 7–1 CHEMICAL CLASSIFICATION OF ACE INHIBITORS. COMPARATIVE DATA ON ACE ACTIVITY, LIPID SOLUBILITY, AND EXCRETORY PATTERNS OF ACTIVE FORMS

Agent	ACE activity IC_{50} nM		Molecular weight of parent compound	Lipid solubility	Excretion
	Rabbit lung	Human plasma			
Sulfhydryl-containing agents					
Captopril	23	22	217	+	K
Zofenoprilat	8	ND	325	+ + +	K,B
Nonsulfhydryl-containing agents					
Benazeprilat	2	1	424	+	K (B)
Cilazaprilat	2	1	389	?	
Delaprilat (OH)	40	ND	424	+ +	K (B)
Enalaprilat	1–5	3	348	+	K
Lisinopril	1	5	405	0	K

	Lung ACE	Human ACE	MW	log P	Excretion
Perindoprilat	2	2	340	++	K
Quinaprilat	3	6*	396	++	K (B)
Ramiprilat	4	2	388	++	K (B)
Spiraprilat	1	1	521	?	B (K)
Trandolaprilat	(2)**	2**	430	+++	B (K)
Phosphoryl-containing agent					
Fosinoprilat	11	ND	453	+++	K,B

*Kaplan et al. Angiology 1989; 40: 335. **Roussel Investigators Brochure; rat not rabbit lung.

Lung ACE data from Thind (1990). Human ACE data from MacFadyen et al (1991).

IC_{50} = active ACE inhibitor concentration required for 50% inhibition of rabbit lung or human plasma ACE.

Lipid solubility based on log P = logarithm of the octanol: water partition coefficient where + = values between 0.5 and 1.0; ++ = 1.1 to 2.0; and +++ = 2.1 or more.

For original data, see Thind (1990) and Duc and Brunner (1992). It is proposed that the higher the lipid solubility and molecular weight, the greater the biliary excretion.

K, kidney; B, biliary; ND, no data; Delaprilat = both delaprilat and hydroxy (OH) form

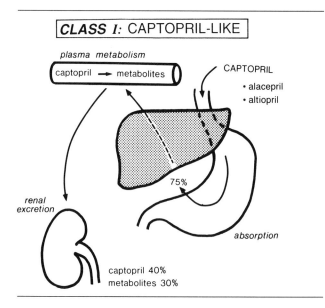

Figure 7–1. *Class I. Pharmacokinetic pattern of captopril-like drugs of which only captopril is generally available. Note conversion of captopril to metabolites and renal excretion. Fig. © LH Opie.*

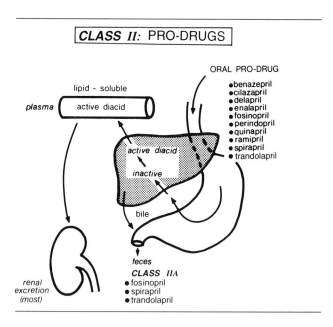

Figure 7–2. *Class II. Pharmacokinetic patterns of prodrugs that are converted to active diacids and then excreted. The predominant pattern for most is renal excretion but in Class IIA drugs, especially fosinopril, biliary and fecal excretion may be as important. Fig. © LH Opie.*

Such compounds do not need any further metabolic conversion to be activated. They circulate unbound to plasma protein and undergo renal elimination in the unchanged form. The only determinants of the plasma levels are, therefore, the oral dose, the rate of absorption, and the rate of renal excretion.

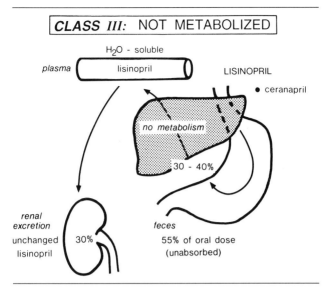

Figure 7–3. Class III. Pharmacokinetic patterns of lisinopril-like drugs that are water-soluble. At present the only compound clinically available is lisinopril. It undergoes no metabolism and is excreted unchanged in the urine. There is no plasma protein binding. That portion of the dose not absorbed is excreted in the feces. Fig. © LH Opie.

It is this pharmacokinetic classification here presented for the first time that will be followed in this chapter.

ALACEPRIL

Although alacepril is strictly a prodrug, it has a unique feature in that its active metabolite is captopril. Thus, it is in effect a long-acting captopril preparation.

Pharmacokinetics

Absorption and metabolism. There is relatively rapid absorption and metabolism so that the peak value of free captopril is reached in 2.5 hours and of total captopril in 3 hours. Total captopril includes mixed disulfides.

Plasma levels. The maximum concentration of free captopril is about 30 ng/ml after a single dose and about 40 ng/ml after consecutive doses. Corresponding values for total captopril are 150 and 190 ng/ml.

Plasma protein binding. This is similar to captopril (30%).

Elimination, distribution and clearance. The area under the curve is about 200 to 400 ng.h/ml for free captopril and about 1700 to 1800 ng.h/ml for total captopril. Elimination half-life for total captopril is about 8 hours. Most of the free captopril is eliminated in the urine within 8 to 10 hours, while the elimination of total captopril first has a fast phase up to about 8 to 10 hours, and then a slow phase up to 24 hours when about 40% of the dose has been eliminated in that form (Shionoiri et al., 1985a).

Pharmacodynamics

In *hypertensive* patients, a single dose of 12.5 mg reduces blood pressure maximally for 2 to 8 hours and then less for the remaining 24 hour period when the dose is given twice daily (Shionoiri et al., 1985a). Plasma ACE inhibition is significantly reduced at 4 to 8 hours after dosage.

Dose and concurrent disease

In *hypertension,* the dose varies from 6.25 mg to 25 mg twice daily with an average dose of 12.5 mg twice daily (Shionoiri et al., 1985a).

In the *elderly,* in those with *renal failure,* and in those with *hepatic failure,* similar precautions should be taken as for captopril.

ALTIOPRIL (MOVELTIPRIL)

Altiopril (moveltipril) contains the captopril structure. It is a prodrug and is converted to captopril or to a similar sulfhydryl-containing compound (Salvetti, 1990). In animals, its hypotensive effect is about twice as long as that of captopril.

BENAZEPRIL

Benazepril, a prodrug, is converted to benazeprilat chiefly by hepatic metabolism and gives a high degree of inhibition of tissue ACE activity (Johnston et al., 1988).

Pharmacokinetics

After oral administration, the active metabolite benazeprilat starts to appear in the blood within 30 minutes and reaches peak values after 1 hour. The plasma half-life is approximately 11 hours with a terminal half-life of 21 to 22 hours. Conversion of benazepril to benazeprilat occurs in the liver. Both compounds are then excreted by the kidneys. Plasma protein binding is 95–97%.

Pharmacodynamics

Plasma converting enzyme activity is very substantially inhibited within 1 hour of administration of benazepril 2 to 20 mg or more. Nearly complete and prolonged (up to 24 hours) inhibition is obtained with all doses above 5 mg (Schaller et al., 1985). Tissue ACE inhibition may be an important pharmacodynamic site of action of ACE inhibitors. According to Johnston et al. (1988), benazeprilat is about as effective in the inhibition of plasma ACE activity as most other prodrugs, and there is also a substantial degree of inhibition of renal ACE activity (over 60%). Benazeprilat is claimed to prevent left ventricular dilation following coronary artery occlusion in the rat (Smith et al., 1988).

Dose and concurrent disease

In *hypertension,* the dose can vary from an initial response at 5 mg to maximal response at 80 mg given once daily. In the majority of studies 20 mg has been chosen (Whalen, 1989), as also justified by peak-trough relationships (Lees, 1992). In a double-blind crossover study, benazepril given as 10 mg twice daily had a better antihypertensive effect than 20 mg once daily, plasma renin increased more while plasma ACE activity decreased more (Guyene et al., 1989).

In *heart failure,* a mean dose of 12 mg daily improved exercise tolerance and decreased mortality over 12 weeks (Colfer et al., 1992).

In *elderly subjects* (MacDonald et al., 1988), the area under the curve increased by 38% compared with young subjects, the dose being 10 mg daily. There were no significant differences between young and elderly for peak concentrations. Only a slight dose reduction appears appropriate in the elderly.

In *black patients,* benazepril 10 mg twice daily reduced blood pressure adequately in 44%, which rose to 72% when combined with nifedipine 20 mg twice daily (Loock et al., 1990).

In *renal disease,* the glomerular filtration rate has to drop below 30 ml/min before the dose of benazepril needs reduction (Kaiser et al., 1989). Even in very severe renal disease there is some nonrenal mechanism of clearance (Kaiser et al., 1989), possibly by biliary excretion.

In patients with *cirrhosis* of the liver, no dose alteration is required (Kaiser et al., 1989).

Side-effects

The agent appears well tolerated. There is no evidence for an incidence of side-effects any different from that of other ACE inhibitors.

Combination therapy and drug interactions

When combined with furosemide the plasma concentrations of benazepril and benazeprilat are unchanged but that of furosemide falls by about one-third (DeLepeleire et al., 1988). When combined with the calcium antagonist nicardipine, the concomitant tachycardia induced by nicardipine is reduced (Bellet et al., 1987), suggesting that benazepril was able to minimize reflex sympathetic stimulation induced by the calcium antagonists.

CAPTOPRIL

Captopril, the first of the ACE inhibitors and still the "gold standard," was originally thought to be a drug with a high incidence of adverse side-effects. Particularly feared were serious complications, such as neutropenia and renal impairment. Today, paradoxically, the drug is being promoted for absence of side-effects and for a good "quality of life." This major difference has come about because it is now known that many adverse side-effects were related to excess captopril doses in the initial studies. However, in addition, the presence of the SH-group was originally thought to be harmful and specifically to cause side-effects such as skin rashes, neutropenia, and loss of taste (ageusia). Now with the lower doses currently used, these side-effects seem rare. Furthermore, consideration is being given to the possibility that the SH-groups of captopril may act to scavenge free radicals, the formation of which is thought to be an adverse side-effect of postischemic reperfusion. Furthermore, the SH-group may specifically account for the benefit of captopril therapy in rheumatoid arthritis. Nonetheless, for practical purposes there is little or no clinical proof that captopril has a greater therapeutic range than other drugs not containing SH-groups.

Pharmacokinetics

Absorption. Absolute absorption for captopril is about 70% and absolute bioavailability is about 60% (Duchin et al., 1982). Absorption is rapid, and blood levels are detected within 15 minutes (Kripalani et al., 1980). Despite the delay in absorption when captopril is taken together with food, from the practical point of view food does not influence the kinetics or pharmacodynamics (Salvetti et al., 1985). *Sublingual captopril* has been used in patients with severe hypertension. However, the availability of the sublingual form is only marginally better than the oral form when judged by the peak effects on blood pressure and peripheral hemodynamics (Longhini et al., 1990).

Metabolism. Captopril is partially metabolized, apparently in liver and in blood, to the disulfide and to polar metabolites.

Plasma levels. In plasma, captopril is partially free, partially bound covalently to plasma proteins, and partially in the form of mixed disulfides with endogenous thiols, such as cysteine and glutathione (Ohman et al., 1985). One proposal is that the bound forms of captopril form a reservoir to replenish free captopril as it distributes to tissues. Total captopril levels are higher and stay elevated for much longer than those of free captopril. Hence kinetic parameters depend on the form of captopril measured (Table 7–2). Noteworthy is the much longer half-life of total captopril than of free captopril. There is also evidence that during chronic administration captopril blood levels are higher and the area under the curve greater (Jarrott et al., 1982).

Plasma protein binding. This is about 30% (Laragh, 1990).

Elimination, distribution, and clearance. About two-thirds of an oral single 100 mg dose is excreted within 4 hours in the urine either unchanged or converted to polar metabolites (Kripalani et al., 1980). Within 24 hours 95% of the oral dose is excreted either unchanged or as metabolites. In volunteers, the elimination half-life of the terminal phase is less than 2 hours (Duchin et al., 1982). The volume of distribution in volunteers is 0.7 L/kg for the steady state (Duchin et al., 1982).

Pharmacodynamics

Captopril is already in the active form and does not require metabolic conversion (see Fig. 7–1). The onset of the blood pressure lowering effect is within 15 minutes with a peak effect at 1 to 2 hours and a total duration of effect of 6 to 10 hours. Serum ACE activity falls to about 40% of control values for 1 to 3 hours after a single dose of 12.5 mg captopril, and large doses will have a more significant effect (Shionoiri et al., 1986a).

Dose and concurrent disease

There have been numerous studies with captopril in patients with *hypertension*, the majority of early studies using what would now be regarded as excessively high doses, such as 50 to 100 mg three times daily. Today, a standard dose would be 25 mg twice daily, as confirmed by ambulatory intraarterial blood pressure measurements in patients with essential hypertension (Shionoiri et al., 1987a). With a sufficiently high dose of captopril (100 mg) in patients on dietary salt restriction, a single daily dose is effective, although it does not reduce blood pressure to normotensive levels (Reyes et al., 1985).

In *congestive heart failure*, captopril kinetics are virtually unchanged (Cody et al., 1982). Concentrations of free captopril rise and fall rapidly as in normals, but plasma renin activity stays elevated much longer suggesting that it is the total and not the free captopril level that is more relevant from the pharmacological point of view. Optimal hemodynamic responses may require plasma levels of free captopril of the order of 100 to 120 ng/ml (Rademaker et al., 1986). In a clinical dose-ranging study where the maximum permitted dose was 75 mg daily, the mean effective captopril dose was 53 mg (Schofield et al., 1991). However, in another study, higher doses were permitted, and the usual mean daily dose was close to 100 mg (Powers et al., 1987). Doses lower than 75 mg daily (25 mg three times daily) may be associated with inadequate control of heart failure and a greater than expected mortality (Pouleur et al., 1991).

In *acute myocardial infarction*, oral captopril added to fibrinolysis by streptokinase and antiplatelet therapy decreased mortality by a nonsignificant 0.46% at the cost of increased hypotension in the massive ISIS-IV study (see Table 11–3).

In *postinfarct* patients with asymptomatic left ventricular dysfunction, captopril 25 mg three times daily was more effective than furosemide 40 mg daily in preventing an increase in left ventricular volume (Sharpe et al., 1988). In the very large-scale SAVE trial, captopril (usual dose 50 mg three times daily) decreased mortality and the development of severe heart failure in postinfarct patients with left ventricular dysfunction as shown by left ventricular ejection fraction values of 40% or less (see Table 5–6). In the United

TABLE 7–2 SOME PHARMACOKINETIC PROPERTIES OF CAPTOPRIL

Author	Captopril dose	Subjects	Conc max ng/ml	Tmax h	Elim T1/2 h	AUC ng.h/ml
Kripalani et al. (1980)	100 mg	Normal	Free 800	1.0	1.7	1150
			Total 1580	No data	4	7160
Creasey et al. (1986)	100 mg	Healthy elderly	Free 803	1.0	1.4	1390
			Total 3350	1.4	—	17320
Ohman et al. (1985)	25 mg	Essential hypt, diuretic treated	Total 400–650	1–2	6.2 3.4*	—

				T_{max}	Elim $T_{1/2}$	AUC
Shionoiri et al. (1986a)	25 mg	Essential hypt	Free 120	1.5	1.2	275
Richer et al. (1984)	1 mg/kg orally	Hypertension	Free 1310	1.0	0.7	—
Cody et al. (1982)	25 mg	Severe CHF	Free 122–142	0.9–1.4	1–1.4	250
			Total 510–840	1.2–1.7	>4	2350–4000
Onoyama et al. (1981)	50 mg	Chronic renal failure	Free 430	0.9	Prolonged from 0.4 to 0.7	793

Conc, concentration; T_{max}, time for maximal concentration; Elim $T_{1/2}$, elimination (terminal) half-life; AUC, area under the curve; Hypt, hypertension; CHF, congestive heart failure

*Non-protein bound

States and in several European countries, captopril is now licensed for postinfarct left ventricular dysfunction.

In *renal failure,* the captopril dose may need reduction by half or more (Sica, 1992) not only because of the decreased urinary excretion of the compound and its metabolites (Onoyama et al., 1981) but also because of the inherently greater risk of neutropenia in patients with collagen vascular disease. During *dialysis,* captopril is still eliminated (Sica, 1992).

In *hepatic failure,* no change in dose is required.

In *elderly patients,* no change in dose is required unless there is decreased renal function.

The *pediatric dose* is 0.3 to 1.3 mg/kg every 8 hours (Lewis and Chabot, 1993).

In *black subjects,* captopril is not recommended as monotherapy for hypertension but works well in combination with a diuretic (Veterans Administration Co-operative Study Group on Antihypertensive Agents, 1982).

In *diabetic patients,* there is no adverse effect on glucose metabolism (Shionoiri et al., 1987b).

Combination therapy and drug interactions

As in the case of all ACE inhibitors, there is an additive therapeutic effect with diuretics, and low-dose initial treatment is required in such circumstances. Potassium-retaining diuretics or potassium supplements should be used with caution, particularly in the presence of renal failure. NSAIDs, such as indomethacin, may reduce the antihypertensive effect of captopril especially in cases of low-renin hypertension. Even aspirin may have this effect. Increased serum lithium levels and even lithium toxicity have been reported in patients receiving lithium and ACE inhibitor therapy together. *Concomitant beta-blockade,* although thought not to have a full additive antihypertensive effect according to the package insert, is often used without proof of full efficacy.

CERANAPRIL

Ceranapril is a phosphinic acid, like fosinopril, but not a prodrug and active as the free acid in the absence of esterification. It has some properties resembling lisinopril. It is excreted by the kidneys in unchanged form. This compound may have a unique effect on brain ACE activity (Cushman et al., 1989). At present, it is in the very early stages of testing in humans.

CILAZAPRIL

Cilazapril is a prodrug, being converted to its active form, cilazaprilat, which has a long terminal half-life with a longer duration of action than enalapril (Natoff et al., 1985; Deget and Brogden, 1991).

Pharmacokinetics

Absorption. The drug is rapidly absorbed with peak plasma levels of cilazapril reached within 1 to 2 hours (Shionoiri et al., 1988).

Metabolism. Cilazapril is rapidly metabolized by deester-ification to its active form, cilazaprilat, mainly in the liver and blood.

Plasma levels. The peak plasma concentration of cilazapril is about 120 ng/ml after a single dose and about 145 ng/ml after consecutive doses; the respective values for cilazaprilat are about 25 and 30 ng/ml (Shionoiri et al., 1988).

Plasma protein binding. Not known (Deget and Brogden, 1991).

Elimination, distribution, and clearance. Both cilazapril and cilazaprilat are found in the urine following dosage of the compound to patients. Cilazaprilat is eliminated almost entirely by the kidneys, possibly in part by active tubular secretion (Deget and Brogden, 1991). Almost all the cilazapril has been excreted by 6 to 8 hours, whereas there is progressive excretion of cilazaprilat in two phases, first an early phase and then a later phase from approximately 8 to 24 hours of much slower excretion (Louis et al., 1992a). The calculated terminal half-lives vary greatly (Francis et al., 1987; Shionoiri et al., 1988). Much depends on the exact elimination phases under consideration and the techniques used. Despite the prolonged terminal phase, there is no accumulation of cilazaprilat with repeated administration (Nussberger et al., 1987).

Pharmacodynamics

Following a single dose of cilazapril, peak inhibition of serum ACE activity is reached at 2 hours (90% or more), levels stayed down for 8 hours, then 24 hours after the initial dose there was only about 30% inhibition (Fasanella d'Amore et al., 1987). The percentage inhibition and drop of blood pressure is very closely related to the plasma levels of cilazaprilat (Shionoiri et al., 1988; Louis et al., 1992a). When the blood pressure of volunteers was increased by an intravenous infusion of angiotensin-I, then the effects of cilazapril declined with an elimination half-life of about 4 hours, very similar to enalapril (Wellstein et al., 1987).

Dose and concurrent disease

In *hypertension*, the initial dose is 1.25 mg (Deget and Brogden, 1991) which suppresses systolic pressure at 24 hours and during consecutive dosing suppresses both systolic and diastolic pressures at 24 hours (Shionoiri et al., 1988). A dose of 2.5 mg/day is the antihypertensive equivalent of propranolol 120 mg/day (Kleinbloesem et al., 1989). Doses of 2.5 to 5.0 mg/day reduced blood pressure over 24 hours when compared with concurrent placebo therapy, tested over a period of 8 weeks (Guntzel et al., 1991). Doses above 5 mg appear to achieve no greater benefit (Lees, 1992).

In *congestive heart failure,* the initial dose is 0.5 mg (Deget and Brogden, 1991) and about two-thirds of patients require 5 mg during sustained therapy (Drexler et al., 1989).

Renal failure. As the renal function and creatinine clearance falls, the area under the curve (AUC) for cilazaprilat increases (Shionoiri et al., 1988), especially with repeated doses (Table 7–3). If the average dose for hypertension is 2.5 mg, then, in patients with severe renal failure, only half that dose, i.e., 1.25 mg, inhibits serum ACE activity by nearly 70% 24 hours after the initial dose (Shionoiri et al., 1988). During *dialysis,* elimination of cilazapril and cilazaprilat is very low, so that a dose of 0.5 mg cilazapril after alternate hemodialysis sessions is recommended (Deget and Brogden, 1991).

Hepatic failure. Plasma clearance of cilazapril and cilazaprilat is reduced in hepatic cirrhosis, so that the dose may need reduction (Deget and Brogden, 1991).

Impaired glucose tolerance. Cilazapril causes no significant changes in the insulinogenic index in patients with normal or impaired glucose tolerance (Shionoiri et al., 1990a).

Elderly patients. The initial dose for hypertension is 1.25 mg daily.

Combination therapy and drug interactions

As for other ACE inhibitors, there should be caution when combining with potassium-retaining diuretics or potassium supplements (risk of hyperkalemia especially in renal failure). The dose should be reduced during concurrent diuretic therapy. Indomethacin impairs the antihypertensive effect (Deget and Brogden, 1991). There are no other known adverse drug interactions.

Combination therapy with beta-blockade. Although the benefits of this combination are controversial, as in the case of many other ACE inhibitors, added beta-blockade does, in fact, give additive blood pressure lowering in the case of cilazapril (Belz et al., 1989). The percentage response (diastolic blood pressure below 90 mmHg) in hypertensive patients rises from <50% with either cilazapril or propranolol alone, to about 75–80% with the drug combination (Belz et al., 1989). The doses used in that study were cilazapril 2.5 mg once daily and propranolol 120 mg once daily. Blood pressure measurements were made at about the peak of drug action about 2 hours after ingestion, and there is no guarantee that the combination gave better reductions over 24 hours.

TABLE 7–3 CILAZAPRIL. SOME PHARMACOKINETIC PROPERTIES OF CILAZAPRILAT

Author	Cilazapril dose	Subjects	Conc max ng/ml	Tmax h	Elim T1/2 h	AUC* ng.h/ml
Francis et al. (1987)	2.5 mg	Volunteers	36	2.1	37	170
	10 mg		165	—	86	550
Shionoiri et al., (1988)	1.25 mg	Hypertension	25	3.2	8.4	227
	1.25 mg repeated	Hypertension	31	3.2	7.5	305
	1.25 mg repeated	Hypertension with CRF	117	4.3	8.2	1541
Louis et al. (1992)	2.5 mg	Hypertension	—	3.0	40	—

For abbreviations, see Table 7–2. CRF, chronic renal failure. *0–24 hours

DELAPRIL

Delapril is a prodrug with *two* active metabolites, the first being the diacid derivative, which can then form, the 5-hydroxy delapril diacid.

Pharmacokinetics

Absorption and metabolism. After oral administration of delapril, peak concentrations of delapril and delaprilat are reached within 1 hour, and of the metabolite 5-hydroxy delaprilat within 2 hours (Shionoiri et al., 1987c). Delapril is an ester-type prodrug with an indane ring instead of the proline ring in enalapril. The conversion to metabolites presumably occurs in liver and blood. After a single dose of 15 mg of delapril, peak plasma concentrations (ng/ml) are about 120 for delapril, 375 to 390 for delaprilat, and 170 to 190 for 5-hydroxy delaprilat, and these concentrations are reached at about 1 to 2 hours (Minamisawa et al., 1990).

Plasma protein binding. Not known.

Elimination, distribution and clearance. The elimination half-lives following single doses are 0.3 hours for delapril, 1.2 hours for delaprilat, and 1.4 hours for 5-hydroxy delaprilat (Shionoiri et al., 1987c) with, however, the latter value rising to 6.2 hours during consecutive dosing (Minamisawa et al., 1990). Elimination is largely renal because the area under the curve increases in renal failure (Minamisawa et al., 1990).

Pharmacodynamics

After a single dose the blood pressure falls significantly in hypertensive patients for 12 hours (Shionoiri et al., 1987c, 1987d). Plasma ACE activity is significantly reduced for 24 hours, while plasma renin activity rises for 24 hours with the peak occurring between 1 and 8 hours (Shionoiri et al., 1987c).

Dose and concurrent disease

In *hypertension,* a single dose of 15 mg lowers the blood pressure for 1 to 8 hours and, just as significantly, up to 24 hours (Shionoiri et al., 1987d). Similar patterns are found during prolonged dosing with 15 mg twice daily. In another study with a single 15 mg dose of delapril, 24 hour blood pressure reduction was not found (Minamisawa et al., 1990), although it became evident with repeated doses.

In *renal failure,* the excretion of delapril and its metabolites is impaired, and the drop is proportional to the fall in creatinine clearance (Minamisawa et al., 1990). The peak values of metabolites and their area under the curve (AUC) values are higher (Shionoiri et al., 1987c). A dose of 15 mg twice daily in patients with mean creatinine clearance values of 37 nl/min/1.73m^2 led to increased values for the maximal concentration reached in the plasma (Cmax) and the area under the curve (Table 7–4). Therefore, dose reduction is required in renal failure.

TABLE 7-4 DELAPRIL. SOME PHARMACOKINETIC PROPERTIES OF DELAPRILAT (DT) AND 5-HYDROXY-DELAPRILAT (5-OH-D)

Author	Delapril dose	Subjects	Metabolite	Conc max ng/ml	Tmax h	Elim T1/2 h	AUC ng.h/ml
Shionoiri et al. (1987a, 1987b)	Single dose 30 mg	EHT	DT 50HD	635 229	1.2 1.9	1.2 1.4	1859 948
		CRF	DT 50HD	797 435	1.4 2.5	4.7 12.9	6400 5068
Minamisawa et al. (1990)	Single dose 15 mg	EHT	DT 50HD	377 170	1.2 2.6	1.2 1.8	918 477
		CRF	DT 50HD	477 281	1.0 1.5	2.3 3.2	2111 1836
	15 mg daily 7 days	CRF	DT 50HD	493 378	1.2 1.6	3.2 22.7	2259 3648

For abbreviations, see Table 7–2.
EHT, essential hypertension; CRF, chronic renal failure; DT, deliprilat = delapril diacid; 50HD, 5-hydroxy delapril

In *elderly patients*, analogy with other prodrugs suggests that no dose reduction is required unless there is an associated decrease in renal function.

ENALAPRIL

This compound was the first of the prodrug ACE inhibitors clinically available. Like the others, it is a prodrug that only becomes active after conversion to the active diacid form by metabolism. Enalaprilat, the resulting active compound, is excreted by the kidneys and has a considerably longer half-life than the parent (Table 7–5). Thus the onset of action is delayed when compared with captopril, but these compounds are correspondingly longer acting. Like most other prodrugs, enalapril is nonsulfhydryl containing. Enalapril is the most widely tested drug in all degrees of heart failure, having been used in trials involving about 4,000 patients (Tables 5–6 and 5–7).

Pharmacokinetics

Absorption. Absorption is rapid with peak concentrations of unchanged enalapril reached at about 1 hour and peak serum concentrations of enalaprilat reached after 3 to 4 hours. About 40% of oral enalapril becomes available as enalaprilat. Absorption is not altered by food (Todd and Heel, 1986), however, enalapril-induced vasodilation may be enhanced by meals (Herrlin et al., 1990). The chief site of metabolism, which occurs by deesterification, is in the liver.

Plasma levels. Following a single 20 mg dose, the peak plasma concentration of enalaprilat is about 70 ng/ml at 2 to 4 hours after administration, dropping to about 20 ng/ml at 12 hours (Davies et al., 1984). Values exceeding 10 ng/ml are required for adequate inhibition of plasma ACE activity in volunteers (Biollaz et al., 1982). The maximum concentration of enalaprilat is linearly related to the enalapril dose, but the area under the curve (AUC) is only closely related when the prolonged terminal phase is omitted in the calculation.

Plasma protein binding. Less than 50% is bound to human protein with two binding sites, one with high affinity and low capacity, which may represent the binding of enalaprilat to circulating ACE. It is thought that such binding accounts for the prolonged terminal phase of the plasma concentration profile.

Elimination, distribution, and clearance. The accumulation half-life is approximately 11 hours as calculated from urine data (Till et al., 1984), whereas the elimination half-life is approximately 6 hours as measured from plasma concentrations (Shionoiri et al., 1985b). A very long terminal phase with a half-life of approximately 30 to 35 hours probably represents about 1 mg of enalaprilat bound to circulating serum ACE (Abrams et al., 1984). Elimination is chiefly renal by glomerular filtration. However, 27% of an oral

TABLE 7–5 ENALAPRIL. SOME PHARMACOKINETIC PROPERTIES OF ENALAPRILAT

Author	Enalapril dose	Subjects	Conc max ng/ml	Tmax h	Elim T1/2	AuUC ng.h/ml
Till et al. (1984)	10 mg orally	Normal volunteers	34	—	11*	—
Shionoiri et al. (1985b; 1985c)	10 mg	Hypertension	35	4	6	452
	10 mg	Hypertension	32	4	8	414
		Chronic RF	110	9	11	1708
Schwartz et al. (1985)	20 mg	Hypertension	about 60	5	—	865
	40 mg	Hypertension	about 80	5.5	2	1615
	5 mg	CHF	about 22	5	3.5	265
	10 mg	CHF	—	4.5	6	420

For abbreviations, see Table 7–2.

CHF, congestive heart failure; RF, renal failure; *From urine data.

Note other reports of terminal half-life of 30–35 hours (Todd and Heel, 1986; Louis et al., 1992).

dose of enalapril can be recovered as fecal enalaprilat (Ulm et al., 1982), presumably the result of biliary excretion.

Pharmacodynamics

After a single 10 mg dose of enalapril given to patients with essential hypertension (Johnston et al., 1983), the peak enalaprilat concentration is reached between 2 and 8 hours at the same time that serum ACE activity is maximally depressed and the blood pressure falls most. Following the 10 mg dose, serum enalaprilat has reverted to normal at 24 hours (Davies et al., 1984) and the blood pressure decrease is very much less than at 8 hours (Gavras et al., 1981). To obtain truly prolonged antihypertensive effect in humans requires a 20 mg dose (Gavras et al., 1981).

Dose and concurrent disease

In *hypertension,* there is a dose-response relationship across the range of 2.5 to 40 mg once daily (Bergstrand et al., 1985). The latter dose also gives the best peak-trough relationship (Lees, 1992). A mean single daily dose of 31 mg reduced blood pressure over 24 hours as shown by ambulatory blood pressure monitoring in 28 patients with hypertension and left ventricular hypertrophy (Gosse et al., 1990). In the Italian Multicenter Study, 40 mg of enalapril given once daily was somewhat more effective than 10 mg given once daily in reducing the blood pressure measured 24 hours after the last dose (Salvetti and Arzilli, 1989). Despite such evidence for once daily dosing, enalapril 10 mg twice daily gives even better overall control than does 20 mg once daily (Meredith et al., 1990).

In *congestive heart failure,* the standard protocol dose has been 10 mg twice daily with mean doses of 16.7 mg in SOLVD-II, 18.4 mg in CONSENSUS-I, and 16.6 mg in SOLVD-I (see Tables 5–6 and 5–7). The initial test dose is 2.5 mg (Hasford et al., 1991) which can, however, still cause significant prolonged hypotension (see Fig. 8–2). Single daily doses of enalapril 5 mg have beneficial hemodynamic effects over 3 months (Brilla et al., 1989), and the acute hemodynamic effects of 5 mg and 10 mg in patients with congestive heart failure are similar (DiCarlo et al., 1983). Sharpe et al. (1984) showed multiple hemodynamic benefits and improved exercise time in patients treated by enalapril 5 mg twice daily for 3 months. Logically, the dose could be geared to the severity of heart failure.

In *acute myocardial infarction,* a study with early intravenous enalaprilat was terminated because of an adverse effect of drug-induced hypotension (Swedberg et al., 1992).

In the *elderly,* the area under the curve (AUC) is increased and the systemic clearance is reduced in proportion to the fall in creatinine clearance (Hockings et al., 1985). Thus, in elderly patients with normal renal function, enalapril in standard doses is an effective antihypertensive agent (Arr et al., 1985).

In *black subjects,* ACE inhibitors are not recommended as monotherapy for hypertension but work well in combination with a diuretic (Freier et al., 1984).

In *chronic renal failure,* the plasma concentrations of enalaprilat are very much higher, the area under the curve is very much greater, and the plasma half-life is prolonged (Shionoiri et al., 1985c). The dose should be reduced by half when the creatinine clearance falls below 30 ml/min (Sica, 1992).

In *hepatic failure,* the appearance of enalaprilat in the plasma is reduced (Johnston et al., 1984) so that, if anything, the dose should be increased. In general, however, prodrug compounds are given in unchanged dose to patients with hepatic cirrhosis.

Combination therapy and drug interactions

These are the same as for all the other ACE inhibitors. Note the increased efficacy when given with diuretics, the capacity to combine with calcium antagonists in the therapy of hypertension, the risk of hyperkalemia with potassium-retaining diuretics or with potassium supplements, and attenuation of the antihypertensive effect by NSAIDs, such as indomethacin.

FOSINOPRIL

Fosinopril is a long-acting prodrug with the active form being the diacid (fosinoprilat). Chemically, this compound differs from other ACE inhibitors chiefly in that it is a phosphinic acid (DeForrest et al., 1990). It belongs to Class II (see Fig. 7–2). It is long-acting, highly protein bound, and has dual routes of excretion, hepatic and renal (Singhvi et al., 1988). The latter, an unusual pharmacokinetic feature, separates it off into Class IIA. The result is that in chronic renal failure, the active fosinoprilat form accumulates less in the blood than does enalaprilat or lisinopril (Sica et al., 1991). The reason is that the hepatic excretion of fosinoprilat increases as the renal elimination lessens (Hui et al., 1991).

Pharmacokinetics

Absorption, metabolism, and elimination. About one-third is absorbed after an oral dose and metabolized in the liver and gut wall almost completely to the active diacid, fosinoprilat (Hui et al., 1991). Fosinoprilat is excreted almost equally in urine and in the bile, hence appearing in the feces.

Plasma levels, half-life, and area under the curve. Following a single oral dose of 20 mg, the plasma level at about 24 hours is 250 ng/ml (Table 7–6) of which about 75% or more is bound to plasma proteins (Sica, 1992). The plasma terminal half-life is about 12 to 14 hours (Table 7–6). The area under the curve is not increased in renal failure because of the dual renal and fecal elimination routes.

Pharmacodynamics

Inhibition of serum ACE in humans is complete for 24 hours after a single dose of 80 mg fosinopril, and after 20

TABLE 7-6 FOSINOPRIL. SOME PHARMACOKINETIC PROPERTIES OF FOSINOPRILAT

Author	Fosinopril dose	Subjects	Conc max ng/ml	Tmax h	Elim T1/2 h	AUC ng,h/ml
Duchin et al. (1991)	20 mg	Young healthy	251	2.4	—	2000
Hui et al. (1991)	7.5 mg IV	Normal	—	—	12.4	4971
Hui et al. (1991)	10 mg	Renal failure				
		Mean CCl 60	165	4.0	14.0	2135
		Mean CCl 32	136	4.0	14.1	2052
		Mean CCl 16	127	4.2	16.9	2405

For abbreviations, see Table 7–2.

IV, intravenous, CCl, creatinine clearance, ml/min.

mg the ACE activity returns slightly to 20% of baseline at 24 hours (Duchin et al., 1991). A single dose of 10 mg reduced blood pressure at 3 hours with a fall in peripheral vascular resistance and a rise in plasma norepinephrine and renin, together with a decreased aldosterone level (Oren et al., 1991). After 12 weeks of administration, the fall in blood pressure was less marked, and plasma epinephrine did not rise. Left ventricular mass fell by 11%.

Dose and concurrent disease

In *hypertension,* the proposed dose is 10 to 40 mg once daily in hypertension, with 20 mg being the usual maintenance dose. In a large clinical trial with concurrent placebo controls, 40 to 80 mg was effective when compared with placebo in mild hypertension (Anderson et al., 1991). A fosinopril dose of 10 mg was less effective, and the dose of 20 mg was not tested (see Figs. 2–3 and 2–4). The optimal response required diuretic addition in about half the patients. In combination with a diuretic, doses of 5, 10 and 20 mg all reduced the blood pressure more than diuretic monotherapy (manufacturer's information). In another study on 418 patients, daily doses of 5, 10, 20 and 40 mg fosinopril were compared with concurrent placebo (Pool, 1990). Fosinopril 20 mg daily gave the best decrease in sitting blood pressure, whereas, for the standing blood pressure, 20 mg and 40 mg doses were about equi-effective. A dose of 5 mg fosinopril was significantly different from placebo.

In *congestive heart failure,* there appear to be no studies and the drug is not licensed for this indication in the United States.

In the *elderly,* the major reason for decreasing doses of other ACE inhibitors is renal impairment. In the case of fosinopril, no dosage adjustment is required.

In *black subjects,* no specific studies have been reported. As for other ACE inhibitors, decreased efficacy may be expected (see Chapter 2).

In *renal failure,* no dosage adjustments are required because the plasma area under the curve remains the same (Table 7–6). During *dialysis* the clearance of fosinoprilat is minimal because of the high degree of binding to the plasma proteins (Sica, 1992).

In *hepatic failure,* the plasma area under the curve approximately doubles (U.S. package insert), so that the dose should be halved.

Comparative studies

In a small study, captopril, lisinopril, and fosinopril all reduced the blood pressure at mean doses of 113 mg, 47 mg, and 52 mg daily, respectively (Zusman, 1992). Only fosinopril increased stroke volume, cardiac output, and filling parameters. The explanations could be (1) a lower systemic vascular resistance with a greater reflex adrenergic stimulation after fosinopril or (2) a greater uptake of fosinoprilat into the myocardium, as favored by the author.

Drug combinations and interactions

These are similar to those of other ACE inhibitors. In addition, co-administration of antacids may impair absorption of fosinopril (U.S. package insert).

LISINOPRIL

Lisinopril is thus far the only clinically available representative of the type III class of nonmetabolized and water-soluble ACE inhibitors (see Fig. 7–3). Thus, its salient pharmacokinetic features are that it has very low lipid solubility, does not undergo metabolism, and is largely excreted as such in the urine.

Pharmacokinetics

Absorption. This is slower than with other ACE inhibitors reaching peak plasma concentrations about 6 hours after administration of 10 to 20 mg (Lancaster and Todd, 1988). About 30% to 50% of lisinopril becomes systemically available. Food appears not to influence the bioavailability.

Metabolism. Because the urinary recovery of an intravenous dose is essentially complete, it can be assumed that lisinopril does not undergo metabolism, in keeping with its very low lipophilicity.

Plasma levels. After a single oral dose of 10 mg the serum lisinopril concentration is about 40 ng/ml in hypertensive patients with normal renal function (Table 7–7) in whom the maximum concentration was reached 6 hours after dosage (Shionoiri et al., 1990b).

Plasma protein binding. The drug is not at all bound to plasma proteins, being entirely water soluble (Gomez et al., 1987).

Elimination, distribution, and clearance. Elimination of the absorbed dose is by the kidneys without metabolism. Most of the drug is eliminated in the early phase with, however, a delayed terminal phase that is thought to represent binding to the angiotensin-converting enzyme (Lancaster and Todd, 1988). The terminal half-life is 6.8 hours (Shionoiri et al., 1990b), although longer half-lives are often reported such as 12 hours (Thind, 1990).

Pharmacodynamics

After a single 10 mg dose, the inhibition of plasma ACE activity exceeds 80% at 4 hours, stays even higher until 5 hours, and then gradually declines to 20% at 24 hours (Millar et al., 1982). In hypertensive patients, such a single dose reduces the blood pressure most over the 4 to 10 hours after the dose. With consecutive dosing, the 24 hours blood pressure reduction is also significant although marginal when allowing for the more complex statistics required for multiple comparisons (Shionoiri et al., 1990b). In patients with

TABLE 7–7 LISINOPRIL. SOME PHARMACOKINETIC DATA

Author	Lisinopril dose	Subjects	Conc max ng/ml	Tmax h	Elim T1/2 h	AUC ng.h/ml
Cirillo et al, (1986)	20 mg	Young healthy	78	ND	ND	1380
		Elderly healthy	143	ND	ND	2379
Shionoiri et al, (1990b)	10 mg single dose	Hypt, normal renal function	42	6	7	524
		Hypt, CRF	74	9	10	1109
Sica et al, (1991)	5 mg for 10 days	CRF Day 1	47	13	ND	816
		CRF Day 10	106	9	ND	2164

For abbreviations, see Table 7–2.
CRF, chronic renal failure; Hypt, hypertension; ND, no data.

congestive heart failure, single doses of 1.25 to 10 mg shows inhibition of the renin-angiotensin system for at least 24 hours (Dickstein et al., 1986).

Dose and concurrent disease

In *hypertension*, in a randomized blinded parallel group study, lisinopril 10 mg reduced the diastolic blood pressure to 90 mmHg or below in 77% of the first group of patients, 20 mg was required in 48% of the second group of patients, and 40 mg in 14% of the third group of patients (Beevers et al., 1991). However, it may not be clear from the paper whether the lisinopril was given before or after the blood pressure was measured in the morning, nor was there concurrent placebo control. In another study (Pannier et al., 1991), the top lisinopril dose chosen was 80 mg and the mean dose was 50 mg daily, chosen after titration; here there was also only a placebo run-in period. Although doses above 20 mg once daily produced little extra effect according to Gomez et al. (1985) and Cirillo et al. (1988), the peak-trough ratio for effects on blood pressure was better at 40 mg (Lees, 1992).

In *congestive heart failure*, the dose is 5 to 20 mg once daily (Chalmers et al., 1987; Powers et al., 1987). With dose titration, the mean dose in patients mostly in New York Heart Association Class III and most treated by both digoxin and furosemide, was 12 mg (Chalmers et al., 1987). The initial dose of lisinopril should be no more than 2.5 mg because of the possibility of prolonged excess hypotensive reactions, although 5 mg has been recommended by Powers et al. (1987). In the United States, lisinopril is now licensed for once daily therapy of congestive heart failure.

In the *elderly*, the rate of absorption of lisinopril is the same, but the maximum serum concentration and the area under the curve are higher, which can be explained by decreased renal function (Lancaster and Todd, 1988). In a number of fairly large trials, however, the lisinopril dose in elderly hypertensives has not been changed (Lancaster and Todd, 1988).

In *black subjects*, lisinopril is less antihypertensive than in nonblacks, even after addition of a diuretic (Pool et al., 1987).

In *renal failure* in hypertensives, for the same dose of lisinopril the peak plasma level is higher (Table 7–7) as is the area under the curve, and there is an inverse correlation between the creatinine clearance and the area under the curve (Shionoiri et al., 1990b); hence the dose should be reduced by 50% in moderate and by 75% in severe renal failure (Sica, 1992). During *dialysis*, lisinopril is eliminated so the dose may have to be increased postdialysis (Sica, 1992).

In *hepatic failure*, there should be no dose adjustment required as the drug is not metabolized in any way by the liver.

In *glucose intolerance*, lisinopril may be given without concern for increasing the impairment (Shionoiri et al., 1990c).

Comparative studies

In hypertension, lisinopril plus hydrochlorothiazide is generally better than lisinopril, or hydrochlorothiazide (Lancaster and Todd, 1988). Compared with atenolol, the effects on seated diastolic blood pressure are similar, but lisinopril is better than atenolol in decreasing seated systolic blood pressure (Beevers et al., 1991), possibly because of the increase in arterial compliance (Pannier et al., 1991). Compared with nifedipine, lisinopril is equieffective (Morline et al., 1987) with, however, a better tolerability (Richardson et al., 1987).

PERINDOPRIL

The ACE inhibitor, perindopril, belongs to the category of ester prodrugs, being converted to the active form perindoprilat chiefly in the liver. Perindoprilat has a long pharmacological half-life. Perindopril has been particularly well studied, both experimentally and clinically, for effects on the vascular changes of hypertension.

Pharmacokinetics

Absorption and metabolism. After rapid absorption from the gastrointestinal tract, perindopril undergoes metabolism by two main pathways, chiefly by cyclization (30% to 40%) to inactive forms, but 15% undergoes hydrolysis in the liver to form the active form, perindoprilat. Other relatively less important routes are excretion in the unchanged form (5%) and conjugation to a glucuronic acid conjugate (5%). Thus the major elimination of perindopril is by metabolic conversion, with renal excretion playing a small part (Todd and Fitton, 1991).

    Perindoprilat itself is eliminated in a biphasic manner, the free fraction rapidly eliminated by renal excretion with a half-life of only 1 hour and the bound fraction (bound to ACE) is eliminated much more slowly (Table 7–8). Perindoprilat does not accumulate with dosing reaching a state of equilibrium (formation versus elimination) in about 4 days. Such data suggest, as in the case of other ACE inhibitors with a long half-life, that the slow phase of elimination of the active drug results from tight binding to the active site of the enzyme or to other tissue sites.

Plasma concentration and kinetics. The peak perindoprilat concentration is about 6 to 7 ng/ml, with a time to peak plasma concentration of about 3 hours, a terminal half-life of 27 to 33 hours or even longer (see Table 7–8). The area under the plasma concentration-time curve is about 90 ng.h/ml. When considering peak and trough blood levels, the inhibitory effects on plasma ACE are similar, which is a desirable indication of sustained activity over 24 hours (Lees, 1992).

Plasma binding and distribution. The percentage binding of perindoprilat to plasma proteins is low, about 20%.

TABLE 7–8 PERINDOPRIL. SOME PHARMACOKINETIC PROPERTIES OF PERINDOPRILAT

Author	Perindopril dose	Subjects	Conc max ng/ml	Tmax h	Elim T1/2 h	AUC ng.h/ml
Lees and Reid (1987)	4 mg IV	Normals	—	—	31	—
Lees et al, (1988)	8 mg orally	Normals	—	—	—	120
		Elderly normals	—	—	—	295
Drummer et al, (1987)	2 mg	Hypertension	2	6.5	60	—
	4 mg	Hypertension	6			
	8 mg	Hypertension	20			
Brown et al, (1990)	4 mg	Hypertension	15	3.6	35	252

Louis et al, (1992b)	4 mg chronic dosing	Hypertension	15	2.5	35–50	143
Servier data on file: see Coversyl product monograph, 1989	4 mg	Hypertension (H)	7	3.3	27	87
		H; mild CRF	13	3.6	—	217
		H; severe CRF	33	12.0	increased	1106
		Heart failure	5	8.2	42	181
Tsai et al, (1989)	8 mg	Mild cirrhosis	29	2.3	—	321

For abbreviations, see Table 7–2.
CRF, chronic renal failure; H, hypertension; IV, intravenous

The volume of distribution is about 9 to 10 liters following an intravenous dose.

Pharmacodynamics

As expected, perindopril is active against animal models of hypertension and in human hypertension. Single oral doses of perindopril produce a dose-dependent inhibition of plasma ACE varying from 80% at peak values with a 2 mg dose to 95% with an 8 mg dose, whereas 24 hours after dosing the inhibition varies from 60% with the 2 mg dose to 79% with the 8 mg dose (Bussien et al., 1986). By contrast, in another study (Louis et al., 1992), perindopril 4 to 8 mg produced about 45% inhibition of plasma ACE at 24 hours. Perindopril reduces left ventricular hypertrophy in humans (Grandi et al., 1991). In animals, it favorably alters the vascular alterations found in chronic hypertension, while in humans it improves the peripheral hemodynamics of the large blood vessels (see Chapter 10).

Dose and concurrent disease

In *hypertension,* the majority of studies have used a single dose of 4 mg daily. In a parallel placebo dose-response multicenter study over 16 weeks, the response curve flattened after 8 mg and a single daily dose was as good as two (Chrysant et al., 1993). Peak-trough relationships also suggest a flattening of effect at 8 mg (Lees, 1992). In a second parallel placebo controlled study over 4 weeks, with automatic blood pressure monitoring, the percentage of blood pressure readings still above 95 mmHg was 83% with placebo, 73% with 2 mg perindopril, 54% with 4 mg perindopril, and 42% with 8 mg perindopril (Luccioni et al., 1988). In a third study using conventional blood pressure recording techniques, in which 2 week treatment periods were used to compare perindopril 2 mg with perindopril 4 mg daily and with placebo, the lower dose (2 mg) failed to reduce the blood pressure, whereas 4 mg did (Luccioni et al., 1989). Approximately 65% of the antihypertensive effect occurs within 10 days, 78% after 1 month, and the full effect after 3 months (Leary et al., 1989).

In *congestive heart failure,* perindopril 2–4 mg daily improved exercise tolerance by 27% versus 5% in placebo-treated subjects over 3 months (Metcalfe and Dargie, 1990). Background therapy was by a loop diuretic and in about half, also by digoxin. Similar benefits were shown in another trial, also double-blinded, with similar doses of perindopril (Bounhoure et al., 1989). The delayed formation of perindoprilat with an increase of the area under the curve (see Table 7–8) means that the dose should be reduced by about half when compared with that required for hypertension. An initial dose of 2 mg seems safe (MacFadyen et al., 1991).

In the *elderly,* there is apparently an increased rate of formation of perindoprilat and a reduction in its renal clearance so that the starting dose should be reduced by about half (e.g., from 4 to 2 mg daily)(Lees et al., 1988).

In *black subjects,* ACE inhibitors as a group are not recommended as monotherapy for hypertension, but work well in combination with a diuretic.

In *renal failure*, there is a reduction in the renal clearance of perindoprilat in proportion to the fall in creatinine clearance (Table 7–8). When the clearance is reduced down to 30 to 60 ml/min, the dose should be reduced by half (from 4 mg to 2 mg daily). With severe renal failure (clearance below 30 ml/min), the dose should be about 2 mg on alternate days. During *dialysis,* when the creatinine clearance falls below 15 ml/min, then perindopril 2 mg should be given on the day of dialysis. Perindoprilat is effectively removed by dialysis, probably because of its low plasma protein binding (Sica, 1992).

In *hepatic failure and cirrhosis,* it may be expected that the conversion of perindopril to perindoprilat is decreased. However, in mild compensated hepatic cirrhosis, the rate of formation of perindoprilat is nonetheless unaltered so that the dose should stay unchanged (Tsai et al., 1989).

Side-effects and cautions

As with other ACE inhibitors, the major problems relate to bilateral renal artery stenosis (contraindicated), unilateral renal artery stenosis (relatively contraindicated for long-term administration), and risk of first-dose hypotension. However, in congestive heart failure in elderly patients, there appears to be relatively little risk of first-dose hypotension (see Fig. 8–2).

Drug combinations and interactions

Perindopril can safely be combined with a diuretic with an enhanced antihypertensive effect (Brown et al., 1990). In general, combination of any ACE inhibitor with a beta-blocker shows less than the expected additive antihypertensive response (Zanchetti and Desche, 1989). Combination with calcium antagonists and methyldopa may produce increased antihypertensive effects. As in the case of all ACE inhibitors, combination with potassium supplements or potassium-sparing diuretics can lead to increased plasma potassium particularly in patients with renal failure.

Quinapril

Quinapril belongs to the group of prodrugs that become active by conversion to the diacid metabolite, in this case quinaprilat. Quinapril is highly lipophilic, which may have some advantage for tissue penetration and for its effects on the tissue renin-angiotensin system.

Pharmacokinetics

Absorption. Quinapril is rapidly absorbed (approximately 60%) and its absorption not influenced by food intake.

Metabolism and plasma levels. There is rapid hydrolysis of quinapril to quinaprilat, chiefly in the liver (Olson et al., 1989), so that the peak plasma concentration of quinapril is achieved within 1 hour and the peak concentration of quinaprilat 2 hours after a single oral dose (Olson et al., 1989).

Plasma protein binding. This is very high, about 97% (Wadworth and Brogden, 1991).

Elimination, distribution, and clearance. Quinaprilat is excreted by the kidneys largely by tubular secretion (Sica, 1992) with an accumulation half-life of about 3 hours (Table 7–9). The elimination half-life of quinaprilat is approximately 2 hours (Olson et al., 1989).

Pharmacodynamics

It is proposed that the prolonged antihypertensive effect, exceeding the plasma half-life of quinaprilat, is because of tissue binding of quinaprilat. Thus, the dissociation time of quinaprilat from human atrial ACE was over 20-fold longer than that of enalaprilat (Kinoshita et al., 1993).

Dose and concurrent disease

In *hypertension,* the dose recommended by the manufacturers is initially 10 mg/day up to a maximum of 40 mg/day; when combined with a diuretic, the initial dose should be 5 mg/day. The dosage can be either once or twice daily; the latter gives a somewhat better effect although the difference is not clearcut (Frank et al., 1990). Quinapril 20 mg twice daily reduced the blood pressure, decreased the systemic vascular resistance, and reduced renal vascular resistance when compared with placebo (Gupta et al., 1990).

In *congestive heart failure,* the initial dose of 5 mg daily is titrated upwards to the usual maintenance dose of 10 to 20 mg daily. A frequent dose is 5 mg twice daily or 10 mg twice daily (Kromer et al., 1990) or in total daily doses of 5 to 30 mg/day given in at least two divided doses (Northridge and Dargie, 1990). Nonetheless, once daily administration is as effective as twice daily (Northridge et al., 1993). In a parallel placebo-controlled blinded study, a dose of 5 mg twice daily did not significantly improve exercise time over 3 months of treatment, whereas 10 mg twice daily and 20 mg twice daily did so in a dose-response manner (Riegger, 1991). An improvement between 6 weeks and 3 months of therapy occurred only in the group given 40 mg daily. During a one year open-label study, however, the majority of patients appeared to respond to 5 mg twice daily (Riegger, 1991).

In *elderly patients,* quinapril appears to be as effective as in younger patients (Schnaper, 1990) although it is not specifically stated that it was given as monotherapy without concurrent diuretic. Because of the risk of reduction in renal clearance, the initial recommended starting dose is 5 mg daily up to 10 mg daily with a peak dose of 40 mg daily.

In *black subjects,* ACE inhibitors as a group are usually not recommended as monotherapy for hypertension. However, quinapril may be more effective than expected (Wadworth and Brogden, 1991).

TABLE 7–9 QUINAPRIL. SOME PHARMACOKINETIC PROPERTIES OF QUINAPRILAT

Author	Quinapril dose	Subjects	Conc max ng/ml	Tmax h	Elim T1/2 h	AUC* ng.h/ml
Olson et al, (1989)	Single dose	Normal volunteers				
	10 mg		223	1.6	1.8	803
	40 mg		923	23	1.9	3380

For abbreviations, see Table 7–2.
*Total AUC

In *renal failure,* the dose should be reduced in relation to the decrease in creatinine clearance.

In *liver disease,* conversion of quinapril to quinaprilat is delayed and the maximum quinaprilat concentration decreased (Wadworth and Brogden, 1991). Thus, the dose may need to be increased.

Drug interactions

As with other ACE inhibitors, diuretics and other antihypertensive drugs increase sensitivity to quinapril, and the dose should, therefore, be reduced. Potassium-sparing diuretics or supplements may seriously elevate plasma potassium levels, especially in patients with renal impairment. A specific interaction is that between quinapril and tetracyclin. When given simultaneously, the absorption of tetracyclin is reduced by about one-third, possibly due to the high magnesium content of quinapril tablets (U.S. package insert).

RAMIPRIL

Ramipril is a prodrug that is converted to the active diacid, ramiprilat, which is very long-acting.

Pharmacokinetics

Absorption, metabolism, and elimination. About 60% is absorbed. Ramipril is converted in the liver to ramiprilat, which is chiefly eliminated by the kidneys with a clearance of about 80–130 ml/min. There is also some fecal excretion (Todd and Benfield, 1990).

Plasma levels, half-life, and area under the curve. These have been studied in hypertensive patients with normal renal function (Shionoiri et al., 1986b). After 5 mg ramipril the peak plasma concentration reached is 18 ng/ml at 1.2 hours. On the other hand, the peak plasma concentration of ramiprilat is 4.7 ng/ml reached at 3.2 hours. The terminal half-life is 34 $\pm$ 13 hours and the area under the curve for ramiprilat is 87 ng.h/ml. These and other studies are shown in Table 7–10. Plasma protein binding is 56% (Todd and Benfield, 1990).

Pharmacodynamics

In normal volunteers, a 5 mg dose of ramipril can achieve nearly total and prolonged (48 hours) inhibition of plasma ACE activity (Vasmant and Bender, 1989). The fall of systolic and diastolic blood pressure in hypertensive subjects reaches significance at 3 hours, with maximal values round about 5 to 12 hours, and is still detectable 24 to 48 hours after administration. There is no change in the pulse. An analysis of peak-trough dose-effect relationships suggests that optimal inhibition of ACE activity would require a dose of 10 mg (Lees, 1992).

TABLE 7–10 RAMIPRIL. SOME PHARMACOKINETIC PROPERTIES OF RAMIPRILAT

Author	Ramipril dose	Subjects	Conc max ng/ml	Tmax h	Elim T1/2 h	AUC* ng.h/ml
Meyer et al, (1987)	10 mg	Young Healthy	33.6	2.1	ND	217
		Elderly healthy	40.6	2.0	ND	186
Witte et al, (1984)	10 mg	Hypt, healthy	24.0	3.0	113	414
Debusmann et al, (1987)	10 mg	Hypt, normal renal function	49.6	3.3	(4.9)*	314
		Hypt, CRF	65.0	5.3	(15.4)*	927
Shionoiri et al, (1986b)	5 mg	Hypt, normal RF	4.7	3.2	34	87
	5 mg	Hypt, CRF	33.6	3.6	39	325

For abbreviations, see Table 7–2.
CRF, chronic renal failure; Hypt, hypertension; ND, no data; RF, renal failure
*Half-life, early phase alpha

Dose and concurrent disease

In patients with *hypertension,* a single dose of 2.5 mg did not significantly reduce the blood pressure, whereas doses of 5 or 10 mg did (de Leeuw et al., 1985; Bauer et al., 1989). On the other hand, in a double-blind parallel-group placebo-controlled study, the supine diastolic blood pressure dropped significantly by approximately 7 mmHg when the ramipril dose was 2.5 mg with greater falls at 5 and 10 mg (Vasmant and Bender, 1989). Thus, the lowest starting dose should be regarded as 2.5 mg. In patients with congestive heart failure, 5 mg of ramipril is the approximate equivalent of 25 mg captopril three times daily (Manthey et al., 1987) with, however, a much more prolonged action; the risk of severe prolonged hypotension means that the starting dose should be 2.5 mg or less (deGraeff et al., 1987).

In *heart failure,* the plasma levels of the drug and of ramiprilat are higher with a greater area under the curve so that titration should start with lower doses (1.25 to 2.5 mg) and doses above 5 mg are rarely required (Gerckens et al., 1989).

In *postinfarct heart failure* (AIRE Study Investigators, 1993), ramipril was highly effective in an initial dose of 2.5 mg twice daily, increasing to 5 mg once daily in most patients.

In *elderly patients,* circulating concentrations of ramiprilat were 20% to 100% higher even when serum creatinine was normal, when compared with younger subjects (Meyer et al., 1987; Gilchrist et al., 1987).

In *black subjects,* there have been no special studies on ramipril. In general, ACE inhibitors are not recommended as monotherapy for hypertension but work well in combination with a diuretic.

In patients with *renal failure,* the area under the curve of ramiprilat increases in relation to the fall in creatinine clearance (Shionoiri et al., 1986b). Peak plasma levels are higher and decline more slowly (Debusmann et al., 1987). Therefore, dose reduction should be considered in patients with renal failure (Schunkert et al., 1989; Kindler et al., 1989). For example a 50% reduction in dose is needed when the creatinine clearance falls below 40 ml/min (Sica, 1992).

In patients with *hepatic cirrhosis,* the dose is unchanged as is the case with other prodrug type ACE inhibitors (Class II).

Drug combinations and interactions

These resemble those for other ACE inhibitors including contraindication in the case of bilateral renal artery stenosis, relative contraindication with unilateral renal artery stenosis and the major side-effects include cough and hypotension.

SPIRAPRIL

Spirapril belongs to Class II and is rapidly hydrolyzed to the active diacid, spiraprilat. Spiraprilat achieves the maximal blood concentration about 2 hours after oral administration to volunteers and disappears with a half-life of under 2 hours. Plasma ACE inhibition is found up to 6 hours after doses up to 0.3 mg/kg and 24 hours after 1 mg/kg. After rapid absorption, spirapril is transformed in the liver mainly to spiraprilat, which appears in the blood within 2 hours and then disappears with a relatively short half-life of about 2 hours or less. Elimination in rats and dogs is chiefly by the liver (biliary). Therefore, it should belong to Class IIA (Fig. 7–2). Plasma ACE inhibition after a 12.5 mg dose lasts for 4 to 6 hours and after a 25 mg dose lasts for 6 to 8 hours (Salvetti, 1990).

In *hypertension*, spirapril 12 to 24 mg once daily reduced blood pressure as monotherapy in about half the patients; the average dose was 20 mg daily. In the remaining patients, combination with hydrochlorothiazide was usually effective (Carlsen et al., 1991).

In *left ventricular hypertrophy*, spirapril reduces left ventricular mass (Steensgaard-Hansen et al., 1990).

TRANDOLAPRIL

Trandolapril is the most recent addition to the growing list of Class II inhibitors. It appears to be one of those with the longest duration of action.

Pharmacokinetics

Trandolapril is converted to the active form, trandolaprilat, by hepatic metabolism. After fast absorption (40% to 60% of the oral dose) and high first-pass metabolism, trandolaprilat is rapidly formed and reaches peak plasma levels at 6 hours. Its binding to plasma proteins depends on the concentration, being 94% at low concentrations and 80% at higher concentrations. Approximately twice as much trandolaprilat is found in the feces as in the urine, suggesting a high rate of biliary elimination, so that the drug may belong to sub-Class IIA. After an initial fast half-life of about 3.5 hours, there is a prolonged terminal elimination phase as in the case of many other ACE inhibitors. The effective terminal half-life is 16 to 24 hours (Duc and Brunner, 1992).

Pharmacodynamics

In humans, after a single oral dose of 2 mg, there is rapid onset of ACE inhibition, starting at 30 minutes, with a peak at 2 to 4 hours and at 24 hours there is still 80% inhibition (Duc and Brunner, 1992). Doses of 0.5 to 8 mg for 10 days give a dose-dependent decrease of ACE activity (Duc and Brunner, 1992).

Dose and concurrent disease

In *hypertension*, there is a dose-response fall in blood pressure over the range of 0.5 to 2 mg (Duc and Brunner, 1992). Higher doses give a flat dose-response curve (manufacturer's information). Trandolapril 1 to 4 mg once daily reduced blood pressure effectively in 64% of patients in one study (Duc and Brunner, 1992).

In the *elderly* with normal renal function, dose adjustment is not needed.

In *chronic renal failure*, despite the predominant biliary excretion, there is some accumulation of trandolaprilat. The dose should be reduced when the creatinine clearance falls below 30 ml/min/1.73m^2, i.e., 17 ml/min uncorrected (Duc and Brunner, 1992).

In *early (3 to 7 days) postinfarct left ventricular dysfunction*, trandolapril is being evaluated in 1,749 patients in the TRACE (Trandolapril Cardiac Evaluation) study.

ZOFENOPRIL

This prodrug has a prolonged duration of action. Its novel feature is that it would appear to be one of the very few compounds that is both a prodrug and contains a sulfhydryl group. Owing to a prolonged duration of action of zofenoprilat, once daily dosing is possible, and the proposed dose in humans is 5 to 10 mg daily in patients with hypertension. It is still in the early stages of testing in humans.

SUMMARY

From the pharmacokinetic point of view, there are three classes of ACE inhibitors. Class I consists of captopril and allied agents, already in the active form but undergoing further metabolism. Class II has as its prototype enalapril, together with all the other agents that are metabolized to the active diacid form. Class IIA is a subclass with biliary excretion. The metabolite of fosinopril is excreted equally by the liver and kidney. This confers an advantage in renal failure when biliary excretion is increased. This advantage does not appear to hold for other Class IIA drugs, although the data are incomplete. Class III consists of lisinopril, a water-soluble drug not metabolized at all.

The majority of ACE inhibitors now available are Class II prodrugs, most of which are converted to active diacid that is then renally excreted. Dose reduction is usual in renal failure or in the elderly (except for fosinopril Class IIA, which is excreted increasingly in bile in chronic renal failure). Of the prodrugs, those with the longest terminal half-life are ramipril and perindopril, and these are agents that can undoubtedly be given once daily for hypertension. Even agents with a shorter terminal half-life, such as cilazapril, fosinopril and quinapril, however, may also be given once daily because the biological half-life exceeds the pharmacological half-life. In general, it is difficult to measure the terminal half-life exactly because of the low plasma concentrations involved. It is likely that ACE inhibitors as a group bind to a tissue site, probably the angiotensin-converting enzyme, which would explain discrepancies between biological and pharmacological half-lives. A more current way of assessing the ideal dose and frequency of drug administration is by consideration of plasma ACE inhibition at peak and trough plasma drug concentrations.

Even captopril has a longer therapeutic action than its

rather short half-life would predict, in this case because it is found in the plasma in multiple forms and there may be an equilibrium between the bound and free forms. While captopril twice daily is established therapy for hypertension, in heart failure the drug should be given three times daily and in adequate doses.

Lisinopril is the prototype of group III drugs. It is entirely water-soluble, metabolized, and has, therefore, simple pharmacokinetic pattern with total renal excretion. In renal failure, corresponding dose adjustment is required.

Despite the major chemical and pharmacokinetic differences between the drugs, they are all active in hypertension and most of them have been tested in heart failure (exception: fosinopril). Thus, different pharmacokinetic properties and durations of action may be among the factors influencing the choice of drug.

REFERENCES

Abrams WB, Davies RO, Gomez HJ. Clinical pharmacology of enalapril. *J Hypertens* 1984; 2 (Suppl 2): 31–36.

AIRE study—The Acute Infarction Ramipril Efficacy (AIRE) Study Investigators. Effect of ramipril on mortality and morbidity of survivors of acute myocardial infarction with clinical evidence of heart failure. *Lancet* 1993; 342: 821–828.

Anderson RJ, Duchin KL, Gore RD, et al. Once-daily fosinopril in the treatment of hypertension. *Hypertension* 1991; 17: 636–642.

Arr SM, Woollard ML, Fairhurst G, et al. Safety and efficacy of enalapril in essential hypertension in the elderly. *Br J Clin Pharmacol* 1985; 20: 279P–280P.

Bauer B, Lorenz H, Zahlten R. An open multicenter study to assess the long-term efficacy, tolerance, and safety of the oral angiotensin converting enzyme inhibitor ramipril in patients with mild to moderate essential hypertension. *J Cardiovasc Pharmacol* 1989; 13 (Suppl 3): S70–S74.

Beevers DG, Blackwood RA, Garnham S, et al. Comparison of lisinopril versus atenolol for mild to moderate essential hypertension. *Am J Cardiol* 1991; 67: 59–62.

Bellet M, Sassano P, Guyenne T, et al. Converting-enzyme inhibition buffers the counter-regulatory response to acute administration of nicardipine. *Br J Clin Pharmacol* 1987; 24: 465–472.

Belz GG, Essig J, Erb K, et al. Pharmacokinetic and pharmacodynamic interactions between the ACE inhibitor cilazapril and beta-adrenoceptor antagonist propranolol in healthy subjects and in hypertensive patients. *Br J Clin Pharmacol* 1989; 27: 317S–322S.

Bergstrand R, Herlitz H, Johansson S, et al. Effective dose range of enalapril in mild to moderate essential hypertension. *Br J Clin Pharmacol* 1985; 19: 605–611.

Biollaz J, Schelling JL, Jacot des Combes B, et al. Enalapril maleate and a lysine analogue (MK-521) in normal volunteers; relationship between plasma drug levels and the renin angiotensin system. *Br J Clin Pharmacol* 1982; 14: 363–368.

Bounhoure JP, Bottineau G, Lechat P, et al. Value of perindopril in the treatment of chronic congestive heart failure. Multicenter double-blind placebo-controlled study. *Clin Exper Theory Pract* 1989; A11 (Suppl 2): 575–586.

Brilla CG, Kramer B, Hoffmeister HM, et al. Low-dose enalapril in severe chronic heart failure. *Cardiovasc Drugs Ther* 1989; 3: 211–218.

Brown CL, Backhouse CI, Grippat JC, Santoni JPh. The effect of perindopril and hydrochlorothiazide alone and in combination on blood pressure and on the renin-angiotensin system in hypertensive subjects. *Eur J Clin Pharmacol* 1990; 39: 327–332.

Bussien JP, d'Amore TF, Perret L, et al. Single and repeated dosing of the converting enzyme inhibitor perindopril to normal subjects. *Clin Pharmacol Therap* 1986; 39: 554–558.

Carlsen JE, Galloe A, Kober L, et al. Comparison of efficacy and tolerability of spirapril and nitrendipine in arterial hypertension. *Drug Invest* 1991; 3: 172–177.

Chalmers JP, West MJ, Cyran J, et al. Placebo-controlled study of lisinopril in congestive heart failure: a multicentre study. *J Cardiovasc Pharmacol* 1987; 9 (Suppl 3): S89–S97.

Chrysant SG, McDonald RH, Wright JT, et al for the Perindopril Study Group. Perindopril as monotherapy in hypertension: a multicenter comparison of two dosing regimens. *Clin Pharmacol Ther* 1993; 53: 479–484.

Cirillo VJ, Gomez HJ, Salonen J, et al. Lisinopril: dose-peak effect relationship in essential hypertension. *Br J Clin Pharmacol* 1988; 25: 533–538.

Cirillo VJ, Till AE, Gomez HJ, et al. Effect of age on lisinopril pharmacokinetics (abstr). *Clin Pharmacol Ther* 1986; 39: 187.

Cody RJ, Schaer GL, Covit AB, et al. Captopril kinetics in chronic congestive heart failure. *Clin Pharmacol Ther* 1982; 32: 721–726.

Colfer HT, Ribner HS, Gradman A, et al. for the Benazapril Heart Failure Study Group. Effects of once-daily benazapril therapy on exercise tolerance and manifestations of chronic congestive heart failure. *Am J Cardiol* 1992; 70: 354–358.

Coversyl (Perindopril) product monograph. Manchester, UK: ADIS International; 1989: Chapter 3.

Creasey WA, Funke PT, McKinstry DN, Sugerman AA. Pharmacokinetics of captopril in elderly healthy male volunteers. *J Clin Pharmacol* 1986; 26: 264–268.

Cushman DW, Wang FL, Fung WC, et al. Differentiation of angiotensin-converting enzyme (ACE) inhibitors by their selective inhibition of ACE in physiologically important target organs. *Am J Hypertens* 1989; 2: 294–306.

Davies RO, Gomez HJ, Irvin JD, Walker JF. An overview of the clinical pharmacology of enalapril. *Br J Clin Pharmacol* 1984; 18 (Suppl 2): 215S–229S.

Debusmann ER, Pujadas JO, Lahn W, et al. Influence of renal function on the pharmacokinetics of ramipril (HOE 498). *Am J Cardiol* 1987; 59: 70D–78D.

DeForrest JM, Waldron TL, Harvey C, et al. Blood pressure lowering and renal hemodynamic effects of fosinopril in conscious animal models. *J Cardiovasc Pharmacol* 1990; 16: 139–146.

Deget F, Brogden RN. Cilazapril. A review of its pharmacodynamic and pharmacokinetic properties, and therapeutic potential in cardiovascular disease. *Drugs* 1991; 41: 799–820.

deGraeff PA, Kingma JH, Dunselman PHJM, et al. Acute hemodynamic and hormonal effects of ramipril in chronic congestive heart failure and comparison with captopril. *Am J Cardiol* 1987; 59: 164D–170D.

deLeeuw PW, Lugtenburg PL, van Houten H, et al. Preliminary experiences with HOE 498, a novel long-acting converting enzyme inhibitor, in hypertensive patients. *J Cardiovasc Pharmacol* 1985; 7: 1161–1165.

DeLepeleire I, Van Hecken A, Verbesselt R, et al. Interaction between furosemide and the converting enzyme inhibitor benazepril in healthy volunteers. *Eur J Clin Pharmacol* 1988; 34: 465–468.

DiCarlo L, Chatterjee K, Parmley WW, et al. Enalapril: a new angiotensin-converting enzyme inhibitor in chronic heart failure: acute and chronic hemodynamic evaluations. *J Am Coll Cardiol* 1983; 2: 865–871.

Dickstein K, Aarsland T, Woie L, et al. Acute hemodynamic and hormonal effects of lisinopril (MK-521) in congestive heart failure. *Am Heart J 1986; 112: 121–129.*

Drexler H, Banhardt U, Meinertz T, et al. Contrasting peripheral short-term and long-term effects of converting enzyme inhibition in patients with congestive heart failure. A double-blind, placebo-controlled trial. *Circulation* 1989; 79: 491–502.

Drummer CH, Rowley K, Johnson H, et al. Metabolism and pharmacodynamics of angiotensin converting enzyme inhibitors with special reference to perindopril. In: Rand MJ, Raper C (eds.), *Pharmacology.* Elsevier Science Publishers, Amsterdam, 1987, 545–550.

Duc LNC, Brunner HR. Trandolapril in hypertension: overview of a new angiotensin-converting enzyme inhibitor. *Am J Cardiol* 1992; 70: 27D–34D.

Duchin KL, Singhvi SM, Willard DA, et al. Captopril kinetics. *Clin Pharmacol Ther* 1982; 31: 452–458.

Duchin KL, Waclawski AP, Tu JI, et al. Pharmacokinetics, safety, and pharmacologic effects of fosinopril sodium, in angiotensin-converting enzyme inhibitor in healthy subjects. *J Clin Pharmacol* 1991; 31; 58–64.

Fasanella d'Amore T, Bussein JP, Nussberger J, et al. Effects of single doses of the converting enzyme inhibitor cilazapril in normal volunteers. *J Cardiovasc Pharmacol* 1987; 9: 26–31.

Francis RJ, Brown AN, Kler L, et al. Pharmacokinetics of the converting enzyme inhibitor cilazapril in normal volunteers and the relationship to enzyme inhibition: development of a mathematical model. *J Cardiovasc Pharmacol* 1987; 9: 32–38.

Frank GJ, Knapp LE, Olson SC, et al. Overview of quinapril, a new ACE inhibitor. *J Cardiovasc Pharmacol* 1990; 15 (Suppl 2): S14–S23.

Freier PA, Wollam GL, Hall WD, et al. Blood pressure, plasma volume, and catecholamine levels during enalapril in blacks with hypertension. *Clin Pharmacol Ther* 1984; 36: 731–737.

Gavras H, Biollaz J, Waeber B, et al. Antihypertensive effect of the new oral angiotensin converting enzyme inhibitor MK-421. *Lancet* 1981; 2: 543–547.

Gerckens U, Grube E, Mengden T, et al. Pharmacokinetic and pharmacodynamic properties of ramipril in patients with congestive heart failure (NYHA III-IV). *J Cardiovasc Pharmacol* 1989; 13 (Suppl 3): S49–S51.

Gilchrist WJ, Beard K, Manhem P, et al. Pharmacokinetics and effects on the renin angiotensin system of ramipril in elderly patients. *Am J Cardiol* 1987; 59: 28D–32D.

Gomez HJ, Sromovsky J, Kristianson K, et al. Lisinopril dose response in mild to moderate hypertension. Abstract No C48. *Clin Pharmacol Ther 1985; 37: 198.*

Gomez HJ, Cirillo VJ, Moncloa F. The clinical pharmacology of lisinopril. *J Cardiovasc Pharmacol* 1987; 9 (Suppl 3): 527–534.

Gosse P, Roudaut R, Herrero G, Dallocchio M. Beta-blockers vs angiotensin-converting enzyme inhibitors in hypertension: effects on left ventricular hypertrophy. *J Cardiovasc Pharmacol* 1990; 16 (Suppl 5): S145–S150.

Grandi AM, Venco A, Barzizza F, et al. Double-blind comparison of perindopril and captopril in hypertension. Effects on left ventricular morphology and function. *Am J Hypertens* 1991; 4: 516–520.

Guntzel P, Kobrin I, Pasquier C, et al. The effect of cilazapril, a new angiotensin converting enzyme inhibitor, on peak and trough blood pressure measurements in hypertensive patients. *J Cardiovasc Pharmacol* 1991; 17: 8–12.

Gupta RK, Kjeldsen SE, Krause L, et al. Hemodynamic effects of quinapril, a novel angiotensin-converting enzyme inhibitor. *Clin Pharmacol Ther* 1990; 48: 41–49.

Guyene TT, Bellet M, Sassano P, et al. Crossover design for the dose determination of an angiotensin converting enzyme inhibitor in hypertension. *J Hypertens* 1989; 7: 1005–1012.

Hasford J, Bussmann W-D, Delius W, et al. First dose hypotension with enalapril and prazosin in congestive heart failure. *Int J Cardiol* 1991; 31: 287–294.

Herrlin B, Sylven C, Nyquist O, Edhag O. Short term haemodynamic effects of converting enzyme inhibition before and after eating in patients with moderate heart failure caused by dilated cardiomyopathy: a double-blind study. *Br Heart J* 1990; 63: 26–31.

Hockings N, Ajayi LAA, Reid JL. The effects of age on the pharmacokinetics and dynamics of the angiotensin converting enzyme inhibitors enalapril and enalaprilat. *Br J Clin Pharmacol* 1985; 20: 262P–263P.

Hui KK, Duchin KL, Kripalani KJ, et al. Pharmacokinetics of fosinopril in patients with various degrees of renal function. *Clin Pharmacol Ther* 1991; 49: 457–467.

Jarrott B, Drummer O, Hooper R, et al. Pharmcokinetic properties of captopril after acute and chronic administration to hypertensive subjects. *Am J Cardiol* 1982; 49: 1547–1549.

Johnston CI, Jackson B, McGrath B, et al. Relationship of antihypertensive effect of enalapril to serum MK-422 levels and angiotensin converting enzyme inhibition. *J Hypertens* 1983; 1 (Suppl 1): 71–75.

Johnston CI, Jackson BJ, Larmour I, et al. Plasma enalapril levels and hormonal effects after short- and long-term administration in essential hypertension. Br J Clin Pharmacol 1984; 18 (Suppl 2): 233S–239S.

Johnston CI, Mendelsohn FAO, Cubela RB, et al. Inhibition of angiotensin converting enzyme (ACE) in plasma and tissues: studies ex vivo after administration of ACE inhibitors. *J Hypertens* 1988; 6 (Suppl 3): S17–S22.

Kaiser G, Ackermann R, Sioufi A. Pharmacokinetics of a new angiotensin-converting enzyme inhibitor, benazepril hydrochloride, in special populations - part 1. *Am Heart J* 1989; 117: 746–751.

Kindler J, Schunkert H, Gassmann M, et al. Therapeutic efficacy and tolerance of ramipril in hypertensive patients with renal failure. *J Cardiovasc Pharmacol* 1989; 13 (Suppl 3): S55–S58.

Kinoshita A, Urata H, Bumpus FM, Husain A. Measurement of angiotensin-I converting enzyme inhibition in the heart. *Circ Res* 1993; 73: 51–60.

Kleinbloesem CH, Erb K, Essig J, et al. Haemodynamic and hormonal effects of cilazapril in comparison with propranolol in healthy subjects and in hypertensive patients. *Br J Clin Pharmacol* 1989; 27: 309S–315S.

Kripalani KJ, McKinstry DN, Singhvi SM, et al. Disposition of captopril in normal subjects. *Clin Pharmacol Ther* 1980; 27: 636–641.

Kromer EP, Elsner D, Riegger GAJ. Digoxin, converting-enzyme inhibition (quinapril), and the combination in patients with congestive heart failure functional Class II and sinus rhythm. *J Cardiovasc Pharmacol* 1990; 16: 9–14.

Lancaster SG, Todd PA. Lisinopril. A preliminary review of its pharmacodynamic and pharmacokinetic properties, and therapeutic use in hypertension and congestive heart failure. *Drugs* 1988; 35: 646–669.

Laragh JH. New angiotensin converting-enzyme inhibitors. Their role in the management of hypertension. *Am J Hypertens* 1990; 3: 257S–265S.

Leary WP, Reyes AJ, van der Byl K, Santoni JP. Time course of the hypotensive effect of the converting enzyme inhibitor perindopril. *Curr Ther Res* 1989; 46: 308–316.

Lees KR. The dose-response relationship with angiotensin-converting enzyme inhibitors: effects on blood pressure and biochemical parameters. *J Hypertens* 1992; 10 (Suppl 5): S3–S11.

Lees KR, Reid JL. Effects of intravenous S-9780, an angiotensin-converting enzyme inhibitor, in normotensive subjects. *J Cardiovasc Pharmacol* 1987; 10: 129–135.

Lees KR, Green ST, Reid JL. Influence of age on the pharmacokinetics and pharmacodynamics of perindopril. *Clin Pharmacol Ther* 1988; 44: 418–425.

Lewis AB, Chabot M. The effect of treatment with angiotensin-converting enzyme inhibitors on survival of pediatric patients with dilated cardiomyopathy. *Pediatr Cardiol* 1993; 14: 9–12.

Longhini C, Ansani L, Musacci GF, et al. The effect of captopril on peripheral hemodynamics in patients with essential hypertension: comparison between oral and sublingual administration. *Cardiovasc Drugs Ther* 1990; 4: 751–754.

Loock ME, Rossouw DS, Venter CP, et al. Benazepril and nifedipine alone and in combination for the treatment of essential hypertension in black patients (abstr). *Eur Heart J* 1990; 11: 420.

Louis WJ, Conway EL, Krum H, et al. Comparison of the pharmacokinetics and pharmacodynamics of perindopril, cilazapril and enalapril. *Clin Exp Pharmacol Physiol* 1992a; 19 (Suppl 19): 55–60.

Louis WJ, Workman BS, Conway EL, et al. Single-dose and steady-state pharmacokinetics and pharmacodynamics of perindopril in hypertensive subjects. *J Cardiovasc Pharmacol* 1992b; 20: 505–511.

Luccioni R, Frances Y, Gass R, et al. Evaluation of the dose-effect relationship of a new ACE inhibitor (perindopril) by an automatic blood pressure recorder. *Eur Heart J* 1988; 9: 1131–1136.

Luccioni R, Frances Y, Gass R, Gilgenkrantz JM. Evaluation of the dose-effect relationship of perindopril in the treatment of hypertension. *Clin Exp Theory Pract* 1989; A11 (Suppl 2): 521–534.

MacDonald NJ, Elliott HL, Howie CA, Reid JL. Age and the pharmacodynamics and pharmacokinetics of benazepril. *Br J Clin Pharmacol* 1988; 27: 707P–708P.

MacFayden RJ, Lees KR, Reid JL. Differences in first dose response to ACE inhibition in congestive cardiac failure—a placebo-controlled study. *Br Heart J* 1991; 66: 206–211.

Manthey J, Osterziel J, Rohrig N, et al. Ramipril and captopril in patients with heart failure: effects on hemodynamics and vasoconstrictor systems. *Am J Cardiol* 1987; 59: 171D–175D.

Meredith PA, Donnelly R, Elliott HL, et al. Prediction of the antihypertensive response to enalapril. *J Hypertens* 1990; 8: 1085–1090.

Metcalfe M, Dargie HJ. Contribution of perindopril in the treatment of congestive heart failure. *JAMA 1990 (Suppl): 23–27.*

Meyer BH, Muller O, Badian M, et al. Pharmacokinetics of ramipril in the elderly. *Am J Cardiol* 1987; 59: 33D–37D.

Millar JA, Derkx FHM, McLean K, Reid JL. Pharmacodynamics of converting enzyme inhibition: the cardiovascular endocrine and autonomic effects of MK 421 (enalapril) and MK 521. *Br J Clin Pharmacol* 1982; 14: 347–355.

Minamisawa K, Shionoiri H, Sugimoto K, et al. Depressor effects and pharmacokinetics of single and consecutive doses of delapril in hypertensive patients with normal or impaired renal function. *Cardiovasc Drugs Ther* 1990; 4: 1417–1424.

Morlin C, Baglivo H, Boeijinga JK, et al. Comparative trial of lisinopril and nifedipine in mild to severe essential hypertension. *J Cardiovasc Pharmacol* 1987; 9 (Suppl 3): S48–S52.

Natoff IL, Nixon JS, Francis RJ, et al. Biological properties of the angiotensin-converting enzyme inhibitor cilazapril. *J Cardiovasc Pharmacol* 1985; 7: 569–580.

Northridge DB, Dargie HJ. Quinapril in chronic heart failure. *Am J Hypertens* 1990; 3: 283S–287S.

Northridge DB, Rose E, Raftery ED, et al. A multicentre, double-blind, placebo-controlled trial of quinapril in mild, chronic heart failure. *Eur Heart J* 1993; 14: 403–409.

Nussberger J, Fasanella d'Amore T, Porchet M, et al. Repeated administration of the converting enzyme inhibitor cilazapril to normal volunteers. *J Cardiovasc Pharmacol* 1987; 9: 39–44.

Ohman KP, Kagedal B, Larsson R, Karlberg BE. Pharmacokinetics of captopril and its effects on blood pressure during acute and chronic administration and in relation to food intake. *J Cardiovasc Pharmacol* 1985; 7: S20–S24.

Olson SC, Horvath AM, Michniewicxz BD, et al. The clinical pharmacokinetics of quinapril. *Angiology* 1989; 40: 351–359.

Onoyama K, Hirakata H, Iseki K, et al. Blood concentration and urinary excretion of captopril (SQ 14,225) in patients with chronic renal failure. *Hypertension* 1981; 3: 456–459.

Oren S, Messerli FH, Grossman E, et al. Immediate and short-term cardiovascular effects of fosinopril, a new angiotensin-converting enzyme inhibitor, in patients with essential hypertension. *J Am Coll Cardiol* 1991; 17: 1183–1187.

Pannier BE, Garabedian VG, Madonna O, et al. Lisinopril versus atenolol: decrease in systolic versus diastolic blood pressure with converting enzyme inhibition. *Cardiovasc Drugs Ther* 1991; 5: 823–829.

Pool JL. Antihypertensive effect of fosinopril, a new angiotensin-converting enzyme inhibitor: findings of the Fosinopril Study Group II. *Clin Therap* 1990; 12: 520–533.

Pool JL, Gennari J, Goldstein R, et al. Controlled multicentre study of antihypertensive effects of lisinopril, hydrochlorothiazide, and lisinopril plus hydrochlorothiazide in the treatment of 394 patients with mild to moderate essential hypertension. *J Cardiovasc Pharmacol* 1987; 9 (Suppl 3): S36–S42.

Pouleur H, Rousseau MF, Oakley C, Ryden L for the Xamoterol in Severe Heart Failure Study Group. Difference in mortality between patients treated with captopril or enalapril in the Xamoterol in Severe Heart Failure Study. *Am J Cardiol* 1991; 68: 71–74.

Powers ER, Chiaramida A, DeMaria AN, et al. A double-blind comparison of lisinopril with captopril in patients with symptomatic congestive heart failure. *J Cardiovasc Pharmacol* 1987; 9 (Suppl 3): S82–S88.

Rademaker M, Shaw TRD, Williams BC et al. Intravenous captopril treatment in patients with severe cardiac failure. *Br Heart J* 1986; 55: 187–190.

Reyes AJ, Leary WP, Acosta-Barrios TN. Once-daily administration of captopril and hypotensive effect. *J Cardiovasc Pharmacol* 1985; 7: S16–S19.

Richardson PJ, Meany B, Breckenridge AM, et al. Lisinopril in essential hypertension: a six month comparative study with nifedipine. *J Human Hypertens* 1987; 1: 175–179.

Richer C, Giroux B, Plouin PF, et al. Captopril: pharmacokinetics, antihypertensive and biological effects in hypertensive patients. *Br J Clin Pharmacol* 1984; 17: 243–250.

Riegger GAJ. Effects of quinapril on exercise tolerance in patients with mild to moderate heart failure. *Eur Heart J* 1991; 12: 705–711.

Salvetti A. Newer ACE inhibitors: A look at the future. *Drugs* 1990; 40: 800–828.

Salvetti A, Arzilli F. Chronic dose-response curve of enalapril in essential hypertensives. An Italian Multicenter Study. *Am J Hypertens* 1989; 2: 352–354.

Salvetti A, Pedrinelli R, Magagna A, et al. Influence of food on acute and chronic effects of captopril in essential hypertensive patients. *J Cardiovasc Pharmacol* 1985; 7: S25–S29.

Schaller M, Nussberger J, Waeber B, et al. Haemodynamic and pharmacological effects of the converting enzyme inhibitor benazepril HCL in normal volunteers. *Eur J Clin Pharmacol* 1985; 28: 267–272.

Schnaper HW. Use of quinapril in the elderly patient. *Am J Hypertens* 1990; 3: 278S–282S.

Schofield PM, Brooks NH, Lawrence GP, et al. Which vasodilator drug in patients with chronic heart failure? A randomised comparison of captopril and hydralazine. *Br J Clin Pharmacol* 1991; 31: 25–32.

Schunkert H, Kindler J, Gassmann M, et al. Steady-state kinetics of ramipril in renal failure. *J Cardiovasc Pharmacol* 1989; 13 (Suppl 3): S52–S54.

Schwartz JB, Taylor A, Abernethy D, et al. Pharmacokinetics and pharmacodynamics of enalapril in patients with congestive heart failure and patients with hypertension. *J Cardiovasc Pharmacol* 1985; 7: 767–776.

Sharpe N, Murphy J, Coxon R, Hannan SF. Enalapril in patients with chronic heart failure: a placebo-controlled, randomized, double-blind study. *Circulation* 1984; 70: 271–278.

Sharpe N, Murphy J, Smith H, Hannan S. Treatment of patients with symptomless left ventricular dysfunction after myocardial infarction. *Lancet* 1988; 1: 255–259.

Shionoiri H, Miyazaki N, Yasuda G, et al. Pharmacokinetics and antihypertensive effects of single and consecutive dosing of alacepril (DU-1219) in patients with severe hypertension. *Curr Ther Res* 1985a; 38: 537–547.

Shionoiri H, Gotoh E, Miyazaki N, et al. Serum concentration and effects of a single dose of enalapril maleate in patients with essential hypertension. *Jpn Circ J* 1985b; 49: 46–51.

Shionoiri H, Miyazaki N, Yasuda G, et al. Blood concentration and urinary excretion of enalapril in patients with chronic renal failure. *Jpn J Nephrol* 1985c; 27: 1291–1297.

Shionoiri H, Yasuda G, Sugimoto K, et al. The antihypertensive effect and the pharmacokinetic profile of captopril retard (CS-522-R) in patients with essential hypertension. *Jpn J Nephrol* 1986a; 28: 73–78.

Shionoiri H, Ikeda Y, Kimura K, et al. Pharmacodynamics and pharmacokinetics of single-dose ramipril in hypertensive patients with various degrees of renal function. *Curr Ther Res* 1986b; 40: 74–85.

Shionoiri H, Miyazaki N, Ochiai H, et al. The effects of twice daily captopril and once daily enalapril on ambulatory intraarterial blood pressure in essential hypertension. *Clin Exp Theory Pract* 1987a; A9: 599–603.

Shionoiri H, Iino S, Inoue S. Glucose metabolism during captopril mono- and combination therapy in diabetic hypertensive patients: a multiclinic trial. *Clin Exp Theory Pract* 1987b: A9: 671–674.

Shionoiri H, Yasuda G, Abe Y, et al. Pharmacokinetics and acute effect on the renin-angiotensin system of delapril in patients with chronic renal failure. *Clin Nephrol* 1987c; 27: 65–70.

Shionoiri H, Yasuda G, Ikeda A, et al. Pharmacokinetics and depressor effect of delapril in patients with essential hypertension. *Clin Pharmacol Ther* 1987d; 41: 74–79.

Shionoiri H, Gotoh E, Takagi N, et al. Antihypertensive effects and pharmacokinetics of single and consecutive doses of cilazapril in hypertensive patients with normal and impaired renal function. *J Cardiovasc Pharmacol* 1988; 11: 242–249.

Shionoiri H, Sugimoto K, Minamisawa K, et al. Glucose and lipid metabolism during long-term treatment with cilazapril in hypertensive patients with or without impaired glucose metabolism. *J Cardiovasc Pharmacol* 1990a; 15: 933–938.

Shionoiri H, Minamisawa K, Ueda S, et al. Pharmacokinetics and antihypertensive effects of lisinopril in hypertensive patients with normal and impaired renal function. *J Cardiovasc Pharmacol* 1990b; 16: 594–600.

Shionoiri H, Ueda S, Gotoh E, et al. Glucose and lipid metabolism during long-term lisinopril therapy in hypertensive patients. *J Cardiovasc Pharmacol* 1990c; 16: 905–909.

Sica DA. Kinetics of angiotensin-converting enzyme inhibitors in renal failure. *J Cardiovasc Pharmacol* 1992; 20 (Suppl 10): S13–S20.

Sica DA, Cutler RE, Parmer RJ, Ford NF. Comparison of the steady-state pharmacokinetics of fosinopril, lisinopril and enalapril in patients with chronic renal insufficiency. *Clin Pharmacokinet* 1991; 20: 420–427.

Singhvi SM, Duchin KL, Morrison RA, et al. Disposition of fosinopril sodium in healthy subjects. *Br J Clin Pharmacol* 1988; 25: 9–15.

Smith EF, Egan JW, Goodman FR, et al. Effects of two nonsulfhydryl angiotensin-converting enzyme inhibitors, benazeprilat and abutapril, on myocardial damage and left ventricular hypertrophy following coronary artery occlusion in the rat. *Pharmacology* 1988; 37: 254–263.

Steensgaard F, Kober L, Torp-Pedersen C, et al. Effect of a new ACE inhibitor, spirapril, and nitrendipine on left ventricular mass and function in essential hypertension (abstr). *Eur Heart J* 1990; 11: 420.

Swedberg K, Held P, Kjekshus J, Rasmussen K, et al on behalf of the CONSENSUS II Study Group. Effects of the early administration of enalapril on mortality in patients with acute myocardial infarction. Results of the Cooperative New Scandinavian Enalapril Survival Study II (CONSENSUS II). *N Engl J Med* 1992; 327: 678–684.

Thind GS. Angiotensin converting enzyme inhibitors: Comparative structure, pharmacokinetics, and pharmacodynamics. *Cardiovasc Drugs Ther* 1990; 4: 199–206.

Till AE, Gomez HJ, Hichens M, Bolognese JA. Pharmacokinetics of repeated oral doses of enalapril maleate (MK-421) in normal volunteers. *Biopharmaceutics and Drug Disposition* 1984; 5: 273–280.

Todd PA, Heel RC. Enalapril. A review of its pharmacodynamic and pharmacokinetic properties, and therapeutic use in hypertension and congestive heart failure. *Drugs* 1986; 31: 198–248.

Todd PA, Benfield P. Ramipril. A review of its pharmacological properties and therapeutic efficacy in cardiovascular disorders. *Drugs* 1990; 1: 110–135.

Todd PA, Fitton A. Perindopril - a review of its pharmacological properties and therapeutic use in cardiovascular disorders. *Drugs* 1991; 42: 90–114.

Tsai HH, Lees KR, Howden CW, et al. The pharmacokinetics and pharmacodynamics of perindopril in patients with hepatic cirrhosis. *Br J Clin Pharmacol* 1989; 28: 53–59.

Ulm EH, Hichens M, Gomez HJ, et al. Enalapril maleate and a lysine analogue (MK-521): disposition in man. *Br J Clin Pharmacol* 1982; 14: 357–362.

Vasmant D, Bender N. The renin-angiotensin system and ramipril, a new converting enzyme inhibitor. *J Cardiovasc Pharmacol* 1989; 14 (Suppl 4): S46–S52.

Veterans Administration Co-operative Study Group on Antihypertensive Agents. Racial differences in response to low-dose captopril are abolished by the addition of hydrochlorothiazide. *Br J Clin Pharmacol* 1982; 14: 97S–101S.

Wadworth AN, Brogden RN. Quinapril. A review of its pharmacological properties, and therapeutic efficacy in cardiovascular disorders. *Drugs* 1991; 41: 378–399.

Wellstein A, Essig J, Belz GG. Inhibition of angiotensin-I response by cilazapril and its time course in normal volunteers. *Clin Pharmacol Ther* 1987; 41: 639–644.

Whalen JJ. Definition of the effective dose of the converting-enzyme inhibitor benazapril. *Am Heart J* 1989; 117: 728–734.

Witte PU, Irmisch R, Hajdu P, Metzger H. Pharmacokinetics and pharmacodynamics of a novel orally active angiotensin converting enzyme inibitor (HOE 498) in healthy subjects. *Eur J Clin Pharmacol* 1984; 27: 577–581.

Zanchetti A, Desche P. Perindopril: first-line treatment for hypertension. *Clin Exp Theory Pract* 1989; A11 (Suppl 2): 555–573.

Zusman RM. Left ventricular hypertrophy and performance: therapeutic options among the angiotensin-converting enzyme inhibitors. *J Cardiovasc Pharmacol* 1992; 20 (Suppl 10): S21–S28.

CHAPTER 8

ACE Inhibitors: Side Effects and Contraindications

"Rates of withdrawal appear to be too crude a marker for the more subtle side-effects and symptoms experienced by the patient." (Testa et al., 1993)

SIDE-EFFECTS

Initially the godfather ACE inhibitor, captopril, was thought to have such serious side-effects that it could only be used in exceptional circumstances. Near-fatal neutropenia, serious renal disease with increased proteinuria, as well as less lethal side-effects such as skin rashes, loss of taste (ageusia), and angioedema, came to be recognized. Most of these serious side-effects of captopril appear to be dose-related and at the doses currently used, neutropenia, for example, is hardly an issue, although there are still warnings in the package insert. On the other hand, angioedema remains a truly serious although rare risk, and a class side-effect. Strangely enough, the possession of the SH-group once thought to be so harmful and the cause of several of the serious side-effects including neutropenia, is now promoted as being beneficial because of its potential for free radical scavenging. Currently the ACE inhibitors as a whole are regarded as a rather safe category of drugs with only occasional side-effects (Fig. 8–1), although with serious risk to the fetus if given during the second or third trimesters of pregnancy.

CLASS SIDE-EFFECTS

Angioedema

Although rare, when it does occur, this reaction can be near-fatal. It usually follows the first does or else develops within 48 hours of starting therapy (Ferner et al., 1987). In a large Swedish study, 77% of cases occurred within 3 weeks of starting the drug (Hedner et al., 1992). Emergency intravenous adrenaline may be required to relieve vocal cord edema. Lesser degrees of the same phenomenon may

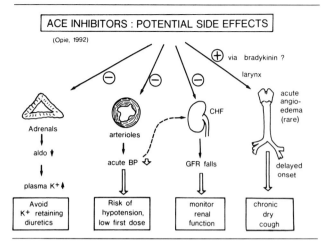

Figure 8–1. Potential side-effects of ACE inhibitors include cough, hypotension and renal impairment. To avoid hypotension, a low first test dose is usually given (see Fig. 8–2). CHF, congestive heart failure; aldo, aldosterone; GFR, glomerular filtration rate. Fig. © LH Opie.

occur after a delay. The mechanism of the angioedema seems to involve potentiation of the subcutaneous effects of bradykinin (Ferner et al., 1987).

Cough

Cough is probably the most common and, literally, the most irritating side-effect of ACE inhibitors. It is thought to occur in a variable percentage of the population from about 3% to 22%. In one retrospective study, the incidence was 43% (Reisin and Schneeweiss, 1992). Much depends on the method used to detect cough (Yeo and Ramsay, 1990). Not all patients are susceptible; rather it seems that there is a specific subgroup in whom ACE inhibitors increase the sensitivity of the cough reflex (McEwan et al., 1989).

"The cough usually starts with a tickling sensation in the throat and is persistent, dry and on occasions severe enough to cause vomiting" (Yeo and Ramsay, 1990). It seems as if the incidence of cough may have been grossly underestimated in some earlier studies, and it is not even commented on in the "quality of life" study by Croog et al. (1986) nor is it sufficiently frequently commented on in postmarketing surveys (Yeo and Ramsay, 1990). The incidence is greater in women than in men, and the onset of this side-effect may be delayed for up to 24 months after the onset of ACE inhibitor therapy (Yeo et al., 1991). Using a visual analog scale in a carefully controlled study, enalapril (mean daily dose 33 mg) had an incidence of associated cough of 29% versus 10% in nifedipine-treated patients, so that the excess incidence associated with enalapril was 19% (Yeo et al., 1991). In the same study, the incidence of cough assessed by spontaneous reporting was only 6%.

The mechanism remains poorly understood, but appears to be related to prostaglandin formation (McEwan et al., 1990), which in itself is thought to follow increased bradykinin activity. The relation of the cough to ACE inhibitor use is not always clear, the cough sometimes appearing at the start of therapy and sometimes later on (Yeo et al., 1991).

How should the cough be dealt with? The simplest is to persuade the patient to stay on the ACE inhibitor, as the cough may wane over 4 months in about half the cases (Reisin and Schneeweiss, 1992). A clinical impression is that switching from one ACE inhibitor to another may sometimes benefit, a practice that is supported by imperfect evidence (Coulter and Edwards, 1987; Goldszer et al., 1988; Lees et al., 1989).

While the addition of *sulindac* (200 mg daily) in two doses will limit the symptom of cough and inhibit the cough reflex (McEwan et al., 1990), the effect on blood pressure control may not be desirable. Sulindac, a nonsteroidal anti-inflammatory drug, may theoretically impair blood pressure control in patients treated by ACE inhibitors. Also, sulindac has a small risk of peptic ulcers.

Therefore, it is of interest that *inhaled sodium cromoglycate* gave benefit in an isolated case report (Keogh, 1993).

Hypotension

Hypotension is a feared complication of ACE inhibitor therapy reported both in patients with congestive heart failure (Webster et al., 1985) and also in severe hypertension, especially in those with high-renin values (Postma et al., 1992). Patients at risk include those with severe renal artery stenosis (Webster, 1987) or severe heart failure, especially if treated by high doses of diuretics. Patients over the age of 60 years are at greater risk of hypotension, presumably because of impaired circulatory reflexes. The current use of low test doses of ACE inhibitors, however, has substantially reduced the incidence of excess hypotension. In an outpatient setting, it is possible to give 6.25 mg captopril to patients, to observe the blood pressure for one or two hours, and then to go ahead with higher doses. A fall of mean blood pressure of more than 30% can be expected in 3% to 4% of patients (Postma et al., 1992). In hospital practice, a large prospective study on 599 patients with moderatly severe congestive heart failure (chiefly New York Heart Association Classes II and III) showed that only three experienced severe hypotension in response to an initial does of enalapril 2.5 mg, the maximum fall being 4 to 5 hours after the dose (Hasford et al., 1991).

In a comparative placebo-controlled study, the possible hypotensive effects of captopril (6.25 mg), enalapril (2.5 mg), and perindopril (2 mg) were compared in unselected elderly patients with congestive heart failure (MacFadyen et al., 1991). Captopril produced early hypotension, maximal at 1.5 hours, whereas enalapril decreased blood pressure maximally 4 to 5 hours after the dose, an effect still manifest at 10 hours (Fig. 8–2). Surprisingly, perindopril did not decrease the blood pressure when compared with control. Means of peak individual blood pressure falls were: placebo −16mmHg, perindopril −15mmHg, captopril −22mmHg, and enalapril −26mmHg. Because both

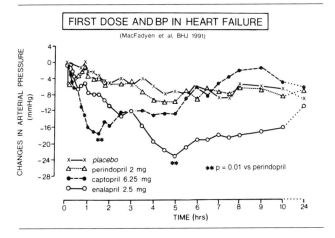

Figure 8–2. Effect of placebo, perindopril (2 mg), captopril (6.25 mg), and enalapril (2.5 mg) on blood pressure (BP) of elderly patients with congestive heart failure in a double-blind randomized parallel group study. Diuretic therapy had been withdrawn for 24 to 48 hours. Note similar fall of blood pressure with placebo and perindopril. Despite dissimilar effects on blood pressure, perindopril and enalapril produced similar degrees of inhibition of plasma ACE activity. Reproduced from MacFadyen et al. (1991) with permission.

perindopril and enalapril equally inhibited plasma ACE activity, the possibility was raised that changes in tissue and not plasma ACE were responsible for differences in the degree of hypotension resulting from these two agents. A further abstract from the same center confirmed a similar hypotension with the second dose of enalapril (p. 145). If the absence of first-dose hypotension with perindopril is confirmed in a larger series including younger patients and both genders, this agent could become the drug of choice for the initial therapy of congestive heart failure. Why perindopril differs from captopril and enalapril is not clear, because the active form, perindoprilat, decreases blood pressure as much as enalaprilat (MacFayden et al., 1993). Hypothetically, the parent drug, perindopril, interacts with the active diacid, perindoprilat, to delay the effect of the latter on tissue ACE activity.

The *mechanism* for the hypotension seems to involve venodilation (Capewell and Capewell, 1991). The absence of a compensatory tachycardia suggests a parasympathomimetic action (Webster, 1987), resembling vasovagal syncope.

Temporary exaggeration of renal failure

Renal failure as a class effect of ACE inhibitors is completely different from captopril-induced kidney damage (see Chapter 3). Found most commonly in heart failure and profoundly in the case of bilateral renal artery stenosis, the mechanism is that ACE inhibition removes efferent glomerular arteriolar tone and thereby decreases the glomerular filtration rate. In the presence of bilateral renal artery stenosis, renal blood flow is fixed, and compensation cannot occur. Sometimes a similar phenomenon occurs in the presence of unilateral renal artery stenosis especially when in a single kidney. In patients with severe congestive heart failure where the renal perfusion is bilaterally decreased, again a similar phenomenon can occur because of excess hypotension (Pierpont et al., 1981), so that the introduction of an ACE inhibitor may be followed by increasing blood urea and creatinine values which, if serious, would require reduction of the ACE inhibitor, as well as a temporary lessening of the diuretic dosage. The mechanism of the renal impairment can be related to the degree of arterial hypotension (Crozier et al., 1987), as also confirmed in CONSENSUS-I (Ljungman et al., 1992).

Practical policy. Thus, in severe congestive heart failure where renal function is already limited by poor renal blood flow, it may be a difficult decision to know whether or not to introduce ACE inhibitor therapy. The danger of exaggeration of the heart failure must be balanced against the possible benefit from an improved cardiac output and decreased renal afferent arteriolar vasoconstriction resulting from ACE inhibitor therapy. Problems can be expected especially when the glomerular filtration is already low and the renin-angiotensin axis highly stimulated (Ljungman et al., 1992). The best policy is to reduce the diuretic dose temporarily and to add the ACE inhibitor in very low doses and to work up, watching blood pressure, plasma creatinine, and urea. Provided that hypotension is avoided, it makes no difference whether a long-acting or short-acting ACE inhibitor is used (Osterziel et al., 1992).

Pre-existing renal failure. Sometimes ACE inhibitor therapy can precipitate temporary acute on chronic renal failure (Verbeelen and de Boel, 1984). The presumed mechanism is either the hypotensive effect or a reduction in efferent glomerular arteriolar tone.

Hyperkalemia

Because ACE inhibitors act to inhibit the release of aldosterone, they tend to increase plasma potassium. Hence, combination with potassium supplement therapy or potassium-containing diuretics may lead to hyperkalemia (Burnakis and Mioduch, 1984). Such combination therapy should, therefore, generally be avoided. For example, in the management of hypertension, it is not appropriate to combine an ACE inhibitor with hydrochlorothiazide-triamterene (Dyazide) or hydrochlorothiazide-amiloride (Moduretic) unless the measure plasma potassium is low.

SIDE-EFFECTS INITIALLY DESCRIBED WITH HIGH-DOSE CAPTOPRIL THERAPY

Neutropenia. Although most firmly linked to the use of high-dose captopril, it is of interest that the FDA-approved package inserts for nonsulfhydryl-containing agents, such as enalapril and quinapril, also mention the risk of neu-tropenia. Thus, there is a suggestion (but no proof) that such effects may be in part a class side-effect. It should be considered that the incidence of neutropenia is ex-tremely low and that the reported cases linking this con-dition to drugs such as enalapril are very few indeed and could have arisen by chance. Nonetheless, these conditions are listed in the package insert and attention must be paid to the possibility that there could also be very rare side-effects of nonsulfhydryl-containing ACE inhibitors.

Proteinuria. Proteinuria occurs in about 1% of patients re-ceiving captopril, especially in the presence of pre-existing renal disease or high doses of captopril (more than 150 mg/day) (Jenkins et al., 1985).

Impaired taste and buccal ulcers. Impaired taste is dose-related and was reported to occur in 2% to 7% of patients treated by captopril. Although it is still found, it now seems rare with the low doses of captopril currently used. Both apthous and tongue ulcers have occurred.

Scalded mouth syndrome. This very rare syndrome is de-scribed as being similar to scalding by very hot coffee or pizza. It is not specific to captopril and has been found with enalapril and lisinopril (Savino and Haushalter, 1992). It seems not to be related to impaired taste.

Precautions with high-dose captopril

Because the side-effects thought to be immune-based were largely found in patients with either collagen vascular dis-ease or already taking other drugs likely to alter the im-mune response, it may still be sensible to caution that all patients who may need high doses of captopril should have a pre-captopril renal evaluation, test for nuclear antibodies, and a white cell count. In practice, many physicians dis-pense with these precautions.

Captopril versus other agents

Should any of the above side-effects, thought to be im-mune-based, occur during captopril therapy, it would make sense cautiously to change to one of the nonsulfhy-dryl-containing agents. However, there is no assurance that the alternate agent would be totally free from any such side-effect, although commonsense would argue the case. In an interesting court decision in the United States, the manufacturers of nonsulfhydryl-containing agents without a significant incidence of any of the above side-effects were unable to refute the claims made by the manufacturers of captopril that there were, in fact, no true differences in the side-effect profiles of the two types of agents. The US pack-age inserts for drugs other than captopril suggest that neu-tropenia and renal damage might still occur, so the issue remains open.

Overdose

Several suicide attempts have been reported with prominent hypotension and sometimes oliguria (Jackson et al., 1993). Therapy consists of intravenous fluids, vasoconstrictors, calcium infusions, and atropine. When these have failed, an angiotensin infusion may be required (Jackson et al., 1993).

CONTRAINDICATIONS TO ACE INHIBITORS

Renal

From the possible renal complications, it follows that bilateral renal artery stenosis is a contraindication to the use of ACE inhibitors, as is unilateral renal artery stenosis in a solitary kidney. Severe congestive heart failure with much decreased glomerular filtration rate is a relative contraindication, as already outlined under side-effects.

Aortic stenosis and severe obstructive cardiomyopathy

ACE inhibitors acting as afterload reducing agents can increase the pressure gradient across the aortic valve or across the obstructed septum. ACE inhibitor therapy is therefore contraindicated in these conditions, unless very carefully given under close supervision, for example, if inoperable aortic stenosis is accompanied by left ventricular failure (Grace et al., 1991).

Pregnancy: prominent warning in US

There is now sound and solid evidence that ACE inhibitors given to the mother during the second and third trimesters of pregnancy are *embryopathic* and can result in severe fetal and neonatal problems, including renal failure, face or skull deformities, and pulmonary hypoplasia (Brent and Beckman, 1991; Hanssens et al., 1991; FDA, 1992). The US Food and Drug Administration now requires a boxed warning on the package. Pharmacists will place a sticker on the prescription bottle reading: "If you become pregnant, consult your doctor promptly about switching to a different drug." The FDA (1992) and Brent and Beckman (1991) state that there is no risk to the fetus from ACE inhibitors given only during the first trimester. Hanssens et al. (1991), however, review a few studies in which captopril and enalapril were stopped before 16 weeks of pregnancy, yet with adverse fetal or neonatal problems.

RELATIVE CONTRAINDICATIONS

Chronic cough

Because of the erratic incidence of cough as a side-effect of ACE inhibitor therapy, patients already coughing prior to the use of such agents should be treated with care. If the seriousness of the coughing augments during ACE inhibitor therapy, then the drug should be stopped, tailed off, or changed. *Asthma* or *bronchospasm* are rarely precipitated though not specific contraindications to ACE inhibitor therapy (Lunde et al., 1994).

Angina, severe congestive heart failure, and hypotension

The combination of heart failure with angina should theoretically be a good setting for the use of ACE inhibitors. The latter agents should relieve the load on the myocardium and thereby decrease the oxygen demand, indirectly relieving angina. The opposite was, however, found by Cleland et al. (1991) in a group of 18 severely ill patients with congestive heart failure and angina. The probable mechanism of the deterioration was failure of the blood pressure to increase during exercise. This adverse effect could be seen as a manifestation of ACE inhibitor-induced hypotension. Such severely ill patients need to be treated with care and caution. Surgical evaluation of the angina is required.

In the SOLVD studies (Chapter 5) on less severely ill patients, most with heart failure of ischemic origin, and about one-third with current angina, enalapril benefitted the group as a whole and lessened the development of unstable angina. Thus, in less critically ill patients also with congestive heart failure and angina, the ACE inhibitors can be used beneficially.

QUALITY OF LIFE

The landmark "quality of life" study by Croog et al. (1986) showed that patients taking captopril felt better and performed better than patients taking equieffective antihypertensive doses of methyldopa or propranolol. In particular, captopril-treated patients had fewer nervous system complaints, performed better sexually, and had a higher general wellbeing score. While it is by no means certain that captopril brought down the blood pressure (because there was no placebo group), this study nonetheless made a profound impact on the choice of an antihypertensive drug to such an extent that all antihypertensive agents now have to be evaluated for their effect on the "quality of life." Subsequently, an important study by Steiner et al. (1990) (see Table 2–5) showed that the quality of life with captopril, enalapril, and atenolol was essentially similar and better than that on propranolol. A reasonable hypothesis is that propranolol and methyldopa, centrally acting agents at least in part, have adverse effects on the quality of life, whereas the other agents do not. For example, the quality of life on enalapril is in reality no better than on placebo (TOMH Study, 1991), although there may be subsets of feelings in which enalapril benefits (Steiner et al., 1990).

Thus, it came as a surprise that Testa et al. (1993), on the basis of a large prospective study, proposed that captopril gave a better quality of life than enalapril. The mean doses used were not stated, but captopril was given as 25–50 mg twice daily and enalapril as 5–20 mg once daily; both top doses could be combined with hydrochlorothiazide. The largest difference in favor of captopril occurred in (1) the combination treatment groups, i.e., those with the least antihypertensive response to ACE inhibitors, but the numbers were not stated and the blood pressure was not given and (2) those with the best pretherapy quality of life (N = 71, for captopril; N = 53 for enalapril). The absence of concurrent blood pressure and quality of life data and full details of the exact doses used means that this study is difficult to assess, especially when compared with the Steiner study (1990), also on large groups of patients. In the latter study, captopril improved a depressed mood when compared with atenolol or propranolol, whereas enalapril gave a better (not worse) index of general health than captopril. It is difficult to avoid the platitude: "More studies are needed."

SUMMARY

In practice, the two major side-effects associated with ACE inhibitor therapy are cough and hypotension. The latter is a major problem in the management of congestive heart failure. Hypotension may be lessened by the use of low initial test doses and by reduction of the diuretic dose. There is evidence that the type of ACE inhibitor used may be important in avoiding first-dose hypotension.

The incidence of cough seems to be increasing in recent reports using more subtle means, such as visual analog analysis, to detect it. The onset of cough may be delayed for up to 24 months after the start of ACE inhibitor therapy. The simplest policy is to wait to see whether the cough spontaneously passes over, which occurs in about half the patients. Then, addition of sulindac or inhaled sodium cromoglycate may help.

Contraindications to ACE inhibitor therapy include bilateral renal artery stenosis, unilateral renal artery stenosis in a solitary kidney, significant aortic stenosis, severe obstructive cardiomyopathy, and pregnancy or risk thereof. Pre-existing chronic cough is a relative contraindication.

REFERENCES

Brent RL, Beckman DA. Angiotensin-converting enzyme inhibitors, an embryopathic class of drugs with unique properties: information for clinical teratology counselors. *Teratology* 1991; 43: 543–546.

Burnakis TG, Mioduch HJ. Combined therapy with captopril and potassium supplementation. A potential for hyperkalemia. *Arch Intern Med* 1984; 144: 2371–2372.

Capewell S, Capewell A. 'First dose' hypotension and venodilation. *Br J Clin Pharmacol* 1991; 31: 213–215.

Cleland JGF, Henderson E, McLenachan J, et al. Effect of captopril, an angiotensin-converting enzyme inhibitor, in patients with angina pectoris and heart failure. *J Am Coll Cardiol* 1991; 17: 733–739.

Coulter DM, Edwards IR. Cough associated with captopril and enalapril. *Br Med J* 1987: 294: 1521–1523.

Croog SH, Levine S, Testa MA, et al. The effect of antihypertensive therapy on the quality of life. *N Engl J Med* 1986; 314: 1657–1664.

Crozier IG, Ikram H, Nicholls G, Jans S. Acute hemodynamic, hormonal and electrolyte effects of ramipril in severe congestive heart failure. *Am J Cardiol* 1987; 59: 155D–163D.

Ferner RE, Simpson JM, Rawlins MD. Effects of intradermal bradykinin after inhibition of angiotensin converting enzyme. *Br Med J* 1987; 294: 1119–1120.

FDA (Food and Drug Administration) 1992. *Health and Human Services News*. Pregnancy warnings strengthened on ACE inhibitors (13 March 1992).

Goldszer RC, Lilly LS, Solomon HS. Prevalence of cough during angiotensin-converting enzyme inhibitor therapy. *Am J Med* 1988; 85: 887.

Grace AA, Brooks NH, Schofield PM. Beneficial effects of angiotensin-converting enzyme inhibition in severe symptomatic aortic stenosis (abstr). *Circulation* 1991; 84 (Suppl II): II–146.

Hanssens M, Keirse MJNC, Vankelcom F, Van Assche FA. Fetal and neonatal effects of treatment with angiotensin-converting enzyme inhibitors in pregnancy. *Obstet Gynecol* 1991; 78: 128–135.

Hasford J, Bussmann W-D, Delius W, et al. First dose hypotension with enalapril and prazosin in congestive heart failure. *Int J Cardiol* 1991; 31: 287–294.

Hedner T, Samuelsson O, Lunde H, et al. Angio-oedema in relation to treatment with angiotensin-converting enzyme inhibitors. *Br Med J* 1992; 304: 941–946.

Jackson T, Corke C, Agar J. Enalapril overdose treated with angiotensin infusion. *Lancet* 1993; 341: 703.

Jenkins AC, Dreslinski GR, Tadros SS, et al. Captopril in hypertension: seven years later. *J Cardiovasc Pharmacol* 1985; 7: S96–S101.

Keogh A. Sodium cromoglycate prophylaxis for angiotensin-converting enzyme inhibitor cough. *Lancet* 1993; 341: 560.

Lees KR, Reid JC, Scott MG, et al. Captopril versus perindopril: a double-blind study in essential hypertension. *J Human Hypertens* 1989; 3: 17–22.

Ljungman S, Kjekshus J, Swedberg K for the CONSENSUS Trial Group. Renal function in severe congestive heart failure during treatment with enalapril (the Cooperative North Scandinavian Enalapril Survival Study [CONSENSUS] Trial). *Am J Cardiol* 1992; 70: 479–487.

Lunde H, Hedner T, Samuelsson O, et al. Dyspnoea, asthma, and bronchospasm in relation to treatment with angiotensin-converting enzyme inhibitors. *Br Med J* 1994; 308: 18–21.

MacFadyen RJ, Lees KR, Reid JL. Differences in first dose response to ACE inhibition in congestive cardiac failure—a placebo-controlled study. *Br Heart J* 1991; 66: 206–211.

MacFadyen RJ, Lees KR, Reid JL. Double blind controlled study of low dose intravenous perindoprilat or enalaprilat infusion in elderly patients with heart failure. *BR Heart J* 1993; 69: 293–297.

McEwan JR, Choudry NB, Fuller RW. The effect of sulindac on the abnormal cough reflex associated with dry cough. *J Pharmacol Exp Ther* 1990; 255: 161–164.

McEwan JR, Choudry NB, Street R, Fuller RW. Change in cough reflex after treatment with enalapril and ramipril. *Br Med J* 1989; 299: 13–16.

Osterziel KJ, Dietz R, Harder K, Kubler W. Comparison of captopril with enalapril in the treatment of heart failure: influence on hemodynamics and measures of renal function. *Cardiovasc Drugs Ther* 1992: 6: 173–180.

Pierpont GP, Francis GS, Cohn JN. Effect of captopril on renal function in patients with congestive heart failure. *BR Heart J* 1981; 46: 522–527.

Postma CT, Dennesen PJW, de Boo T, Thien T. First dose hypotension after captopril: can it be predicted? A study of 240 patients. *J Human Hypertens* 1992; 6: 205–209.

Reid JL, MacFadyen RJ, Squire IB, Lees KR. Blood pressure response to the first doses of angiotensin-converting enzyme inhibitors in congestive heart failure. *Am J Cardiol* 1993; 71: 57E–60E.

Reisin L, Schneeweiss A. Complete spontaneous remission of cough induced by ACE inhibitors during chronic therapy in hypertensive patients. *J Human Hypertens* 1922; 6: 333–335.

Savino LB, Haushalter NM. Lisinopril-induced "scalded mouth syndrome." *Ann Pharmacother* 1992; 26: 1381–1382.

SOLVD Investigators. Effect of enalapril on survival in patients with reduced left ventricular ejection fractions and congestive heart failure. *N Engl J Med* 1991; 325: 293–302.

Steiner SS, Friedhoff AJ, Wilson BL, et al. Antihypertensive therapy and quality of life; a comparison of atenolol, captopril, enalapril and propranolol. *J Human Hypertens* 1990; 4: 217–225.

Testa MA, Anderson RB, Nackley JF, et al. Quality of life and antihypertensive therapy in men. A comparison of captopril with enalapril. *N Engl J Med* 1993; 328: 907–913.

Treatment of Mild Hypertension Research Group (TOMH). The treatment of mild hypertension study. A randomized, placebo-controlled trial of a nutritional-hygienic regimen along with various drug monotherapies. *Arch Intern Med* 1991; 151: 1413–1423.

Verbeelen DL, de Boel S. Reversible acute on chronic renal failure during captopril treatment. *Br Med J* 1984; 289: 20–21.

Webster J. Angiotensin converting enzyme inhibitors in the clinic: first-dose hypotension. *J Hypertens* 1987; 5 (Suppl 3): S27–S30.

Webster J, Petrie JC, Robb OJ, et al. A comparison of single doses of bucindolol and oxprenolol in hypertensive patients. *Br J Clin Pharmacol* 1985; 20: 393–400.

Yeo WW, Ramsay LE. Persistent dry cough with enalapril: incidence depends on method used. *J Human Hypertens* 1990; 4: 517–520.

Yeo WW, MacLean D, Richardson PJ, Ramsay LE. Cough and enalapril: assessment by spontaneous reporting and visual analogue scale under double-blind conditions. *Br J Clin Pharmacol* 1991; 31: 356–359.

CHAPTER 9

ACE Inhibitors: Drug Combinations and Interactions

Increasing use of ACE inhibitors has led to consideration of possible combinations with other antihypertensive agents, such as beta-blockers, diuretics, and calcium antagonists. The combination of ACE inhibitors with diuretics is well established and that with calcium antagonists is coming to be accepted practice. Combination with beta-blockade is not yet, however, into the realm of standard practice.

Beta-Blockers

Based on the experience with captopril, it has been commonly thought that beta-blockade added to ACE inhibition might not be an optimal combination in the therapy of hypertension. ACE inhibitors decrease the renin-angiotensin axis through inhibition of the angiotensin-converting enzyme, and beta-blockers act on the same axis by inhibition of renin release. Thus, the addition of beta-blockers to the ACE inhibitor captopril is less effective than diuretic addition (Staessen et al., 1983). It is, therefore, somewhat surprising that a detailed study adding propranolol to the ACE inhibitor cilazapril showed an additive antihypertensive effect (Belz et al., 1989). On the whole, the blood pressure reduction with cilazapril and with propranolol was very similar, and the combination produced approximately additive effects, the drugs being given in doses of 2.5 mg cilazapril and 120 mg propranolol once daily. With cilazapril, the peripheral vascular resistance fell, and the cardiac output rose; opposite changes were found with propranolol and, with the combination, there was no change in either parameter suggesting a hemodynamically ideal combination.

An *important reservation* to the study by Belz et al. (1989), is that blood pressure measurements were made about 2 hours after drug ingestion; confirmation of the additive antihypertensive effect over 24 hours is required by ambulatory blood pressure measurements. Although the combination of ACE inhibitors and beta-blockers still cannot generally be recommended (MacGregor et al., 1985), the cilazapril study by Belz et al. (1989) raises the possibility that careful reevaluation will show that these two types of agents are, after all, additive.

DIURETICS

Advantages of an ACE inhibitor plus diuretic

In the *therapy of hypertension,* the potential advantages of combining diuretics with ACE inhibitors have been succinctly outlined by Johnston (1985). The blood pressure lowering capacity of diuretics is limited by a reactive hyperreninemia (Fig. 9–1). Therefore, the combination with ACE inhibitor therapy becomes logical, and the response rate to the combination is high, possibly over 80% (Degaute et al., 1992). Taking a standard dose of an ACE inhibitor, for example 5 mg ramipril, and doubling it is less effective in reducing the blood pressure than adding a diuretic, hydrochlorothiazide 25 mg daily (Heidbreder et al., 1992).

Second, *in black patients with hypertension,* often held to be a low-renin group, the response to ACE inhibition alone is poor, but the sensitivity is restored by combination with a diuretic (Veterans Administration Cooperative Study Group on Antihypertensive Agents, 1982).

Third, ACE inhibitors decrease the effect of angiotensin-II in releasing aldosterone, so that secondary hyperaldosteronism is lessened with a consequent tendency to potassium retention. Thiazide diuretics, on the other hand, promote potassium loss. Specifically, hydrochlorothiazide

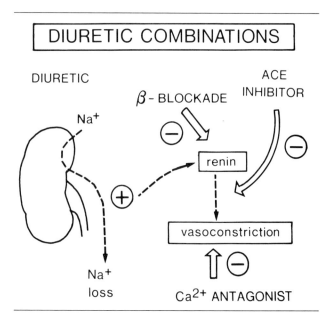

Figure 9–1. Theoretical basis for beneficial interaction between diuretics and ACE inhibitors in the therapy of hypertension. Fig. © LH Opie.

25 mg decreased the mean potassium concentration by 0.47 mmol/L, whereas the addition of ramipril 2.5 to 10 mg almost eliminated the fall (Scholze et al., 1993).

Fourth, the effects of thiazide diuretics in increasing blood uric acid and blood sugar are diminished by concurrent therapy with ACE inhibitors (Weinberger, 1982).

In *heart failure*, ACE inhibitors potentiate the natriuresis of diuretics. Conversely, addition of diuretics to ACE inhibitor therapy lessens the dose of ACE inhibitor required.

Disadvantages of the combination ACE inhibitor-diuretic

First, when there is marked salt retention, there tends to be a considerable reactive hyperreninemia, so that the ACE inhibitor can cause a serious hypotensive first-dose effect. This problem can be overcome by giving a very low first dose of the ACE inhibitor as a test dose, for example 6.25 mg of captopril.

Second, the addition of an ACE inhibitor to a diuretic may decrease the glomerular filtration rate with an increase in the plasma creatinine level, particularly in patients with resistant heart failure (Cleland et al., 1988) or in those with severe hypertension and a fixed renal vascular resistance as in the case of bilateral renal artery stenosis. Thus, patients with severe congestive heart failure need monitoring for some days after the addition of ACE inhibitor therapy and careful dose titration.

Third, when combined with potassium-sparing diuretics or potassium supplements, there is danger of hyperkalemia (Textor et al., 1982). The ideal diuretic to be combined with an ACE inhibitor should not have any potassium-retaining qualities nor built-in or added potassium supplementation (Burnakis and Mioduch, 1984). A standard combination for hypertension could be the usual dose of the ACE inhibitor together with 12.5 mg hydrochlorothiazide daily.

Interaction between ACE inhibitors and diuretics

Captopril—furosemide. There appears to be a specific inhibitory effect of captopril on the diuretic action of furosemide (Toussaint et al., 1989) not shared by ramipril nor enalapril. The mechanism is that captopril interferes with the renal tubular excretion of furosemide. It is this negative interaction that may explain why captopril 1 mg allows a greater diuresis than captopril 25 mg when combined with furosemide (Motwani et al., 1992). Thus, if these agents are given together in standard doses, the times of administration should be spaced.

Captopril—spironolactone. Low doses of captopril may be successfully combined with furosemide and with spironolactone in patients with severe heart failure (Dahlstrom and Karlsson, 1993) despite potential hyperkalemia. This combination may be particularly useful when captopril causes excess hypotension and the dose must be limited.

CALCIUM ANTAGONISTS

Since the initial report by Guazzi et al. (1984), the combination ACE inhibitor/calcium antagonist has been widely used (Fig. 9–2). Calcium antagonists, being vasodilators, tend to increase plasma renin and, therefore, combination with an ACE inhibitor is theoretically sound. Second, ACE inhibitors are better at reducing the blood pressure than calcium antagonists in the lower hypertensive ranges, whereas the reverse is the case in more severe hypertension (Herpin et al., 1992). Furthermore, calcium antagonists of the nifedipine group (dihydropyridines) tend to have a diuretic effect that, again, should combine well with ACE inhibition. Of considerable interest is that diuresis and natriuresis can be invoked by the addition of the calcium antagonist isradipine to captopril (Krusell et al., 1992). Because the efficacy of ACE inhibitors is so dependent on the sodium status (see Fig. 2–2), combining an ACE inhibitor with a calcium antagonist may theoretically have the same improved hypotensive effect as adding a diuretic. More definitive studies are required to clarify this issue.

Thus, nitrendipine and captopril have a synergistic action in the therapy of hypertension (Gennari et al., 1989). Also of interest is the lessening of the tachycardia induced by felodipine during concurrent ACE inhibitor therapy by ramipril (Bainbridge et al., 1991) in keeping with the proposed sympatho-inhibitory effect of ACE inhibitors.

In *hypertension with chronic renal failure,* the combination of nitrendipine and cilazapril reduces blood pressure more than either agent alone (Kloke et al., 1989).

In *diabetic hypertensive nephropathy with microalbuminuria,* the

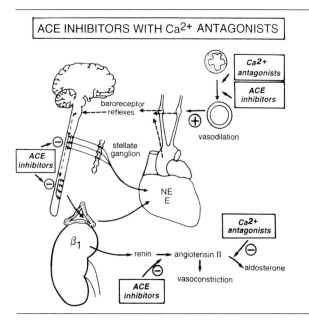

Figure 9–2. *Mechanisms for additive arteriolar dilation induced by calcium antagonists and ACE inhibitors. The latter inhibit two consequences of acute vasodilation: (1) the reflex baroreceptor stimulation and (2) the indirect activation of the renin-angiotensin system. See also Figure 1–9. Fig. © LH Opie.*

combination of verapamil with either cilazapril or lisinopril lessens microalbuminuria more than either agent alone and apparently does so independent of blood pressure changes (see Chapter 12).

More tantalizing are possible long-term preventative effects of the combination, as both ACE inhibitors and calcium antagonists have been claimed to (1) decrease experimental atherosclerosis and (2) improve arterial wall compliance.

As the early studies showing the benefit of captopril-nifedipine combinations used two drugs with relatively short action (Singer et al., 1987), the current tests are to assess the combination of long-acting calcium antagonists together with long-acting ACE inhibitors—an example would be the combination of amlodipine with perindopril or ramipril.

ALPHA-BLOCKERS

Clinically, both alpha$_1$-adrenoceptor blockers and ACE inhibitors are capable of first-dose hypotension. There appears to be an enhancement by an ACE inhibitor of the first-dose hypotension caused by an alpha-blocker (Baba et al., 1990). Experimentally, enalaprilat can nearly double the effect of the alpha$_1$-blocker, doxazosin, on the rat tail artery (Marwood et al., 1991). Thus far the potentially additive antihypertensive effect of the combination ACE inhibitor-alpha$_1$-blocker has apparently not been explored. As both categories of drugs have favorable or neutral metabolic effects, the combination is worthy of testing.

DIGOXIN

Despite earlier data suggesting that captopril increases serum digoxin by about one-quarter (Cleland et al., 1986), a further study showed no effect of captopril on digoxin kinetics (Miyakawa et al., 1991). Also, neither ramipril nor lisinopril altered digoxin levels in volunteers (Morris et al., 1985; Doering et al., 1987), nor did perindopril alter digoxin levels or kinetics in patients with heart failure (Vandenburg et al., 1993). To reconcile these apparently conflicting data, it should be considered that the study of Cleland et al. (1986) was conducted on patients with severe heart failure, whereas the other studies were on normal volunteers or on patients with mild heart failure. In severe heart failure, captopril is more likely to cause renal impairment with a secondary rise in digoxin levels. Thus, in considering the possible interaction between ACE inhibitors and digoxin, it is important to monitor renal function.

NONSTEROIDAL ANTI-INFLAMMATORY AGENTS

In *hypertension*, it is known that nonsteroidal anti-inflammatory drugs (NSAIDs) can blunt the antihypertensive effect of most agents, including ACE inhibitors (Fig. 9–3). The

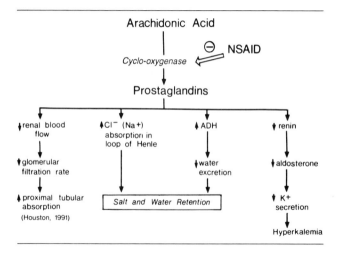

Figure 9–3. Proposed mechanism whereby NSAIDs block cyclo-oxygenase pathway and thereby inhibit formation of vasodilatory prostaglandins. Ultimately salt and water retention decreases the effects of almost all antihypertensives. In addition, NSAIDs decrease renin and aldosterone through an entirely different mechanism. For references, see Houston (1991). Modified from Houston (1991) with permission.

mechanism may include lessened formation of vasodilatory prostaglandins (Witzgall et al., 1982). These agents do not all have the same effects and indomethacin and naproxen appear more consistently to cause a blood pressure increase than sulindac or ibuprofen (Pope et al., 1993). Indomethacin (50 mg twice daily) added to ACE inhibitor therapy in several double-blind trials variably lessened the antihypertensive effect by 3% to 34% (Salvetti, 1990; Abdel-Haq et al., 1991).

Whereas the effects of NSAIDs in decreasing with the control of blood pressure are now well accepted, it is generally less well known that these agents can interfere with the hemodynamic status in congestive heart failure. Acute administration of indomethacin decreased cardiac index, increased left ventricular filling pressure, and increased arterial pressure and systemic vascular resistance in patients with congestive heart failure and hyponatremia (Dzau et al., 1984). The effects of the NSAIDs in lowering renin and decreasing aldosterone can be dissociated from effects on the blood pressure (Houston, 1991). More detailed studies of the interactions between NSAIDs and ACE inhibitors are required.

ASPIRIN

When aspirin (350 mg) was combined with enalapril (10 mg daily), the ACE inhibitor was much less vasodilatory, and the left ventricular filling pressure no longer improved (Hall et al., 1992). Thus, not only NSAIDs but aspirin may also impair the hemodynamic effect of ACE inhibition in heart failure.

LITHIUM

ACE inhibitors may increase blood lithium levels and the risk of toxicity, according to US package inserts. In normal volunteers, however, lithium levels rose in only one of nine subjects after the addition of enalapril (DasGupta et al., 1992). Conceivably, in patients with renal impairment, the ACE inhibitors are more likely to increase lithium levels.

PROBENECID

Many of the ACE inhibitors are organic acids and, therefore, excreted both by glomerular filtration and renal tubular secretion. Probenecid decreases the excretion of captopril and leads to higher blood levels (Singhvi et al., 1982). This possible interaction presumably holds for all ACE inhibitors that are organic acids (and most of them are). An exception is the new ACE inhibitor, fosinopril, which is a sodium salt and another new ACE inhibitor, zofenopril, which is a calcium salt (Kostis, 1989).

INTERACTION WITH DIABETIC THERAPY

ACE inhibitors are thought to improve insulin sensitivity (Chapter 11). Hence, in patients with type II diabetes receiving oral antidiabetic therapy, there is the risk of additive effects of ACE inhibitor therapy leading to symptomatic hypoglycemia (Arauz-Pacheco et al., 1990). The mechanism could include a reduction in glomerular function induced by ACE inhibitor therapy (Buller and Perazella, 1991). To avoid such interactions, it is appropriate to recheck blood sugar levels whenever ACE inhibitors are added to oral hypoglycemics.

SUMMARY

ACE inhibitors have been combined with virtually all other classes of antihypertensive drugs, especially with diuretics. ACE inhibitors blunt the hypokalemic effect of standard diuretics but should not normally be combined with potassium-retaining diuretics.

ACE inhibitors are subject to relatively few adverse drug interactions. Captopril interferes with the diuretic effect of furosemide in healthy volunteers and captopril also increases serum digoxin. Neither of these effects appear to be shared by some of the other ACE inhibitors. Nonsteroidal anti-inflammatory agents lessen the antihypertensive effect of ACE inhibitors; indomethacin appears to be particularly potent in this regard. Not only is the antihypertensive effect of ACE inhibitors blunted by NSAIDs, but the beneficial effect in heart failure may be overcome. In addition, aspirin impairs the vasodilatory effects of ACE inhibition in patients with heart failure.

REFERENCES

Abdel-Haq B, Magagna A, Favilla S, Salvetti A. Hemodynamic and humoral interactions between perindopril and indomethacin in essential hypertensive subjects. *J Cardiovasc Pharmacol* 1991; 18 (Suppl 7): S33–S36.

Arauz-Pacheco C, Ramirez LC, Rios JM, Raskin P. Hypoglycemia induced by angiotensin-converting enzyme inhibitors in patients with non-insulin-dependent diabetes receiving sulfonylurea therapy. *Am J Med* 1990; 89: 811–813.

Baba T, Tomiyama T, Takebe K. Enhancement of an ACE inhibitor of first-dose hypotension caused by an alpha$_1$-blocker. *N Engl J Med* 1990; 322: 1237.

Bainbridge AD, MacFadyen RJ, Lees KR, Reid JL. A study of the acute pharmacodynamic interaction of ramipril and felodipine in normotensive subjects. *Br J Clin Pharmacol* 1991; 31: 148–153.

Belz GG, Breithaupt K, Erb K, et al. Influence of the angiotensin-converting enzyme inhibitor cilazapril, the beta-blocker propranolol and their combination on haemodynamics in hypertension. *J Hypertens* 1989; 7: 817–824.

Buller GK, Perazella M. ACE inhibitor-induced hypoglycemia. *Am J Med* 1991; 91: 104–105.

Burnakis TG, Mioduch HJ. Combined therapy with captopril and potassium supplementation. A potential for hyperkalemia. *Arch Intern Med* 1984; 144: 2371–2372.

Cleland JGF, Dargie HJ, Pettigrew A, et al. The effects of captopril on serum digoxin and urinary urea and digoxin clearances in patients with congestive heart failure. *Am Heart J* 1986; 112: 130–135.

Cleland JGF, Gillen G, Dargie HJ. The effects of frusemide and angiotensin-converting enzyme inhibitors and their combination on cardiac and renal haemodynamics in heart failure. *Eur Heart J* 1988; 9: 132–141.

Dahlstrom U, Karlsson E. Captopril and spironolactone therapy for refractory congestive heart failure. *Am J Cardiol* 1993; 71: 29A–33A.

DasGupta K, Jefferson JW, Kobak KA, Greist JH. The effect of enalapril on serum lithium levels in healthy men. *J Clin Psychiatry* 1992; 53: 398–400.

Degaute J-P, Leeman M, Desche P. Long-term acceptability of perindopril: European Multicenter Trial on 858 patients. *Am J Med* 1992; Suppl 4B: 84S–89S.

Doering W, Maass L, Irmisch R, Konig E. Pharmacokinetic interaction study with ramipril and digoxin in healthy volunteers. *Am J Cardiol* 1987; 59: 60D–64D.

Dzau VJ, Packer M, Lilly LS, et al. Prostaglandins in severe congestive heart failure. Relation to activation of the renin-angiotensin system and hyponatremia. *N Engl J Med* 1984; 310: 347–352.

Gennari C, Nami R, Pavese G, et al. Calcium-channel blockade (nitrendipine) in combination with ACE inhibition (captopril) in the treatment of mild to moderate hypertension. *Cardiovasc Drugs Ther* 1989; 3: 319–325.

Guazzi MD, De Cesare N, Galli C, et al. Calcium-channel blockade with nifedipine and angiotensin-converting enzyme inhibition with captopril in the therapy of patients with severe primary hypertension. *Circulation* 1984; 70: 279–284.

Hall D, Zeitler H, Rudolph W. Counteraction of the vasodilator effects of enalapril by aspirin in severe heart failure. *J Am Coll Cardiol* 1992; 20: 1549–1555.

Heidbreder D, Froer K-L, Breitstadt A, et al. Combination of ramipril and hydrochlorothiazide in the treatment of mild to moderate hypertension: Part I—a double-blind, comparative, multicenter study in nonresponders to ramipril monotherapy. *Clin Cardiol* 1992; 15: 904–910.

Herpin D, Vaisse B, Pitiot M, et al. Comparison of angiotensin-converting enzyme inhibitors and calcium antagonists in the treatment of mild to moderate systemic hypertension, according to baseline ambulatory blood pressure level. *Am J Cardiol* 1992; 69: 923–926.

Houston MC. Nonsteroidal anti-inflammatory drugs and antihypertensives. *Am J Med* 1991; 90 (Suppl 5A): 42S–47S.

Johnston CI. Drug interactions. *ACE Report* 15, April 1985, 1–5.

Kloke JH, Huysmans FThM, Wetzels JFM, et al. Antihypertensive effects of nitrendipine and cilazapril alone, and in combination in hypertensive patients with chronic renal fialure. *Br J Clin Pharmacol* 1989; 27: 289S–296S.

Kostis JB. Angiotensin-converting enzyme inhibitors. Emerging differences and new compounds. *Am J Hypertens* 1989; 2: 57–64.

Krusell LR, Sihm I, Jespersen LT, et al. Combined actions of isradipine and captopril on renal function in hypertension. *J Human Hypertens* 1992; 6: 401–407.

MacGregor GA, Markandu ND, Smith SJ, Sagnella GA. Captopril: contrasting effects of adding hydrochlorothiazide, propranolol, or nifedipine. *J Cardiovasc Pharmacol* 1985; 7 (Suppl 1): S82–S87.

Marwood J, Tierney G, Stokes G. Interactions between enalaprilat and doxazosin at rat tail artery alpha$_1$-adrenoceptors. *J Cardiovasc Pharmacol* 1991; 17: 1–7.

Miyakawa T, Shionoiri H, Takasaki I, et al. The effect of captopril on pharmacokinetics of digoxin in patients with mild congestive heart failure. *J Cardiovasc Pharmacol* 1991; 17: 576–581.

Morris FP, Tamrazian S. Marks C, et al. An acute pharmacokinetic study of the potential interaction of lisinopril and digoxin in normal volunteers. *Br J Clin Pharmacol* 1985; 20: 281P–282P.

Motwani JG, Fenwick MK, Morton JJ, Struthers AD. Furosemide-induced natriuresis is augmented by ultra low-dose captopril but not by standard doses of captopril in chronic heart failure. *Circulation* 1992; 86: 439–445.

Pope JE, Anderson JJ, Felson DT. A meta-analysis of the effects of nonsteroidal anti-inflammatory drugs on blood pressure. *Arch Intern Med* 1993; 153: 477–484.

Salvetti A. Newer ACE inhibitors. A look at the future. *Drugs* 1990; 40: 800–828.

Scholze J for the East Germany Collaborative Trial Group. Short report: ramipril and hydrochlorothiazide combination therapy in hypertension: a clinical trial of factorial design. *J Hypertens* 1993; 11: 217–221.

Singer DRJ, Markandu ND, Shore AC, MacGregor GA. Captopril and nifedipine in combination for moderate to severe essential hypertension. *Hypertension* 1987; 9: 629–633.

Singhvi SM, Duchin KL, Willard DA, et al. Renal handling of captopril: effect of probenecid. *Clin Pharmacol Ther* 1982; 32: 182–189.

Staessen J, Fagard R, Lignen P, et al. A double-blind comparison between propranolol and bendroflumethiazide in captopril treated resistant hypertensive patients. *Am Heart J* 1983; 106: 321–328.

Textor SC, Bravo EL, Fouad FM, et al. Hyperkalaemia in azotemic patients during angiotensin-converting enzyme inhibition and aldosterone reduction with captopril. *Am J Med* 1982; 73: 719–725.

Toussaint C, Masselink A, Gentges A, et al. Interference of different ACE inhibitors with the diuretic action of furosemide and hydrochlorothiazide. *Klin Wochenschr* 1989; 67: 1138–1146.

Vandenburg MJ, Stephens J, Resplandy G, et al. Digoxin pharmacokinetics and perindopril in heart failure patients. *J Clin Pharmacol* 1993; 33: 146–149.

Veterans Administration Cooperative Study Group on Antihypertensive Agents. Captopril: evaluation of low doses, twice-daily doses and the addition of diuretic for the treatment of mild to moderate hypertension. *Clin Sci* 1982; 63 (Suppl 8): 443S–445S.

Weinberger MH. Comparison of captopril and hydrochlorothiazide alone and in combination in mild to moderate essential hypertension. *Br J Clin Pharmacol* 1982; 14: 127–131.

Witzgall H, Hirsch F, Scherer B, Weber PC. Acute haemodynamic and hormonal effects of captopril are diminished by indomethacin. *Clin Sci* 1982; 62: 611–615.

CHAPTER 10

ACE Inhibitors, Vascular Structure, and Arterial Disease in Hypertension

"The increased wall/lumen ratio of the resistance vessels. . . .appears to be crucial for both creating and maintaining true hypertension" (Folkow et al., 1973)

"From cardiac to vascular protection: the next chapter" (The Lancet, 1992)

Until recently, the role of the arterial bed in hypertension was relatively neglected in comparison with the attention given to control of the hypertension itself and the prevention of cardiac and coronary complications. Now a series of recent experiments have focused on vascular disease as a crucial component of hypertension in conformity with the current knowledge that the major benefit thus far achieved in treating the condition has been in reduction of vascular mortality and morbidity, especially in the elderly (Staessen et al., 1990).

Some crucial new concepts are the following. First, it is now recognized that the endothelium has an incredibly active role in controlling vascular tone of normal arterioles. The endothelium is readily damaged by hypertension thus initiating and promoting the process of atherosclerosis. Second, the adverse consequences of vascular smooth muscle hypertrophy and the associated increase in peripheral vascular resistance is now becoming well established. Third, processes leading to degeneration of the matrix of the vascular wall and especially the increase in the collagen/elastin ratio and consequent loss of elasticity lead to altered compliance and properties of the large conduit vessels with, hypothetically, adverse consequences for the arteriolar resistance vessels. Fourth, relatively nonspecific arterial disease, such as that found in ageing or in atherosclerosis, is intimately associated with the hypertensive process and the damages of hypertension on the vascular bed.

This chapter will first review arterial physiology, then discuss the reaction of the arterioles to hypertension, then that of the large conduit arteries, and then propose a hypothesis on the role of the large conduit arteries in perpetuating and increasing the severity of hypertension.

Thereafter the potential role of ACE inhibitors in controlling vascular disease will be critically assessed.

ARTERIAL PHYSIOLOGY

As arterial disease is the basis of ischemic heart disease and hypertensive renal disease and contributes to the deleterious influences of hypertension and ageing on the cerebral circulation, the nature of such arterial disease must be understood before considering the possible protective effects of ACE inhibitors and other antihypertensive treatments on vascular disease. Arterial disease adversely affects the function of normal intima and media and influences a variety of cell types such as the endothelium, the smooth muscle cells, and the elastin and collagen fibers of the matrix. Hence, it is necessary first to review vascular physiology as an introduction to an analysis of three types of vascular damage: (1) endothelial and subintimal disease; (2) medial hypertrophy in response to the increased intraluminal pressure of hypertension; and (3) end-stage arterial disease, which is the dilated stiff and often calcified arterial wall, an end-product of ageing and accelerated by hypertension.

Endothelial structure and function

Arteries consist of three basic layers: the intima, the media, and the adventitia (Fig. 10–1). Each of these can be adversely influenced by hypertension. The endothelium (Fig. 10–2) is the crucial structure in the intimal layer; it consists of a monolayer of thin cells, highly metabolically active in the control of the circulation which it achieves by the production of numerous vasoactive compounds including (1)

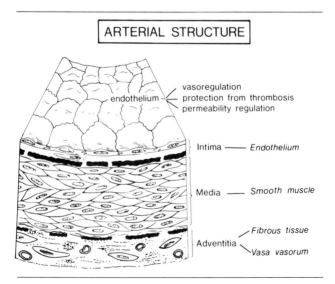

Figure 10–1. Histological structure of normal muscular artery, emphasizing different roles of endothelium, smooth muscle cells and fibrous tissue. Modified with permission from Ross and Glomset (1976).

endothelium-derived relaxation factor (EDRF) now known to be nitric oxide; (2) endothelin that acts to vasoconstrict; and (3) the synthesis of angiotensin-I and possibly angiotensin-II (Veltmar et al., 1991). Some of these important functions are listed in Table 10–1.

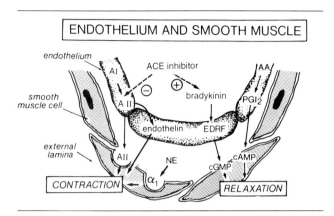

Figure 10–2. *Role of endothelium in producing vasoconstrictor agents including angiotensin-II and endothelin, as well as vasorelaxing agents such as endothelium-derived relaxation factor (EDRF) and prostacyclin (PGI$_2$). ACE, angiotensin-converting enzyme; AI, angiotensin-I; AII, angiotensin-II; α_1, alpha$_1$-adrenergic receptor; NE, norepinephrine; AA, arachidonic acid; cGMP, cyclic GMP; cAMP, cyclic AMP. Fig. © LH Opie.*

TABLE 10–1 PROPOSED FUNCTIONS OF VASCULAR ENDOTHELIUM

1. **Release of vasoactive agents**

   EDRF (endothelium-derived relaxation factor)
   Endothelin
   Angiotensin-I (and possibly angiotensin-II)
   Prostacyclin, thromboxane

2. **Prevention of coagulation**

   Thromboresistant surface
   Formation of antiaggregant prostacyclin

3. **Immune function**

   Supply of antigens to immunocompetent cells
   Secretion of interleukin-I (a T cell inducer)

4. **Enzymatic activity**

   Angiotensin converting enzyme (conversion of angiotensin-I to angiotensin-II)

5. **Growth signal to vascular smooth muscle**

   EDGF secretion (endothelium-derived growth factor)
   Heparin-like inhibitors of growth

6. **Protection of vascular smooth muscle from vasoconstrictory influences**

   Requirement of endothelial integrity for some vasodilator stimuli such as acetylcholine

The concept is that the endothelium is in fact a very active organ, constantly synthesizing and releasing a variety of molecules that can all contribute to the regulation of arterial tone. "The endothelium appears to serve as a mechanoreceptor within the vasculature that senses flow or pressure and modulates vascular tone accordingly" (Gibbons and Dzau, 1990).

Besides these functions, the endothelium protects the arterioles from a number of vasoconstrictory influences, such as serotonin released from damaged platelets. A classic observation made by Furchgott and Zawadzki (1980) was that endothelial integrity was required for acetylcholine, the messenger of parasympathetic activity, to exert its physiologic vasodilatory activity. When endothelial integrity was lost, then acetylcholine became vasoconstrictory. *Thus, endothelial damage can change a vasodilatory stimulus into a vasoconstrictory stimulus* (Vanhoutte, 1989). Following this argument further, the endothelium can be damaged, for example by hypertensive mechanical stress when it is likely to lose its vasodilatory role and to become a vasoconstrictor tissue. Speculatively, hypertensive damage to the endothelium could release vasoconstrictory endothelin or inhibit the release of vasodilatory nitric oxide that could, in turn, increase peripheral vascular resistance and exaggerate the severity of hypertension.

Subendothelial tissue. Endothelial cells rest on a basement membrane, separated from smooth muscle cells by the internal elastic lamina. This consists of sheets of elastic fibers with openings large enough to allow the permeation of metabolites, growth factors, and cells in either direction. In early vascular disease, the intima proliferates and smooth muscle cells from the tunica media move into the lesion to contribute to the developing plaque (Fig. 10–3).

Tunica media and vascular smooth muscle cells

This is the middle layer of the arterial wall (see Fig. 10–1) which basically consists of smooth muscle cells lying within a connective tissue matrix. Thus, the two major components of the medial layer are (1) the smooth muscle cell that upon appropriate stimulation contracts to narrow the diameter of ther arterial wall, and (2) the supporting matrix that binds the muscle cells into bundles and keeps them in the correct orientation in the arterial wall. In the *small muscular arterioles* ("small bore arteries," diameter less than 1 mm), it is these smooth muscle cells that respond to a rise of cytosolic calcium concentration by contracting and thereby decreasing the diameter of the arterioles, which increases the peripheral vascular resistance and causes the blood pressure to rise.

One proposal for the origin of hypertension is that the peripheral vascular resistance is abnormally increased because

$$BP = CO \times PVR$$

where BP is blood pressure, CO is cardiac output, and PVR is peripheral vascular resistance. The cause of the increased

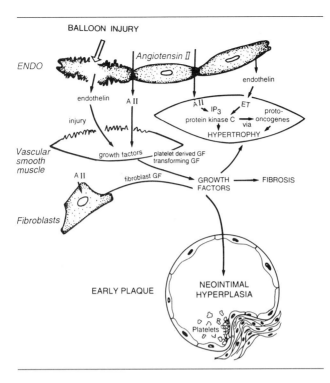

Figure 10–3. *Proposed role of endothelium in response to vascular wall injury. Note role of growth factors (GF) which are also stimulated by angiotensin-II (AII). ET, endothelin; IP$_3$, inositol trisphosphate. Fig. © LH Opie.*

PVR in hypertension could be an excess of vasoconstrictory stimuli, such as alpha$_1$-adrenergic activity and angiotensin-II whether circulating or locally formed. Alternatively, an increased cytosolic calcium could indirectly originate from sodium pump inhibition as a result of the activity of the proposed circulating "natriuretic hormone." Alternatively, there could be a lack of vasodilatory stimulation, such as decreased cholinergic activity.

The *matrix* of the medial layer is that component which determines to a major extent, together with the adventitia, the mechanical properties of the artery. First, the ratio of matrix to muscle cells varies. In the large conduit arteries, like the aorta and its major branches, elastin is the most important component of the matrix and in the largest vessels, such as the aorta, the major component of the arterial wall (Table 10–2). It is the elastin in the aortic wall that allows the aorta to expand in systole as blood is rapidly ejected from the left ventricle, then in diastole the elastic recoil helps to propel the blood flow onwards and hence to maintain the diastolic blood pressure (Fig. 10–4). This is the "pressure-equalizing" function of the elastic layer.

The elasticity of elastin is explained by its hydrophobic properties. When relaxed, crucial hydrophobic regions have minimal contact with the surrounding water of the extracellular space. When stretched, contact with water increases, and the hydrophobic area reacts in such a way that the fibers return to their original length. The synthesis of

TABLE 10–2 DIFFERENCES BETWEEN PROPERTIES OF COMPONENTS OF THE ARTERIAL TREE

	Number	Diameter	Wall thickness	Predominant structure	Function
Aorta	1	2–3 cm	2–3 mm	Elastin	Conduction
Large and mid-sized arteries	10^2	3–8 mm	0.5–1 mm	Muscle	Distribution
Small arteries	10^3	0.5–3 mm	0.5–1 mm	Muscle	Distribution
Arterioles	10^6	10–100 μm	10–100 μm	Muscle	Resistance
Capillaries	10^{10}	4–10 μm	1–3 μm	Endothelium	Exchange

From Camilleri et al. (1989) with permission.

| CONDUIT ARTERIES AS PRESSURE BUFFERS |

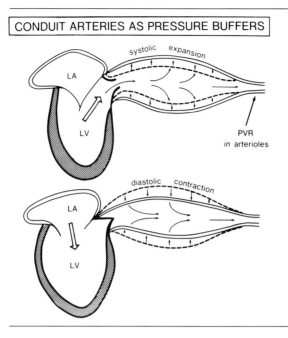

Figure 10–4. The "pressure-equalizing" or "buffering" function of
the aorta. During ventricular systole the stroke volume ejected by the
ventricle results in some forward capillary flow, but most of the
ejected volume is stored in the elastic arteries. During ventricular
diastole the elastic recoil of the arterial wall maintains blood flow
throughout the remainder of the cardiac cycle. From Berne and Levy
(1983) with permission.

elastin from pro-elastin is triggered mechanically, whereas
its breakdown by elastase is accelerated in old age.

Collagen is the other major connective tissue protein
of the matrix and is closely related in structure to the collagen found in the myocardium. Collagen is an important
component of the medial wall, helping it to keep its shape
despite the high intraluminal pressure exerted by the
blood. Hence, collagen has extremely high tensile properties and is distributed in such a way in the medial layer that
the arteries are highly resistant to the intraluminal pressure. When, however, conduit arteries such as the external
carotid or the common iliac are treated by collagenase, then
segments of these arteries readily rupture when subjected
to pressure (Dobrin et al., 1984). Different types of collagen
have different responses to mechanical stress. Types I and
II collagen, the most common in the media, consist of fibrils
about 20 to 90 nm in diameter. Groups of fibrils constitute
fibers. Type III collagen is more elastic, while Type IV collagen is found chiefly in the intima and Type V in the basement membrane of the arterial wall.

Other matrix proteins are the *glycoproteins,* which include fibronectin, a biological "glue," and the *glycosaminog-
lycans* (GAG), which are hydrophilic, forming aggregates
that make up a gel containing electrolytes and small molecules in passage from blood to the various tissues through
the vessel wall.

Adventitia

The adventitia, the external layer, separated from the media by the external elastic lamina, is essentially a vessel bearing and nerve conducting layer. The blood vessels running to the arterial wall are found here (vasa vasorum) as are lymphatics and the autonomic nerves. Histologically, this layer contains collagen, fibroblasts, and a few muscle cells besides the blood vessels. In the large conducting arteries, the adventitia is thin and the elastic layer of the media is dominant. In the small muscular arteries, the site of the peripheral vascular resistance, the adventitia is thicker especially its inner layer.

ENDOTHELIUM IN HYPERTENSION

A recent hypothesis is that the vascular endothelium may be damaged in hypertension, possibly by mechanical shear forces (Shichiri et al., 1990), leading to increased release of vasoconstrictory endothelin or less vasodilatory endothelium-derived relaxation factor (EDRF, nitric oxide). These endothelial changes allow the postulate of a hypertensive vicious circle mechanism (Fig. 10–5), which is, however, very controversial (Vanhoutte, 1993). ACE inhibitors could theoretically protect the endothelium in one of two ways. First, they could diminish the amount of angiotensin-II available to act on the endothelium; angiotensin-II is one of the factors inducing release of the vasoconstrictory endothelin. Second, ACE inhibitors increase formation of bradykinin which, in turn, elicits the release of vasodilators such as nitric oxide from the endothelium. Although still hypothetical, these proposals suggest a further mechanism for a vasoprotective effect of ACE inhibitors (Lüscher, 1993; Farhy et al., 1993).

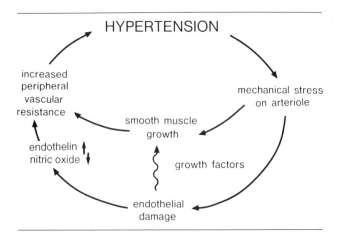

Figure 10–5. Role of mechanical stress on the arteriole both in causing endothelial damage and in stimulating smooth muscle growth. Note the possible release of endothelin during endothelial damage to increase peripheral vascular resistance. Fig. © LH Opie.

Endothelial morphology

In hypertension, the subendothelial layer thickens with in-filtrated cells derived from the media and with the growth of matrix cells. Morphologic changes include roughening of the intimal surface and discontinuity of the intercellular junctions (Berry and Sosa-Melgarejo, 1989). The latter change may account for the increased permeability to mac-romolecules with risk of penetration of blood lipoprotein components and possible initiation of atheroma. The en-dothelium loses much of its vasodilator capacity and under-goes thickening (Gibbons and Dzau, 1990). These endothe-lial changes add to the risk of a reduction in luminal area of the arteriole. Although there is no direct proof of the role of an endothelial renin-angiotensin system in these changes, nonetheless it is of interest that vascular endothe-lial cells have the capacity for renin expression in culture (Re et al., 1982).

ARTERIOLES IN HYPERTENSION

It is the arterioles that are the site of the systemic vascular resistance and hence respond most to an increase in size of the medial wall. The reaction of the arterioles to hyperten-sion can best be understood in terms of the Meerson hy-pothesis applied to the myocardium. This great Russian physiologist, currently still living in Moscow, described the well known three stages of myocardial adaptation. The first stage is the acute adaptation to the mechanical overload, a process involving the transduction of excess wall stress into

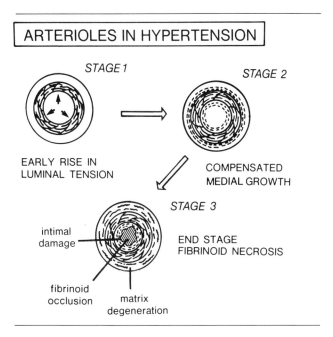

Figure 10–6. The proposed three stages of the medial reaction to hypertension with the ultimate production of irreversible arteriolar damage. Fig. © LH Opie.

protein synthesis, probably by stimulation of mechanore-
ceptors. The second stage is that of compensatory hypertrophy in which the enlarged hypertrophied myocardium
has a wall stress that has reverted to normal. The third is
the stage of decompensation and irreversible myocardial
failure, when an excess prolonged load causes cardiac dilation. The transition from compensation to irreversible decompensation may be linked, hypothetically, to cellular
ischemia and reactive stimulation of fibroblasts with collagen formation and fibrosis.

Similar principles may be applied to the arteries (Fig.
10–6). In the first phase, an excess intraluminal pressure
leads to compensatory protein synthesis, thereby establish-
ing the second phase with the hypertrophied thickened
medial wall, which restores normal wall tension despite the
continued increase in the intraluminal pressure. In the
third phase, the media degenerates and disorganization of
the matrix leads to irreversible damage, often with calcinosis. The two crucial biological steps to understand are (1)
the trigger to smooth muscle growth and (2) the nature of
end-stage degeneration.

ARTERIOLAR GROWTH AND WALL/ LUMEN RATIO

Trigger to vascular smooth muscle growth

According to current concepts, the two major types of stimuli are (1) mechanical, acting by deformation of the smooth
muscle cells, and (2) receptor agonists, acting by intracellular signaling systems.

Mechanical stimulation by stretch. Because stretch of
isolated vascular myocytes leads to enhanced protein synthesis and cell hypertrophy (Leung et al., 1976), hypertension could be acting at least in part through stretch mechanisms to cause medial hypertrophy. The role of pressure
in vascular hypertrophy was proven by an ingenious experiment in which the pressure in the femoral artery was
specifically reduced in spontaneously hypertensive rats by
a partially occluding ligature (Bund et al., 1991). In the distal artery protected from systemic hypertension, the following abnormalities reverted to normal: an increased medial wall thickness and cross-sectional area, and the
increased media-lumen ratio. Thus, in these experiments,
it was not necessary to postulate the operation of any nonmechanical factor in achieving these improvements in vascular structure.

Another way of dissociating the effects of angiotensin-
II and blood pressure is by infusing peridopril-treated hypertensive rats with saline (Harrap et al., 1993). The latter
procedure restored the blood pressure to the previously elevated levels and once again increased wall media-lumen
ratio.

Balloon injury. Endothelial damage is an important initi-
ator of atherosclerosis (see Chapter 11). One method of in-

juring the endothelium and inducing its growth is by balloon injury (see Fig. 10–3). The new growth is called the *neointima* and is accompanied by hypertrophy of the medial layer (Rakugi et al., 1993). Angiotensin-II promotes such growth by the local autocrine production of growth factors.

Receptor stimulation as growth signal

An alternate hypothesis not involving mechanical effects is that *receptor agonists acting as vasoconstrictors might also stimulate the signals to vascular smooth muscle growth* (Fig. 10–7). Among the potential agonists is the local vascular renin-angiotensin system (Table 10–3). The logical explanation would be that cytosolic calcium acts as the common factor with a short-lived calcium rise acting as a vasoconstrictor and a sustained calcium rise acting as a growth promoter. In particular, angiotensin-II promotes both contraction and hypertrophy (Khairallah and Kanabus, 1983; Geisterfer et al., 1988; Gibbons and Dzau, 1990) and angiotensin-II increases cytosolic calcium in vascular smooth muscle cells working in part by activation of voltage-dependent Ca^{2+} channels (Ohya and Sperelakis, 1991) and in part through stimulation of the phosphoinositol pathway (Schelling et

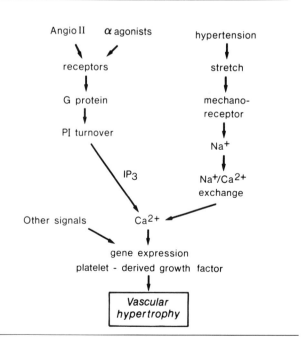

Figure 10–7. Proposed mechanism whereby vasoconstrictive agents such as angiotensin-II and alpha-agonist stimulation could lead to vascular growth. In addition, mechanical stretch can in some experiments be the major or even sole factor that can be related to vascular growth (Bund et al., 1991). For role of PDGF (platelet-derived growth factor), see Naftilan et al. (1989). For role of Angio-II, α agonists, PI and IP_3, see Figure 1–3. For G protein, see Figure 1–2. Fig. © LH Opie.

TABLE 10–3 ANGIOTENSIN-II AND ITS PROPOSED ROLE
IN BLOOD VESSELS

---

1. Evidence for local angiotensin-II production

  a. Induced coexpression of angiotensinogen renin and
     angiotensin-converting enzyme activity in medial layer
     (Dzau, 1988)

  b. Induction of mRNA for angiotensinogen in media and
     neointima after balloon injury (Rakugi et al., 1993)

  c. Increase of aortic, mesenteric and renal artery renin levels
     despite normal circulating renin (Okamura et al., 1986)

  d. Inhibition of angiotensin-II release from perfused
     mesenteric artery by renin and ACE inhibitors
     (Higashimori et al., 1991)

**2. Effects of angiotensin-II on growth factors and
isolated myocytes**

  a. Increased growth of vascular smooth muscle cells
     stimulated by plasma factor (Campbell-Boswell and
     Robertson, 1981)

  b. Hypertrophy of quiescent aortic smooth muscle cells
     (Geisterfer et al., 1988)

  c. Induction of proto-oncogenes and platelet-derived growth
     factor (PDGF) (Kawahara et al., 1988; Moalic et al., 1989;
     Naftilan et al., 1989)

  d. Receptor-mediated stimulation of collagen synthesis in
     cultured vascular smooth muscle cells (Kato et al., 1991)

3. Effects on vascular hypertrophy in vivo

  a. Angiotensin-II infusion induces smooth muscle cell
     proliferation and DNA synthesis when infused into
     normotensive rats (Daemen et al., 1991)

---

al., 1991). Conversely, chronic ACE inhibitor therapy decreases arterial calcium content (Sada et al., 1990). According to some current concepts, angiotensin-II could be a
stimulus to cell growth, acting in part by a sustained increase of cytosolic calcium which, in turn, stimulates
gene expression and formation of proto-oncogenes, which
would lead to increased vascular growth (Fig. 10–8). Thus,
it is not surprising that in animal models of hypertension
captopril and perindopril not only prevent hypertension
but lessen vascular hypertrophy with improved vascular
function (Lee et al., 1991; Christensen et al., 1989).

Consequences of arteriolar changes in hypertension

Although the enlarged hypertrophied arteriole (compensated arteriolar hypertrophy, Stage II) is able to withstand
the increased intraluminal pressure, there are inevitable
disadvantages ("no gain without pain" as is said in sports
medicine). There are two problems. First, the concentric
hypertrophy not only increases the medial thickness but
reduces the internal diameter of the lumen (Mulvany et al.,
1978). At this stage Poiseuille's law (Fig. 10–9) should be
recalled. The vascular resistance (R) is:

$$R = P/Q = (8 \times \text{viscosity} \times \text{length})/\pi r^4$$

ANGIOTENSIN II AND VASCULAR GROWTH

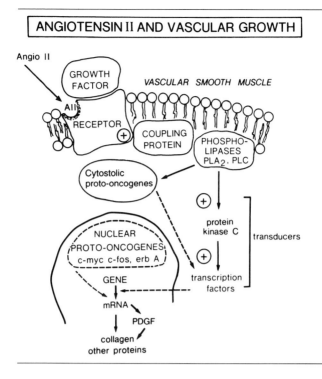

Figure 10–8. *Proposed role of angiotensin-II (Angio-II) as a growth factor in vascular smooth muscle. For role of PDGF (platelet-derived growth factor), see Naftilan et al. (1989). PLA, phospholipase A; PLC, phospholipase C. Fig. © LH Opie.*

where Q is flow, r is radius, and P is pressure drop. Any given fall of radius leads to a much greater increase in resistance. Reduction of the diameter (or radius) of the arteriole by 5% increases the vascular resistance by 23%, whereas a 10% reduction increases the vascular resistance by as much as 70%.

The second disadvantage is that there is still a sustained sensitivity to vasoconstrictor agonists although in some experiments this response is muted (Lee et al., 1991). Starting from a smaller arteriolar lumen, any vasoconstrictor stimulus such as angiotensin-II or alpha$_1$-adrenergic activity will cause a greater rise in the systemic vascular resistance. For example, if the normal lumen is reduced by 5%, then the vascular resistance will increase by 23% as already calculated. However, if the lumen is *already reduced*, then an additional further reduction of another 5% will vastly increase the vascular resistance. Whether there is increased, decreased, or altered arteriolar response to the same degree of vasoconstrictor stimulation is still a matter of controversy.

A third point of note is that there is evidence for enhanced activity of the vasoconstrictor mechanisms in hypertension. For example, vascular renin activity appears to be increased in experimental hypertension (Dzau and Safar, 1988). In mildly hypertensive patients, there are increased circulating levels of catecholamines in response to psychologic stress such as mental arithmetic (Nestel, 1969).

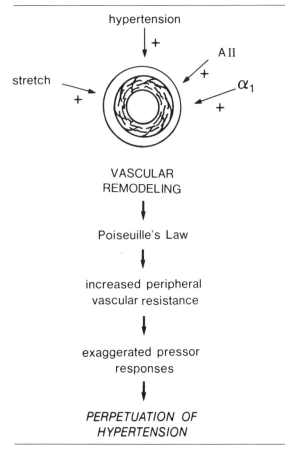

Figure 10–9. *The role of vascular remodeling in perpetuation of hypertension. A decreased luminal size acts by Poiseuille's law to increase peripheral vascular resistance and thereby to allow exaggerated pressor responses. AII, angiotensin-II; α_1, alpha$_1$ adrenergic. Fig. © LH Opie.*

Furthermore, there may be alterations in the intracellular coupling systems. Thus, the alpha-receptor may be better coupled to its messenger system (Papageorgiou and Morgan, 1991). While the experimental vascular data largely relate to aorta and may not be applicable to arterioles, nonetheless the principle of a decreased resting lumen size and an increased reaction to vasoconstrictor stimulation would appear to be firmly established.

Enhanced arteriolar vasoconstriction may therefore perpetuate and exaggerate hypertension (Gibbons and Dzau, 1990), particularly in the presence of structural changes. Thus it is proposed that the arteriolar wall plays a crucial role in the continuation of the hypertensive process.

End-stage arterial disease

The genesis of end-stage arterial disease is not well understood and here the analogy with Meerson's Stage III is not exact. On the one hand, the arterial smooth muscle cells appear to undergo degeneration and to be replaced by an inflammatory infiltrate, as well as collagen fibrosis. This process corresponds reasonably well with Meerson's Stage III for the myocardium. In addition, however, there is marked intimal damage with fibrin deposition and often arteriolar occlusion. The latter process suggests that the hypertensive process has extensively damaged the endothelium and intima which, in turn, has resulted in fibrin deposition and arterial occlusion. The analogy with Meerson's Stage III for the heart can, however, be made by pointing out that end-stage arterial disease in the heart and in the arteriole are the result of unremitting intraluminal wall tension, in the one case from left ventricular dilation and in the other case from sustained intraluminal hypertension.

LARGE CONDUIT (CONDUCTING) ARTERIES IN HYPERTENSION

In hypertension, large conduit arteries, like the small bore arterioles, are exposed to increased intraluminal tension and also undergo an increase in mural thickness. Thus, there are two major sites of vascular damage in hypertension, the large conduit arteries and the arterioles. Because there is relatively less muscle mass than matrix in these large arteries, an increase in the matrix mass becomes relatively more important. Of the two chief matrix components, elastin and collagen, it is the synthesis of collagen that responds to a greater extent, especially in male rats (Wolinsky, 1971). The net result is a fall in the ratio of elastin to collagen with a relative stiffening of the large arteries. Such changes may explain the *loss of arterial wall compliance* (Safar and London, 1987) found not only in the brachial arteries (Safar et al., 1981) but also in the femoral arteries (Liao et al., 1991).

Mechanism of collagen growth

As in the case of the arterioles, the two major proposed stimuli to growth of the elements of the arterial wall are (1) mechanical tension and (2) nonmechanical factors such as renin-angiotensin stimulation. One proposal is that angiotensin-II plays a specific role as a growth factor (see Fig. 10–8). To assess the role of collagen production, Michel et al. (1992) transplanted the aortic wall of normotensive and hypertensive rats, thereby inducing arterial allograft rejection. Perindopril treatment reduced intimal thickening and collagen density. Other data suggest a selective enhancing effect of angiotensin-II on growth signals for collagen growth, including the division of fibroblasts, which are the cells that synthesize collagen (Schelling et al., 1991).

Smooth muscle polyploidy

In large conduit arteries, an increase of the number of polyploid cells (those with more than one nucleus) is proposed as a second major factor causing loss of compliance, because each individual smooth muscle cell would have relatively less contractile element and relatively more nuclear material. Enalapril, when given to spontaneously hypertensive rats during the phase of development of hypertension, leads to a fall of blood pressure and reduced aortic polyploidy (Black et al., 1989). In patients too, polyploid smooth muscle cells have been found in the carotid artery (Barrett et al., 1983). There appears to be an increase in the size of each individual smooth muscle cell rather than a great deal of hyperplasia.

Lumen size

Because of the large size of the lumen of the conduit arteries, it cannot be anticipated that any change in medial hypertrophy will impinge on the luminal diameter. Yet, the larger the vessel, the greater the matrix component of the composition of the wall (p. 243). In patients with sustained uncomplicated essential hypertension, the unchanged internal diameter of the common carotid artery indicates a decreased compliance because there is an increased intraluminal pressure (Safar, 1988). It is this decreased compliance that interferes with the buffering capacity of the large arteries (Dzau and Safar, 1988). In advanced arterial disease, a further factor reducing arterial compliance and increasing the stiffness is deposition of calcium. These changes in the mechanical properties of the conduit arteries lead to a hypothesis, now to be presented, that stresses that these arteries could be of crucial importance in the hypertensive process, at least in some subsets of the population.

HYPOTHESIS: LARGE CONDUIT ARTERIES HAVE A CRUCIAL ROLE IN PERPETUATING AND INCREASING THE SEVERITY OF HYPERTENSION

This hypothesis (Fig. 10–10) rests upon the following proposals:

1. Large conduit arteries increase collagen (Wolinsky, 1971) and lose elasticity in hypertension (Safar, 1988)
2. Therefore, the pressure equalizing and buffering function of the large arteries is diminished (Dzau and Safar, 1988)
3. An increased systolic pressure is increasingly transmitted to the resistance arterioles, a self-evident proposition
4. Pressure-induced stretch, acting as a growth stimulus in the arterioles, would cause medial hypertrophy and intimal damage
5. Such arterioles have a reduced capacity to dilate maximally (Lee et al., 1991), a decreased luminal diameter (Christensen et al., 1989), and a thicker media (Mulvany et al., 1978) so that the systemic vascular resistance is increased
6. An increased peripheral vascular resistance will perpetuate hypertension; this component of the hy-

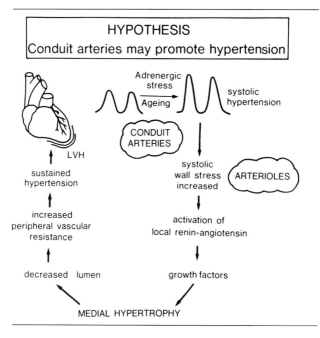

Figure 10–10. Hypothesis emphasizing possible role of conduit arteries in initiating hypertension in certain subsets of the population. For example, ageing by reducing aortic and conduit arterial elasticity causes a systolic hypertension which increases systolic wall stress and either mechanically or through activation of the local renin-angiotensin system causes medial hypertrophy with sustained hypertension. A similar sequence could be invoked to explain why catecholamine-inducing stress reactions can eventually cause sustained hypertension. It is not the intention of this figure to show that this mechanism operates in all patients with hypertension, but rather to point out a possible mechanism operating in some patients. LVH, left ventricular hypertrophy. Fig. © LH Opie.

pothesis has previously been proposed by Lever (1986)

7. Therefore, a predominantly systolic hypertension, as found in conditions with an increased adrenergic drive in the young and during the ageing process, will be transmitted from the conduit to the resistance arteries and thereby converts systolic hypertension into sustained systolic and diastolic hypertension.

It is not proposed that this hypothesis would generally apply to all patients with hypertension. Rather two subsets of the hypertensive population may chiefly be involved. For example, this hypothesis would explain why hypertension in the young tends to be that of a high cardiac output type, whereas later it becomes a high vascular resistance type (Folkow et al., 1973). It would also explain why aged patients with systolic hypertension have diastolic values higher than could be expected solely from the changes in compliance (Randall et al., 1984).

The importance of this hypothesis is that a variety of agents interrupting the vicious circle whereby "hypertension begets hypertension", could become beneficial. The unexpected antihypertensive effects of heparin could thus be explained (Gibbons and Dzau, 1990). This agent which has no direct effect on vascular tone is able both to inhibit vascular smooth muscle cell growth and when given chronically to reduce the blood pressure (Wilson et al., 1981), apparently acting to inhibit renal glomerular fibrinoid lesions. The hypothesis would also explain why the pulsatile pressure (difference between systolic and diastolic values) is so closely linked to the mean arterial pressure (Darne et al., 1989) because increased pulsatile pressure would be followed by increased mean blood pressure.

The hypothesis would also accord special importance to those antihypertensive agents that act not only to reduce blood pressure but also to inhibit directly the growth process in the smooth muscle cells of the tunica media of arterioles. Such agents include the ACE inhibitors and the calcium antagonists, of which the ACE inhibitors are better tested in this situation.

Therapeutic interruption of vascular vicious circle in hypertension

The vicious circle proposed could be interrupted at several points. First of all, any agent acting as a general nonspecific antihypertensive will remove the major initial stimulus to the loss of compliance in the conduit arteries. Agents that reduce early episodes of increased cardiac output and systolic hypertension could likewise be expected eventually to diminish the cycle. Therefore, conventional antihypertensive therapy has a definite place. In addition, agents that specifically reduce systolic hypertension will help to decrease the propagation of the pressure wave to the resistance arterioles. There is provisional evidence that ACE inhibitors are better able to reduce the systolic component of hypertension than, for example, beta-blockers. Lisinopril and enalapril are better able than atenolol to achieve this aim (Helgeland et al., 1986; Beevers et al., 1991; Pannier et al., 1991). A recent careful analysis of the comparative effects of perindopril on systolic and diastolic pressure by Safar's group supports the concept of a relatively greater reduction in the systolic component of the blood pressure (Asmar et al., 1988a). The ACE inhibitors appear to maintain *conduit artery relaxation*. For example, captopril, enalapril and perindopril allow maintained increase in the arterial diameter during prolonged therapy, even when the blood pressure has fallen. In a particularly interesting study, Asmar et al. (1988b) subjected patients with essential hypertension to 1 month of placebo therapy before administration of perindopril (mean dose 6 mg daily) for a period of 3 months and a subsequent placebo washout period also of 1 month. They compared the effects on brachial mechanical properties with the findings in two placebo periods, one before and one after the perindopril treatment. During the active treatment period, the brachial artery compliance increased as the blood pressure fell. Of specific interest is the increase in arterial diameter, the exact opposite of what would be expected from the decreased intraluminal pressure.

It is clear that the blood vessels must be regarded as a valid site for end-organ damage in hypertension, in addition to the conventional end-organs such as brain, retina, heart, and kidneys. Damage to blood vessels could play a crucial role in perpetuating hypertension, as already proposed by Folkow et al. in 1973. It is also clear that the experimental and clinical properties of the actions of ACE inhibitors on the blood vessels (Tables 10–4 and 10–5) need careful appraisal for their potential role in lessening or even reversing hypertensive vascular disease.

TABLE 10–4 SOME VASCULAR EFFECTS OF ACE INHIBITORS IN SPONTANEOUSLY HYPERTENSIVE RATS (SHR) AND OTHER MODELS

1. Experimental effects in aorta and large conduit arteries

a. Perindopril—reduction of aortic cell hypertrophy in renovascular hypertension and increased compliance (Levy et al., 1988a).

b. Perindopril—increase of elastin/collagen ratio in SHR (Levy et al., 1988b). Decrease of collagen (Levy et al., 1993).

c. Perindopril—decreased thickness of media and decreased nuclear density in SHR (Levy et al., 1989; Levy et al., 1991).

d. Captopril—reduction of intimal-medial area and aortic wall hypertrophy in one kidney one clip hypertension (Wang and Prewitt, 1990).

e. Enalapril—reduction of aortic smooth muscle cell polyploidy together with therapy of hypertension in SHR (Black et al., 1989).

2. Experimental effects in medium sized arteries

a. Cilazapril—cerebral arteries of SHR have decreased thickness of media (Clozel et al., 1989).

b. Captopril—mesenteric arteries in SHR have increased lumen size at maximal relaxation (Lee et al., 1991).

c. Captopril—reduction of mesenteric wall/lumen ratio in SHR (Freslon and Guidicelli, 1983).

3. Experimental effects in small sized arteries (arterioles)

a. Perindopril—mesenteric resistance arterioles of SHR have a reduction of media/lumen ratio (Christensen et al., 1989).

b. Perindopril—brief therapy of young SHR results in delayed decrease of media/lumen ratio reversed by concurrent angiotensin-II infusion (Harrap et al., 1991).

c. Captopril—reduces intima/lumen ratio and media/lumen ratio in SHR (Lee et al., 1991).

d. Captopril—reduction of arteriolar wall density in one kidney one clip rats (Wang and Prewitt, 1990).

e. Cilazapril—inhibits unfavorable remodeling of cerebral arterioles and improves their distensibility in stroke-prone SHR; no effect of hydralazine (Hajdu et al., 1991).

TABLE 10–5 Some Clinical Effects of ACE Inhibitors on Carotid, Brachial and Femoral Arteries in Man

1. Normal volunteers

a. Perindopril—marked increase of blood flow and substantial decrease in vascular resistance suggests improved compliance because only minor changes in blood pressure found (Richer et al., 1987).

2. Hypertensive subjects

a. Perindoprilat—in an acute study brachial artery diameter increased and pulse wave velocity decreased especially at the higher dose (2.5 μg/kg/min) (Benetos et al., 1990).

b. Perindopril—in a chronic study there was increased brachial artery diameter and compliance at a time when the blood pressure decreased showing that the changes induced by increased intraluminal tension are reversible (Asmar et al. 1988b). During chronic therapy over 1 year the increased arterial compliance and decreased cardiac mass were maintained in those patients who responded to perindopril monotherapy (Asmar et al., 1988c). Nine months of therapy normalized the increased media/lumen ratio as assessed by subcutaneous biopsy in hypertensive subjects (Sihm et al., 1993).

c. Captopril—when compared with cadralazine there were similar decreases in blood pressure and in carotid bed vascular resistance but only captopril increased arterial diameter and decreased the pulse wave velocity (Lacolley et al., 1989).

d. Trandolapril—when the antihypertensive dose (2 mg) was exceeded, pulse wave velocity fell as the dose increased (Asmar et al., 1992).

EFFECTS OF ACE INHIBITORS ON ARTERIAL DISEASE

Two proposed mechanisms

An important question is the extent to which the changes found in the various studies with ACE inhibitors can be caused purely by intraluminal pressure reduction, or whether there is a more specific effect such as interference with the vascular tissue renin-angiotensin system. On the one hand, mechanical relief of pressure in the arterial tree induced simply by a local ligature can revert almost fully toward normal the abnormalities found in the resistance arterioles of spontaneously hypertensive rats (Bund et al., 1991). On the other hand, there is another factor, independent of changes in intraluminal pressure. In a model of hypertension (one kidney, one clip) that is not renin-dependent, ACE inhibitor therapy decreases the severity of aortic wall hypertrophy. The mean blood pressure only fell from 193 ± 5 mmHg to 183 ± 5 mmHg in captopril treated rats and this small change was most unlikely to account for the decreased aortic wall thickness (Wang and Prewitt, 1990). The most reasonable conclusion is that ACE inhibition in this model has a direct beneficial effect on the aortic wall.

Thus, ACE inhibition potentially acts on arterial disease through both mechanisms, first reducing intraluminal pressure by the general blood pressure lowering effect and, second, by an additional effect independent of any pressure change, possibly related to the effects of angiotensin-II in stimulating vascular growth.

Experimental effects on large arteries (Table 10–4)

In keeping with the basic data showing that angiotensin-II is a specific stimulator of vascular growth (see Table 10–2), it is not surprising that hypertension (renovascular model) leads to an increased thickness of the aorta and a fall in its compliance (Levy et al., 1988a). Treatment by the ACE inhibitor perindopril (1 mg/kg/day for 4 weeks) decreased the medial thickness of the arterial wall. In the spontaneously hypertensive rat model treated by perindopril, the elastin/collagen ratio fell and the thickness of the medial wall decreased (Levy et al., 1988b, 1989 and 1991). Specifically, there were reductions in smooth muscle hypertrophy and in collagen density (Levy et al., 1993).

In a second study, also in spontaneously hypertensive rats, the ACE inhibitor enalapril was given during the growth phase of rats with spontaneous hypertension (Black et al., 1989). Polyploidy is thought to contribute to the loss of compliance in large arteries in hypertension. Enalapril 25 to 30 mg/kg/day prevented the development of hypertension in this model and reduced the number of aortic smooth muscle cells that exhibited polyploidy (an increased number of nuclei in each cell).

Experimental effects on medium sized arteries

In *cerebral arteries* of spontaneously hypertensive rats, there is medial hypertrophy. When such rats were treated by cilazapril 10 mg/kg/day during the growth phase, then the medial hypertrophy diminished, and the capacity of the cerebral arterial tree to undergo maximal vasodilation was increased toward normal (Clozel et al., 1989).

In *mesenteric arteries* of spontaneously hypertensive rats treated by captopril, there was an increased lumen size at maximal relaxation and a decreased number of smooth muscle cell layers (Lee et al., 1991). In another study, captopril treatment also reduced the wall/lumen ratio of the mesenteric arteries and had a greater effect than the nonspecific vasodilator, dihydralizine (Freslon and Guidicelli, 1983).

Effects on arteriolar disease

Both perindopril and captopril reduced the media/lumen ratio in arterioles of spontaneously hypertensive rats (Christensen et al., 1989; Lee et al., 1991). In stroke-prone spontaneously hypertensive rats, cilazapril inhibited the unfavorable remodeling of cerebral arterioles and improved their distensibility (Hadju et al., 1991). In the one model of hypertension (one kidney, one clip), captopril reduced the arterial wall density (Wang and Prewitt, 1990).

During the active phase of treatment of hypertension in spontaneously hypertensive rats, ACE inhibition was more effective than other modalities of treatment in controlling the structural vascular abnormalities because the wall/lumen ratio was lowest, particularly with perindopril (Christensen et al., 1989).

Likewise, in the spontaneously hypertensive rat, captopril treatment reduced the abnormally increased wall/lumen ratio, the intima/lumen ratio, and the media/lumen ratio (Lee et al., 1991).

Effects of withdrawal of therapy on arteriolar disease in experimental hypertension

If arteriolar structural changes are crucial to the development of hypertension, then the therapeutic improvement of the abnormalities involved should be followed by improvement in the blood pressure even when treatment is withdrawn (Fig. 10–11). This proposal has been tested in spontaneously hypertensive rats treated by a variety of agents including the ACE inhibitors perindopril and captopril during the growth phase of the rats from 4 to 24 weeks (Christensen et al., 1989). During the phase of therapy withdrawal, from 24 to 36 weeks, the blood pressure remained controlled in those rats that had been treated by perindopril and captopril but not in those previously treated by the calcium antagonist isradipine, nor by the beta-blocker metoprolol, nor by the non-specific vasodilator hydralazine. The ACE inhibitors were better at normalizing the media/lumen ratio, suggesting that therapeutic control of the arteriolar structural changes in these rats could have led to the sustained post-treatment normalization of blood pressure by the ACE inhibitors (see Fig. 10–11). The post-treatment hypotensive effect is found even at low doses of perindopril (Eriksen et al., 1992).

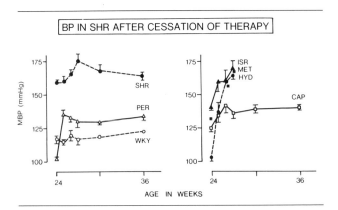

Figure 10–11. Mean blood pressure (MBP) values in spontaneously hypertensive rats (SHR) compared with control rats (WKY) after cessation of therapy by a variety of agents: perindopril (PER), captopril (CAP), isradipine (ISR), metoprolol (MET) and hydralazine (HYD). Note that there is a rapid rebound in the blood pressure values after therapy with all agents except the ACE inhibitors perindopril and captopril. Modified from Christensen et al. (1989) with permission.

In a particularly interesting study, Harrap et al. (1990) gave brief periods of ACE inhibitor therapy (perindopril 3 mg/kg/day) from 6 to 10 weeks and found a reduction in the media/lumen ratio of mesenteric resistance vessels at 32 weeks of age. This reduction was reverted by infusion of angiotensin-II with perindopril over the same time. Thus early perindopril therapy led to a late benefit in vascular structure.

It seems safe to conclude that in models of hypertension, ACE inhibition can have a post-treatment effect in lowering blood pressure and can maintain improvements in vascular structure that appear to exceed the effects achieved by representatives of other types of antihypertensive agents. Although these studies need confirmation in other models of animal hypertension, they do suggest that the hypertensive vicious circle outlined in Fig. 10–10 could be interrupted therapeutically.

While any application to human hypertension remains speculative, Gibbons and Dzau (1990) have proposed that such reversion of vascular structure if found in humans could actually cure hypertension in a subset of patients.

Clinical studies with ACE inhibitors (Table 10–5)

Doppler echocardiographic techniques have led to the establishment of non-invasive measurements of indices of vascular compliance and of blood flow velocity in the major arteries such as the carotids, the brachials, and the femorals. In *normal volunteers*, the ACE inhibitor perindopril markedly increased blood flow and decreased vascular resistance even when the changes in the blood pressure were slight (Richer et al., 1987). Thus the suggestion is that vascular resistance decreased as the compliance increased.

In *hypertensive subjects*, in an acute study, intravenous perindoprilat (the active form of perindopril) increased brachial artery blood flow and diameter as well as compliance at a time when the blood pressure decreased (Benetos et al., 1990). These changes were especially evident at the higher dose used (2.5 μg/kg/min).

In a chronic study, oral perindopril also gave a similar increase in arterial compliance (Asmar et al, 1988b). During chronic therapy over 1 year, the increase in compliance was maintained while cardiac mass decreased in those patients responding to perindopril monotherapy (Asmar et al, 1988c). There was still some increase in brachial artery diameter even when wrist arterial occlusion had been used to reduce the brachial blood flow and hence to lessen any direct effect of the rate of blood flow on the diameter (flow-induced arterial dilation). When subcutaneous arteries are subject to biopsy, the increased media/lumen ratio of hypertensive subjects reverted to normal after 9 months of treatment by perindopril (Sihm et al., 1993).

Vascular changes may also be induced by captopril. When compared with the hydralazine-like compound, cadralazine, there were comparable changes in blood pressure but only captopril increased arterial diameter and decreased pulse wave velocity (Lacolley et al., 1989).

These human studies are still in their infancy. At pre-

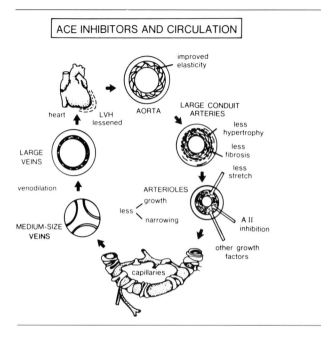

Figure 10–12. *Proposed effects of ACE inhibitors on the circulation include effects on the aorta, large conduit arteries, and arterioles. There are probably two major mechanisms for the action of ACE inhibitors, first indirectly by a decrease of stretch (nonspecific effect of blood pressure reduction) and, second, by inhibition of the effects of angiotensin-II). The loss of elasticity of the aorta and large conduit vessels can to some extent be reverted by ACE inhibitor therapy, as can the abnormal arteriolar changes. AII, angiotensin-II. Fig. © LH Opie.*

sent their importance is twofold. First, they show that the animal data can at least in part be extrapolated to human disease. Second, human data counter the argument that the high doses of all agents used in animal models might have induced vascular changes not achieved at lower doses. Although there is a more marked vascular response to a high dose of perindoprilat in humans (Benetos et al., 1990), vascular changes have been found even at standard oral doses. Overall, the basic and clinical data suggest that the ACE inhibitors have multiple sites of action on the arterial tree (Fig. 10–12) including not only the stretch-induced changes resulting from a reduction of intraluminal pressure, but also specific changes dependent on inhibition of angiotensin-II, possibly independent of any effect on the blood pressure.

REVERSAL OF VASCULAR REMODELING

The prominent role of vascular damage in perpetuating hypertension (see Figs. 10–8 and 10–9) has led to the concept that favorable vascular remodeling should be one of the aims of antihypertensive therapy. Experimentally, subhypertensive doses of perindopril and ramipril were able to improve not only vascular structure but also vascular function (Gohlke et al., 1993). Specifically, indices of endothelial function were also improved.

Strictly speaking, however, the term *remodeling* should be limited to a rearrangement of otherwise normal vascular cells, according to Heagerty et al. (1993). Such remodeling can also be reversed by antihypertensive treatment, though not in full.

Summary

That changes in vascular structure occur in hypertension is not a new concept, dating back at least to Folkow in 1973. The concept has taken a new meaning with the discovery of the prominent role of the vascular endothelium in producing vasoconstrictory endothelin and vasodilatory nitric oxide (endothelium-derived relaxation factor). Hypothetically, endothelial damage could perpetuate or even initiate hypertension.

Recent evidence from molecular biology of arterial tissue and morphometric analysis of the structure of arteries that has shown the complex ways in which angiotensin-II acts as a signal to vascular growth. The other major signal to vascular growth is intraluminal stretch, resulting from the increased blood pressure. Experimental and clinical evidence with the use of ACE inhibitors shows that arterial and arteriolar changes associated with hypertension can at least in part be reverted toward normal. Of particular interest is a carry-over effect found when therapy has been stopped, which experimentally is found with the ACE inhibitors and not with the calcium antagonists, the beta-blockers, or hydralazine. While these effects on vascular structure are likely to be a class effect of ACE inhibitors, it is perindopril that seems best tested for the vascular effects, followed by captopril.

The proposed specific role of angiotensin-II in vascular growth and the delineation of the new site of action of ACE inhibitors on the vascular tree leads to the concept that these agents could interrupt a hypertensive vicious circle mechanism and thereby achieve more benefit than would result only from reduction of the blood pressure.

Viscoelastic properties of the large arteries and the lumen size of small arteries both contribute to the afterload. Hence abnormalities of both types of arteries can contribute to the development of left ventricular hypertrophy.

The clinical implications of these proposals, well supported experimentally, will need careful evaluation in prospective trials.

References

Asmar RG, Pannier B, Santoni JP, Safar ME. Angiotensin converting enzyme inhibition decreases systolic blood pressure more than diastolic pressure as shown by ambulatory blood pressure monitoring. *J Hypertens* 1988a; 6 (Suppl 3): S79–S81.

Asmar RG, Pannier B, Santoni JP, et al. Reversion of cardiac hypertrophy and reduced arterial compliance after converting enzyme inhibition in essential hypertension. *Circulation* 1988b; 78: 941–950.

Asmar RG, Journo HJ, Lacolley PJ, et al. Treatment for one year with perindopril: effect on cardiac mass and arterial compliance in essential hypertension. *J Hypertens* 1988c; 6 (Suppl 3): S33–S39.

Asmar RG, Benetos A, Darne BM, et al. Converting enzyme inhibition: dissociation between antihypertensive and arterial effects. *J Human Hypertens* 1992; 6: 381–385.

Barrett TB, Sampson P, Owens GK, et al. Polyploid nuclei in human artery wall smooth muscle cells. *Proc Natl Acad Sci USA* 1983; 80: 882–885.

Beevers DG, Blackwood RA, Garnham S, et al. Comparison of lisinopril versus atenolol for mild to moderate essential hypertension. *Am J Cardiol* 1991; 67: 59–62.

Benetos A, Santoni JP, Safar ME. Vascular effects of intravenous infusion of the angiotensin converting enzyme inhibitor perindopril. *J Hypertens* 1990; 8: 819–826.

Berne RM, Levy MN. *Physiology.* St. Louis: CV Mosby, 1983.

Berry CL, Sosa-Melgarejo JA. Nexus junctions between vascular smooth muscle cells in the media of the thoracic aorta in normal and hypertensive rats. A freeze-fracture study. *J Hypertens* 1989; 7: 507–513.

Black MJ, Adams MA, Bobik A, et al. Effects of enalapril on aortic smooth muscle cell polyploidy in the spontaneously hypertensive rat. *J Hypertens* 1989; 7: 997–1003.

Bund SJ, West KP, Heagerty AM. Effects of protection from pressure on resistance artery morphology and reactivity in spontaneously hypertensive and Wistar-Kyoto rats. *Circ Res* 1991; 68: 1230–1240.

Camilleri JP, Berry CL, Fiesinger JN, Bariety J. *Diseases of the Arterial Wall.* Berlin: Springer-Verlag, 1989.

Campbell-Boswell M, Robertson AL, Effects of angiotensin-II and vasopressin on human smooth muscle cells in vitro. *Exp Mol Pathol* 1981; 35: 265–276.

Christensen KL, Jespersen LT, Mulvany MJ. Development of blood pressure in spontaneously hypertensive rats after withdrawal of long-term treatment related to vascular structure. *J Hypertens* 1989; 7: 83–90.

Clozel JP, Kuhn H, Hefti F. Effects of cilazapril on the cerebral circulation in spontaneously hypertensive rats. *Hypertension* 1989; 14: 645–651.

Daemen MJAP, Lombardi DM, Bosman FT, Schwartz SM. Angiotensin-II induces smooth muscle cell proliferation in the normal and injured rat arterial wall. *Circ Res* 1991; 68: 450–456.

Darne B, Girerd X, Safar M, et al. Pulsatile versus steady component of blood pressure: a cross-sectional analysis and a prospective analysis on cardiovascular mortality. *Hypertension* 1989; 13: 392–400.

Dobrin PB, Baker WH, Gley WC. Elastolytic and collagenolytic studies of arteries. *Arch Surg* 1984; 119: 405–409.

Dzau VJ. Circulating versus local renin-angiotensin system in cardiovascular homeostasis. *Circulation* 1988; 77 (Suppl I): 14–113.

Dzau VJ, Safar ME. Large conduit arteries in hypertension: role of the vascular renin-angiotensin system. *Circulation* 1988; 77: 947–954.

Eriksen S, Christensen KL, Thybo NK, et al. A negative correlation between perindopril dose and persistent effects on blood pressure in spontaneously hypertensive rats after withdrawal of treatment (Abstr). *Acta Physiol Scand* 1992; 146 (Suppl 608): 74.

Farhy RD, Carretero OA, Ho K-L, Scicli AG. Role of kinins and nitric oxide in the effects of angiotensin-converting enzyme inhibitors on neointima formation. *Circ Res* 1993; 72: 1202–1210.

Folkow B, Hallback M, Lundgren Y, et al. Importance of adaptive changes in vascular design for establishment of primary hypertension, studied in man and in spontaneously hypertensive rats. *Circ Res* 1973; Vols 32 and 33 (Suppl I): I-2–I-16.

Freslon JL, Guidicelli JF. Compared myocardial and vascular effects of captopril and dihydralazine during hypertension in spontaneously hypertensive rats. *Br J Pharmacol* 1983; 80: 533–543.

Furchgott R, Zawadzki JV. The obligatory role of endothelial cells in the relaxation of arterial smooth muscle by acetylcholine. *Nature* 1980; 288: 373–376.

Geisterfer AAT, Peach MJ, Owens GK. Angiotensin-II induces hypertrophy, not hyperplasia, of cultured rat aortic smooth muscle cells. *Circ Res* 1988; 62: 749–756.

Gibbons GH, Dzau VJ. Angiotensin converting enzyme inhibition and vascular hypertrophy in hypertension. *Cardiovasc Drugs Ther* 1990; 4: 237–242.

Gohlke P, Lamberty V, Kuwer I, et al. Vascular remodeling in systemic hypertension. *Am J Cardiol* 1993; 7: 2E–7E.

Hajdu MA, Heistad DD, Baumbach GL. Effects of antihypertensive therapy on mechanics of cerebral arterioles in rats. *Hypertension* 1991; 17: 308–316.

Harrap SB, van der Merwe WM, Griffin SA, et al. Brief ACE inhibitor treatment in young spontaneously hypertensive rats reduces blood pressure long-term. *Hypertension* 1990; 16: 603–614.

Harrap SB, Mitchell GA, Casley DJ, et al. Angiotensin-II, sodium, and cardiovascular hypertrophy in spontaneously hypertensive rats. *Hypertension* 1993; 21: 50–55.

Heagerty AM, Aalkjaer C, Bund SJ, et al. Small artery structure in hypertension. Dual processes of remodeling and growth. *Hypertension* 1993; 21: 391–397.

Helgeland A, Strommen R, Hagelund CH, Tretli S. Enalapril, atenolol and hydrochlorothiazide in mild to moderate hypertension. A comparative multicentre study in general practice in Norway. *Lancet* 1986; 1: 872–875.

Higashimori K, Gante J, Holzemann G, Inagami T. Significance of vascular renin for local generation of angiotensins. *Hypertension* 1991; 17: 270–277.

Kato H, Suzuki H, Tajima S, et al. Angiotensin II stimulates collagen synthesis in cultured vascular smooth muscle cells. *J Hypertens* 1991; 9: 17–22.

Kawahara Y, Sunako M, Tsuda T, et al. Angiotensin-II induces expression of the c fos gene through protein kinase C activation and calcium ion metabilization in cultured vascular smooth muscle cells. *Biochem Biophys Res Commun* 1988; 150: 52–59.

Khairallah PA, Kanabus J. Angiotensin and myocardial protein synthesis. In: Tarazi RC, Dunbar JB (eds.), *Perspectives in Cardiovascular Research,* Vol 8. New York: Raven Press, 1983; 337–347.

Lacolley PJ, Laurent ST, Billaud EB, Safar ME. Carotid arterial hemodynamics in hypertension: acute administration of captopril or cadralazine. *Cardiovasc Drugs Ther* 1989; 3: 859–863.

Lancet Editorial. From cardiac to vascular protection: the next chapter. *Lancet* 1992; 340: 1197–1198.

Lee RMKW, Berecek KH, Tsoporis J, et al. Prevention of hypertension and vascular changes by captopril treatment. *Hypertension* 1991; 17: 141–150.

Leung DYM, Glagov S, Mathews MB. Cyclic stretching stimulates synthesis of matrix components by arterial smooth muscle cells in vitro. *Science* 1976; 191: 475–477.

Lever AF. Slow pressor mechanisms in hypertension. A role for hypertrophy of resistance vessels? *J Hypertens* 1986; 4: 515–524.

Levy BI, Michel JB, Salzmann JL, et al. Effects of chronic inhibition of converting enzyme on mechanical and structural properties of arteries in rat renovascular hypertension. *Circ Res* 1988a; 63: 2227–2239.

Levy BI, Michel JB, Salzmann JL, et al. Arterial effects of angiotensin converting enzyme inhibition in renovascular and spontaneously hypertensive rats. *J Hypertens* 1988b; 6 (Suppl 3): S23–S25.

Levy BI, Michel JB, Salzmann JL, et al. Effects of chronic converting enzyme inhibition on the structure and function of large arteries in the rat. *Clin and Exper Theory and Practice* 1989; All (Suppl 2): 487–498.

Levy BI, Michel JB, Salzmann JL, et al. Remodeling of heart and arteries by chronic converting enzyme inhibition in spontaneously hypertensive rats. *Am J Hypertens* 1991; 4: 240S–245S.

Levy BI, Michel JB, Salzmann JL, et al. Long-term effects of angiotensin-converting enzyme inhibition on the arterial wall of adult spontaneously hypertensive rats. *Am J Cardiol* 1993; 71: 8E–16E.

Liao JK, Bettmann MA, Sandor T, et al. Differential impairment of vasodilator responsiveness of peripheral resistance and conduit vessels in humans with atherosclerosis. *Circ Res* 1991; 68: 1027–1034.

Lüscher TF. Angiotensin, ACE inhibitors and endothelial control of vasomotor tone. *Basic Res Cardiol* 1993; 88 (Suppl I); 15–24.

Michel JB, Plissonnier D, Bruneval P. Effect of perindopril on the immune arterial wall remodeling in the rat model of arterial graft rejection. *Am J Med* 1992; 92 (Suppl 4B): 39S–46S.

Moalic JM, Bauters C, Himbert D, et al. Phenylephrine, vasopressin and angiotensin-II as determinants of protooncogene and heat-shock protein gene expression in adult rat heart and aorta. *J Hypertens* 1989; 7: 195–201.

Mulvany MJ, Hansen PK, Aalkjaer C. Direct evidence that the greater contractility of resistance vessels in spontaneously hypertensive rats is associated with a narrowed lumen, a thickened media, and an increased number of smooth muscle cell layers. *Circ Res* 1978; 43: 854–864.

Naftilan AJ, Pratt RE, Dzau VJ. Induction of platelet-derived growth factor A-chain and c-myc gene expressions by angiotensin-II in cultured rat vascular smooth muscle cells. *J Clin Invest* 1989; 83: 1419–1424.

Nestel PJ. Blood pressure and catecholamine excretion after mental stress in labile hypertension. *Lancet* 1969; 1: 692–694.

Ohya Y, Sperelakis N. Involvement of a GTP-binding protein in stimulating action of angiotensin-II on calcium channels in vascular smooth muscle cells. *Circ Res* 1991; 68: 763–771.

Okamura T, Myazaki M, Inagami T, Toda N. Vascular renin-angiotensin system in two-kidney, one clip hypertensive rats. *Hypertension* 1986; 8: 560–565.

Pannier BE, Garabedian VG, Madonna O, et al. Lisinopril versus atenolol: decrease in systolic versus diastolic blood pressure with converting enzyme inhibition. *Cardiovasc Drugs Ther* 1991; 5: 775–782.

Papageorgiou P, Morgan KG. Increased Ca^{2+} signaling after alpha-adrenoceptor activation in vascular hypertrophy. *Circ Res* 1991; 68: 1080–1084.

Rakugi H, Jacob HJ, Krieger HJ, et al. Vascular injury induces angiotensinogen gene expression in the media and neointima. *Circulation* 1993; 87: 283–290.

Randall OS, Van den Bos GC, Westerhof N. Systemic compliance: does it play a role in the genesis of essential hypertension? *Cardiovasc Res* 1984; 18: 455–462.

Re RN, Fallon TJ, Dzau VJ, et al. Renin synthesis by cultured arterial smooth muscle cells. *Life Sci* 1982; 30: 99–106

Richer C, Thuillez C, Giudicelli JF. Perindopril, converting enzyme blockade, and peripheral arterial hemodynamics in the healthy volunteer. *J Cardiovasc Pharmacol* 1987; 9: 94–102.

Ross R, Glomset J. The pathogenesis of atherosclerosis. *N Engl J Med* 1976; 295: 369–377.

Sada T, Koike H, Ikeda M, et al. Cytosolic free calcium of aorta in hypertensive rats. Chronic inhibition of angiotensin converting enzyme. *Hypertension* 1990; 16: 245–251.

Safar ME. Therapeutic trials and large arteries in hypertension. *Am Heart J* 1988; 115: 702–710.

Safar ME, London GM. Arterial and venous compliance in sustained essential hypertension. *Hypertension* 1987; 10: 133–139.

Safar ME, Peronneau PA, Levenson JA, et al. Pulsed Doppler: diameter, blood flow velocity and volumic flow of the brachial artery in sustained essential hypertension. *Circulation* 1981; 63: 393–400.

Schelling P, Fischer H, Ganten D. Angiotensin and cell growth: a link to cardiovascular hypertrophy? *J Hypertens* 1991; 9: 3–15.

Sihm I, Schroeder AP, Aalkjaer C, et al. Normalization of media to lumen ratio of human subcutaneous arteries during antihypertensive treatment with a perindopril based regimen (abstr). *Eur Heart J* 1993; 14 (abstr suppl): 63.

Shichiri M, Hirata Y, Ando K, et al. Plasma endothelin levels in hypertension and chronic renal failure. *Hypertension* 1990; 15: 493–496.

Staessen J., Fagard R, Lijnen P, et al. Review of the major hypertension trials in the elderly. *Cardiovasc Drugs Ther* 1990; 4: 1237–1248.

Vanhoutte PM. Endothelium and control of vascular function. State of the Art Lecture. *Hypertension* 1989; 13: 658–667.

Vanhoutte PM. Is endothelin involved in the pathogenesis of hypertension? *Hypertension* 1993; 21: 747–751.

Veltmar A, Gohlke P, Unger T. From tissue angiotensin converting enzyme inhibition to antihypertensive effect. *Am J Hypertens* 1991; 4: 263S–269S.

Wang D-H, Prewitt RL. Captopril reduces aortic and microvascular growth in hypertensive and normotensive rats. *Hypertension* 1990; 15: 68–77.

Wilson SK, Solez K, Boitnott JK, Heptinstall RH. The effects of heparin treatment on hypertension and vascular lesions in stroke-prone spontaneously hypertensive rats. *Am J Pathol* 1981; 102: 62–71.

Wolinsky H. Effects of hypertension and its reversal on the thoracic aorta of male and female rats. *Circ Res* 1971; 28: 622–637.

CHAPTER 11

ACE Inhibitors, Coronary Artery Disease, Ischemia, Arrhythmias and Postinfarct Protection. Other Preventative Studies

"We know what we are but we know not what we may be"
Shakespeare (Ophelia, in Hamlet)

The outstanding efficacy of ACE inhibitors in congestive heart failure and the unexpected benefit in prevention of reinfarction in the SAVE (1991) and SOLVD (1991 and 1992) studies has led to an examination of their potential use in preventing a common sequence of events culminating in heart failure (Fig. 11–1). By modifying risk factors for ischemic heart disease, such as hypertension, ACE inhibitors could also act on primary risk factors (Fig. 11–2 and Table 11–1). Recently, more direct effects on the atheromatous process have been postulated.

ACE Inhibitors and Atherosclerosis

The atherosclerotic process

Currently it is hypothesized that endothelial damage plays a prominent role in the early events leading to eventual atherosclerosis (Fig. 11–3). Each of the three primary risk factors, hypercholesterolemia, hypertension, and cigarette smoking, leads through different mechanisms to endothelial damage. For example, in hypercholesterolemic patients, the endothelial-dependent vasodilator response to acetylcholine is pathologically changed into vasoconstriction (Drexler and Zeiher, 1991). The events thereafter leading to plaque formation include neointimal proliferation and lipid deposition. The plaque has several potential fates, including (1) rupture to precipitate arterial thrombosis, (2) growth, (3) regression, and/or (4) irreversible calcinosis. All the above steps except calcinosis are reversible, so that the overall process of atherosclerosis is highly dynamic and not static.

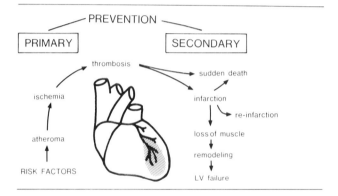

Figure 11–1. *A scheme whereby risk factors for coronary artery disease can lead to left ventricular failure, evolved from that proposed by Dzau and Braunwald (1991) with permission of the authors and the* American Heart Journal. *Note contrasting sites of action of primary and secondary prevention. LV, left ventricular.*

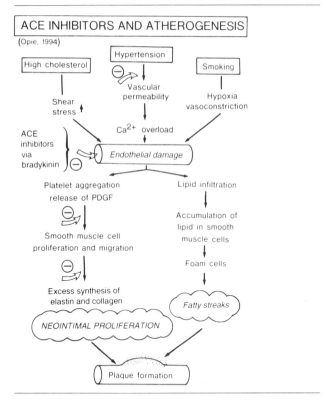

Figure 11–2. *Proposed sites at which ACE inhibitors could modulate or inhibit the atherogenic process. Note that ACE inhibitors have not yet been shown to alter atheroma in clinical studies, although lessening reinfarction in patients. For basic concepts, see text. PDGF, platelet-derived growth factor. Fig. © LH Opie.*

Endothelial damage

Can endothelial damage, for example by one of the three primary risk factors, initiate growth of vascular smooth muscle? Dzau et al. (1991) proposed that the endothelium normally releases growth inhibitors, such as prostacyclin

TABLE 11-1 PROPOSED CARDIOPROTECTION BY ACE INHIBITION

Clinical entity or effect and proposed relevant mechanism	Effects of ACE inhibitors
1. Left ventricular hypertrophy	
Prevention and treatment	Effective (pp 94–97)
a. via blood pressure fall	Yes
b. possible specific antiproliferative and antifibrotic effects	Experimentally effective (Table 4-3; Weber et al., 1994).
2. Postinfarct remodeling	
Prevention and treatment	Effective (p 122)
a. via preload and afterload reduction	Yes (p 123)
b. possible added specific effect	Not known
3. Coronary flow regulation	
(Physiologic role of angiotensin-II not clear)	Probably not major factor in humans
4. Indirect anti-ischemic effect	
LV dysfunction increases circulating catecholamines	Reduction of adrenergic activation (Bartels et al., 1994)

5. Antiarrhythmic effect

a. Indirectly by decrease of left ventricular dilation during therapy of congestive heart failure — May occur in humans

b. Ischemia and reperfusion arrhythmias in isolated hearts — Variable results, many positive

c. Inhibition of arrhythmogenic transient inward current — Shown in myocytes with high concentrations of perindoprilat

d. Acute ischemic arrhythmias in pigs — Perindoprilat prevents fall in ventricular fibrillation threshold (Muller et al., 1992)

e. Protection by pretreatment against acute ischemic arrhythmias in pigs — Shown for trandolapril (Muller et al., 1994)

6. Prevention of congestive heart failure

a. by prevention of adverse remodeling — Enalapril effective in preventing heart failure in LV dysfunction (SOLVD Study 1991; 1992)

b. possibly by indirect antiadrenergic effect

7. Vascular effects

a. endothelial-platelet interaction — a. prevention of reinfarction (SAVE study, 1992)

b. prevention of postinfarct unstable angina (SOLVD study 1991 and 1992)

8. Inhibition of plasminogen activator (PA); other hemostatic effects — Angio-II infusion increases PA inhibitor-1 (Ridker et al., 1993). See also Sbarouni et al (1994).

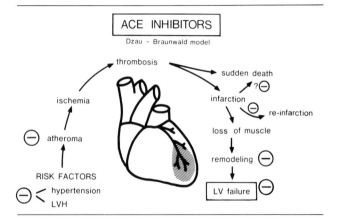

Figure 11–3. *Proposed sites of action of ACE inhibitors in primary and secondary prevention. ACE inhibitors have an indirect effect in primary prevention by lessening hypertension and by decreasing left ventricular hypertrophy. In addition, it is proposed that they may inhibit experimental atherogenesis (see Fig. 11–2). By an antiarrhythmic effect (see Table 11–2), they may act to prevent sudden death, a possibility that is being tested in postinfarct trials. By lessening wall stress (see Chapter 4), they may beneficially improve postinfarct remodeling and decrease the incidence of left ventricular failure. The concept of sequential changes leading to a chain of events from risk factors to left ventricular failure is based on Dzau and Braunwald (Fig. 11-1). LVH, left ventricular hypertrophy. Fig. © LH Opie.*

(PGI$_2$). Endothelial injury, on the other hand, releases fibroblastic growth factor and allows angiotensin-II to activate platelet derived growth factor. Therefore, endothelial injury of whatever source should promote growth of vascular smooth muscle. The Dzau hypothesis further distinguishes between the effects of endothelial damage and vascular smooth muscle hypertrophy, as found in hypertension, and hyperplasia, as found in balloon-induced injury. A relevant consideration may be that because hypertension stimulates stretch receptors (see Fig. 10–7), a consequence may be a series of molecular events resulting in vascular hypertrophy rather than in hyperplasia. Theoretically, the hypertrophic vessel should be better able to cope with increased wall stress as, for example, from catecholamine-induced surges in blood pressure, and may therefore be less likely than the hyperplastic arteriole wall to be associated with plaque rupture.

Neointimal proliferation in balloon injury

Using the model of balloon-induced injury (see Fig. 10–3), there are three phases or ways of neointimal growth (Farhy et al., 1993). First, in the growth phase, the vascular smooth muscle cells of the media become activated and proliferate, apparently driven by the fibroblast factor. Second, vascular smooth muscle cells migrate into the intima, probably under stimulation of the platelet-derived growth factor. Third, the smooth muscle cells proliferate in the intima causing true neointimal hyperplasia. The whole vascular response is enhanced by angiotensin-II, the origin of which is at least in part locally synthesized angiotensinogen (Rakugi et al., 1993). Furthermore, the activity of angiotensin-II receptors (subtype 2) in the lesions is increased (Janiak et al., 1992).

It should not be supposed that these proliferating cells retain normal control of cell calcium. Rather there are markedly depressed responses to depolarization-induced opening of the calcium channels and to the release of calcium from the sarcoplasmic reticulum in response to inositol trisphosphate or external calcium (Masuo et al., 1991). Thus, the plaque is likely to be the site of hypocontractility, which could speculatively increase its susceptibility to wall stress and could promote platelet adhesion to the endothelium.

ACE inhibitors and atherogenesis

Recently a careful consideration of the many processes involved in atherogenesis has led to the suggestion that at least some of these many steps could be susceptible to modulation by ACE inhibitors. Fleckenstein et al. (1989) have called calcium antagonists and ACE inhibitors "two outstandingly effective means of interference with cardiovascular calcium overload, high blood pressure, and arteriosclerosis in spontaneously hypertensive rats." Calcium antagonists, previously thought of as agents only dealing with hypertension or ischemic heart disease, can experimentally inhibit several stages of the arteriosclerotic process with some clinical benefit (Lichtlen et al., 1990; Waters et al., 1990).

In very similar experimental studies, Fleckenstein and his group (1989) have shown that ACE inhibitors too have protective effects on various steps of the atherosclerotic process. In addition, Chobanian et al. (1990) found an anti-atherogenic effect of captopril in rabbits with hereditary hyperlipidemia.

Aberg and Ferrer (1990) studied the effects of captopril therapy on monkeys in whom atherosclerosis was induced by a high cholesterol diet. After 6 months of treatment, there was less progression of arterial disease in monkeys given captopril, especially in the coronary arteries, and of note was the fact that the plasma levels were in the normal expected therapeutic range for captopril.

Rolland et al. (1993) created dietary atheroma in pigs. Four months of oral treatment by perindopril, in a high but still clinically relevant dose, normalized many mechanical and structural abnormalities in the aorta and the number of lipid-laden lesions. The mechanism of action was not an effect on blood lipoprotein patterns.

At present these studies have no support in humans. Yet it seems possible that following in the footsteps of the calcium antagonists, ACE inhibitors would likewise be able to have a clinically relevant primary preventative effect on early atheroma.

Mechanism of possible antiatherosclerotic effects

There are three major contenders for a possible site of action of ACE inhibitors on atherogenesis itself. First, an in-

TABLE 11-2 EFFECT OF ACE INHIBITORS ON BLOOD LIPID PROFILES

Agent	Daily dose	Concurrent placebo	Patient group	Patient number	Duration of trial	Total chol	HDL chol	LDL chol	Triglycerides	Reference
Captopril	50–100 mg	No	Hypertensives	50	12 weeks	0	0	0	0	Pollare et al. (1989)
Captopril	75–450 mg	No	Hypertensives	15	4 weeks	+1	+5	0	−11	Okun and Kraut (1987)
Captopril	100 mg (plus other agents)	No	Hypertensives	14	3 months*	−14	+11	ND	−7	Costa et al. (1988)
Captopril	50–100 mg (± diuretic)	No	Hypertensives + lipidemia	17	6 months	−12	+6	−8	−29	Ghirlanda et al. (1986)
Captopril	50 mg (+ diuretic)	No	Hypertensives + lipidemia	139	16 weeks	−3	0	−3	0	Lacourciere and Gagne (1993)
Enalapril	10–40 mg	No	Hypertensives	21**	1 year	+6	ND	ND	−16	Malini et al. (1984)
Enalapril	10–20 mg	No	Diabetic hypertensives	9	6 weeks	−9	0	ND	0	Prince et al. (1988)
Perindopril	4–8 mg	No	Diabetic hypertensives	17	12 months	ND	+14	ND	ND	Jandrain et al. (1992)

Lipid values represent percentage changes from controls; ND, no data; chol, cholesterol

*Comparing 6 and 3 months of captopril therapy; other controls not valid because of confounding effects of other agents used.

**Protocol not clear

crease of cytosolic calcium promotes calcium overload at many points in the sequence leading to atheroma (see Fig. 11–2). ACE inhibitor therapy may decrease the cytosolic calcium, which is higher than normal in a model of hypertension (Sada et al., 1990). Second, captopril has an antiatherogenic effect in hereditary hyperlipidemic rabbits (Chobanian et al., 1990). The reduced cellularity of the lesions suggests that captopril treatment inhibited cell migration into plaques. Because cell motility is influenced by cytosolic calcium, again an effect of ACE inhibitors in decreasing cytosolic calcium may be responsible. Third, ACE inhibitors are likely to decrease the component of neointimal hyperplasia mediated by angiotensin-II (see Fig. 10–3). Fourth, ACE inhibitors increase local levels of bradykinin which has a protective effect against endothelial damage (Wiemer et al., 1991; Lüscher, 1993). Fifth, the ACE inhibitors appear to have antiplatelet effects (James et al., 1988), which would indirectly lessen the release of platelet-derived growth factor. All these mechanisms, however, are still speculative at present.

Possible effects on the blood lipid profile

ACE inhibitors may have a cholesterol lowering effect that is, however, not very well documented. In an important study by Costa et al. (1988), patients with a relatively high cholesterol value (mean value 287 mg/dL) had their values reduced after 6 months of captopril therapy to a mean of 237 mg/dL. In a subgroup who returned to their previous therapy, the initial cholesterol was 290 mg/dL, the value during captopril therapy was 220 mg/dL, and on return to previous therapy was 282 mg/dL. On the other hand, in a group of patients with a lower initial cholesterol, namely 205 mg/dL, captopril therapy was associated with a minor and insignificant increase in the level (Okun and Kraut, 1987). The data are, therefore, conflicting. Yet it seems safe to conclude that ACE inhibitor therapy does not increase circulating cholesterol and may, at least sometimes, reduce it. Unexpectedly, the combination of captopril 50 mg daily and thiazide 25 mg daily slightly reduced cholesterol levels over 16 weeks, albeit only in those with higher initial values (Lacourciere and Gagne, 1993). Furthermore, in two studies, captopril therapy has been associated with an increase in "beneficial" high density lipoprotein cholesterol (Ghirlanda et al., 1986; Costa et al., 1988). Many more data, including concurrent controls which are absent in most studies, are required before such a potentially beneficial effect of ACE inhibitor therapy on the blood lipid profile can be accepted.

PROTECTION AGAINST CORONARY EVENTS BY ACE INHIBITORS

Thus, it can be concluded that there is reasonable evidence that ACE inhibitors are potentially antiatherosclerotic, that they have indirect antiadrenergic effects, and that they improve the mechanical characteristics of the arterial wall, the latter event occurring in part independently of blood pressure reduction. Because plaque rupture is thought to result from mechanical shear forces, it is not unreasonable to conclude that ACE inhibitors should prevent coronary thrombosis. But, do they really act in this beneficial way? According to recent trials, the answer is yes. Besides the clinical and experimental evidence that they may be beneficial in preventing postinfarct left ventricular dilation, these agents appear to have an additional vascular effect. Indirect evidence suggests that they may alter the endothelial-platelet interaction (Sbarouni et al., 1994). Thus, in patients with past myocardial infarction and left ventricular dysfunction, there are preventative effects of ACE inhibitors on the clinical consequences of coronary artery disease, including the development of reinfarction, left ventricular failure, unstable angina, and coronary mortality. Many of these benefits are similar to those of beta-blockers.

VENTRICULAR ARRHYTHMIAS AND ACE INHIBITORS

There is extensive experimental evidence relating ACE inhibitor therapy to decreased arrhythmias in various experimental preparations. Particularly well studied are the effects of various ACE inhibitors, not only those containing SH-groups but others such as ramipril, on reperfusion arrhythmias. In general, such studies are marred by the suprapharmacologic concentrations of the agents used. For example, the concentration of captopril required to inhibit plasma or lung ACE is only about 10^{-8}M (see Table 7–1), yet experimental studies showing an antiarrhythmic effect for captopril may use concentrations up to 10^{-3}M. In one of the few studies with a dose-effect concentration response, Winterton and Sheridan (1990) found an antiarrhythmic effect in the isolated guinea-pig heart at captopril 10^{-8}M. In another study, a supratherapeutic concentration of enalapril (10^{-4}M) increased cardiac refractoriness (De Mello et al., 1992). This observation may have a clinical counterpart (Bashir et al., 1993).

If such data are to be applied to patients, the effects of oral pretreatment should be known. Muller et al. (1992, 1994) have shown that pretreatment of pigs with perindopril or trandolapril before coronary artery occlusion leads to better maintenance of the ventricular fibrillation threshold soon after coronary occlusion, that is to say the propensity to ventricular fibrillation is diminished. Potentially these data point to an important preventative capacity of ACE inhibitors, possibly limiting sudden death in patients with ischemic heart disease. This possibility is reinforced by the finding that enalapril reduces ventricular arrhythmias and sudden death in patients with severe heart failure in the V-HeFT-II study (Fletcher et al., 1993).

The mechanism of the antiarrhythmic effect of ACE inhibitors is not well understood. First, a general effect in decreasing and modulating sympathetic nervous system activity appears likely, because of the links between such activity and ventricular fibrillation in a variety of experimental preparations (Lubbe et al., 1992).

Second, according to the general hypothesis that an accumulation of intracellular calcium promotes ischemic and reperfusion arrhythmias (Opie and Clusin, 1990), the effects of angiotensin-II in raising cell calcium could be arrhythmogenic (see Fig. 4–7). Enous et al. (1992) showed that perindoprilat in a suprapharmacologic concentration interferes with the transient inward current, which is thought to be crucial in mediating calcium-induced arrhythmias.

It must, however, be emphasized the ACE inhibitors are not antiarrhythmic agents in the conventional sense, nor is there yet convincing clinical evidence for any effect in reducing ischemic arrhythmias. A review of clinical data by Pahor et al. (1994) shows that (1) there was an antiarrhythmic effect in 10 of 16 clinical studies and (2) reduction of sudden death was found in 4 of 8 trials.

ANTI-ISCHEMIC EFFECTS OF ACE INHIBITORS

Besides hypothetically delaying the development of atherosclerosis (see Fig. 11–2), can ACE inhibitors prevent ischemia in established coronary artery disease? There are several pointers in this direction. First, angiotensin-II is vasoconstrictive and positively inotropic (see Chapter 1), so that activation of the renin-angiotensin system should increase the myocardial oxygen demand and lessen the supply, thereby predisposing to ischemia (Rump et al., 1993). Thus, in patients with congestive heart failure, angiotensin-converting enzyme inhibition by cilazapril decreased the coronary vascular resistance and improved myocardial lactate metabolism (Kiowski et al., 1991).

Second, angiotensin-converting enzyme inhibition has indirect antiadrenergic effects (see Chapter 1). During effort angina, there is catecholamine activation as shown by increased plasma norepinephrine levels with systemic vasoconstriction. ACE inhibition by perindoprilat lessens angina and postanginal left ventricular filling pressure, according to a preliminary communication (Bartels et al., 1993). Similarly, enalaprilat ameliorates pacing-induced angina (Remme, 1989).

Third, in the specific postinfarct situation, where the SAVE study showed that captopril could prevent the development of heart failure and reinfarction, captopril is also able to lessen ST-segment depression on the ambulatory ECG (Sogaard et al., 1993). This change, found after 3 months, is coupled to a decreased end-systolic volume, so that the explanation may be a fall in the myocardial oxygen demand.

Fourth, ACE inhibitors may prevent nitrate tolerance and enhance the therapeutic efficacy of nitrates (see Chapter 4).

Thus while ACE inhibitors cannot be regarded as anti-ischemic agents in the conventional sense of the word, they do have several indirect beneficial actions.

TRIALS IN PROGRESS OR RECENTLY REPORTED

There are still several large trials either in progress or recently reported that aim to assess possible benefits of ACE inhibitors on coronary events (Table 11–3). In patients with early phase acute myocardial infarction (within 24 hours of onset), the ISIS-IV trial on over 50,000 patients studied the effects of graded addition of captopril (see Table 5–8). In a preliminary trial, captopril markedly increased cardiac output (Pipilis et al., 1991), which might also have increased cardiac oxygen requirements. In GISSI-3 (see Table 5–8), lisinopril given acutely decreased mortality by 0.9% and reduced the risk of dying by 11%; when combined with transdermal nitrates the reduction was 17%, nearly as impressive as found in the SAVE study (see Table 5–7).

The AIRE (Acute Infarction Ramipril Efficacy) Study Investigators (1993) examined the effects of ramipril 2.5 mg (initial dose) up to 5 mg twice daily or placebo started 3 to 10 days postinfarct in patients with clinical heart failure. There was a highly significant fall in total mortality by 27%. This trial will undoubtedly increase the use of ACE inhibitors in patients with early postinfarct heart failure.

The preliminary data from the Chinese trial (Chinese CEI-AMI Trial Collaborative Group, 1991) are promising in that the trend is towards less development of heart failure and a lower incidence of ventricular fibrillation in captopril-treated patients.

In the QUIET study (Texter et al., 1993), the aim is to follow normolipidemic coronary patients after angioplasty or atherectomy. The end-point is both clinical, including myocardial infarction and sudden death, and angiographic. The test drug is quinapril 20 mg once daily.

RESTENOSIS: A FAILED STUDY

Restenosis following percutaneous transluminal coronary angioplasty (PTCA) occurs in about one-third of patients and is currently a major limiting factor in the success of this important and relatively simple procedure. The hypothesis that angiotensin-converting enzyme inhibition may prevent restenosis is based on the role of angiotensin-II as a growth factor promoting the neointimal lesion (see Fig. 10–3). In the MERCATOR trial (see Table 11–3), the angiotensin-converting enzyme inhibitor cilazapril in an antihypertensive dose of 5 mg twice daily failed to prevent restenosis. The proposed explanations are several and include the following. First, the dose of an ACE inhibitor effective on the vessel wall may exceed the antihypertensive dose by several fold (Asmar et al., 1992); this problem may be overcome in the as yet unpublished North American MARCATOR study in which the dose of cilazapril could be twice as high. Second, the ACE inhibitor should be started some days before the PTCA (Smalling, 1992). Third, the basic process in restenosis may be mural thrombosis rather than neointimal hyperplasia, in which case the hypothesis on which the ACE inhibitor trials is based would be incorrect.

While awaiting further trials, it would be logical to combined high-dose ACE inhibition starting before the PTCA with fish oil supplements (Bairati et al., 1992). Clearly the problem of restenosis has not yet been solved.

IS CARDIOPROTECTION NOW A VALID CONCEPT IN RELATION TO THE USE OF ACE INHIBITORS?

"Can inhibition of the renin-angiotensin system have a cardioprotective effect?" asked Michel et al. in 1985. In 1989, Zanchetti recognized that the term cardioprotection could be criticized as being too vague. He listed three crucial areas that required specific further study, namely the prevention of cardiac dilation which goes hand in hand with the reversal of cardiac hypertrophy; improvement of coronary flow; and prevention of cardiac arrhythmias. His goals have been expanded in Table 11–2, together with an assessment of the effects of ACE inhibitors in relation to each aim. A goal fulfilled is that of restructuring the heart by favorable myocardial remodeling, a logical concept bearing in mind the preload and afterload reducing properties of ACE inhibitors and the possible direct modification of the cardiac hypertrophic process by ACE inhibition. The recent publication of several post-infarct trials (see Tables 5–6 and 5–7) has shown that the experimental benefits and early clinical trials can be translated into improved morbidity and mortality in postinfarct patients. Other trials are examining the potential of ACE inhibitors to prevent cardiovascular complications in hypertension (CAPPP Group, 1990) and their possible anti-ischemic effect (Texter et al., 1993). Clearly the next step is to establish prospectively whether or not ACE inhibitors limit coronary atheroma. The QUIET study (Texter et al., 1993) should go far to establish the truth. Until then, the possible cardiovascular protective role of ACE inhibitors remains controversial (Kloner and Przyklenk, 1992), whereas cardioprotection is established.

Future developments

Another future possibility still to be tested is the possible combination of ACE inhibitors with other "cardioprotective agents." It is already known from the SAVE study (Pfeffer et al., 1992) that at least some of these protective effects of ACE inhibitors are additive to those of aspirin and beta-blockade. A particularly attractive combination is that of ACE inhibitors with beta-blockers. ACE inhibitors could offset the tendency of beta-blockers to cause left ventricular dilation and peripheral arterial constriction. ACE inhibitors potentially have complementary properties, beneficially influencing left ventricular and vascular remodeling, to those of beta-blockers, which are anti-ischemic and prevent sudden death postinfarction (Table 11–4).

Another inevitable speculation is that the proposed cardiovascular protective effects of ACE inhibitors and calcium antagonists could be additive, acting through differ-

TABLE 11–3 LARGE PREVENTATIVE TRIALS IN PROGRESS OR RECENTLY REPORTED WITH ACE INHIBITORS

Acronym or other name	Clinical entry point	Agent tested	Estimated trial population	End-points of study	Estimated end of trial or presentation of data; preliminary results
ISIS-IV (International Study and Infarct Survival)	Clinical diagnosis of acute myocardial infarction within first 24 hours	Captopril 6.25 mg test, then up to 50 mg 2 × daily for 4 weeks; isosorbide mononitrate; magnesium sulphate	58,000	35 day mortality with long-term follow-up	November 1993 (AHA) 0.46% reduction in mortality (p=0.04); risk reduction 6%
GISSI-3[+]	Admission to CCU within 24 hours of onset of AMI	Lisinopril, 2.5–10 mg 1 × daily, nitroglycerin patch or both	18,895	6 weeks morality	November 1993 (AHA) 0.9% reduction in mortality (p=0.03); risk reduction 11%
Chinese CEI-AMI trial	Clinical diagnosis of AMI within 36 hours of symptoms	Captopril 6.25 mg test then 12.5 mg 3 × daily for 4 weeks vs placebo	11,000	Mortality	November 1993 (AHA) 0.4% reduction in mortality (NS)

Trial	Patient population	Drug/dosage	Number	Endpoints	Status/results
AIRE (Acute Infarction Ramipril Efficacy)	Postinfarct clinical left ventricular failure	Ramipril 5–10 mg daily Placebo	2,006	Total mortality; progression to levt ventricular failure; reinfarction; stroke	Total mortality reduced by 6%; risk reduction 27% (Table 5–7)
PTCA (CAP)	Post-PTCA or post-thrombolytic therapy	Captopril Placebo	380	Incidence of reocclusion	Not yet decided
MARCATOR*	Post-PTCA	Cilazapril 1–10 mg 2 × daily Placebo	?1,000	Incidence of reocclusion	European Trial (MERCATOR) negative with 5 mg 2 × daily
CAPPP (Captopril Prevention Project)	Hypertension	Captopril 50–100 mg daily	7,000	Cardiovascular mortality and morbidity; diabetes mellitus	1995
QUIET (QUinapril Ischemic Event Trial)	Previous angioplasty or atherectomy	Quinapril 20 mg 1 × daily	1,740	Infarction, sudden death, coronary angiography	1995

IV, intravenous; AMI, acute myocardial infarction; PTCA, percutaneous transluminal coronary angiogram; CCU, coronary care unit; AHA, American Heart Association.

*MARCATOR, Multicenter American Research Trial with Cilazapril after Transluminal Angioplasty to Prevent Coronary Reocclusion; MERCATOR, similar European trial; + Gruppo Italiano per lo Studio della Sopravvivenza nell'Infarto Miocardico.

TABLE 11–4 Estimated Comparative Cardioprotective Effects of ACE Inhibitors (ACEI), Beta-blockers and Calcium Channel Antagonists (CCA)

	ACEI	Beta-blockers	CCA
Blood pressure reduction	+ +	+ +	+ +
LVH regression	+ +	+ or + +	+ or + +
Postinfarct CHF (prevention)	+ +	no data	0 (+, verapamil)
Early AMI with CHF	+ +	C/I	C/I
Ischemic VT (prevention)	+	+ +	+
Ischemic VT (treatment)	0	+ +	0
Sudden death (prevention)	+ /0	+ +	0 (+, verapamil)
Unstable angina (prevention)	+	no data	no data

+ +, proven use; +, possible use; 0, not used; C/I, contraindicated.

LVH, left ventricular hypertrophy; CHF, congestive heart failure; AMI, acute myocardial infarction; VT, ventricular tachycardia.

Note: In the absence of comparative studies, the above evaluation is strictly objective and the personal opinion of the author.

ent mechanisms, for example on the atherosclerotic process and on large vessel compliance.

In the far future lies possible prophylactic administration of ACE inhibitors to carriers of the DD gene who are at risk of myocardial infarction and have increased levels of circulating ACE (Cambien et al., 1992).

SUMMARY

Cardioprotection is a complex and overused term that includes treatment and prevention of left ventricular hypertrophy, improvement of postinfarct remodeling, beneficial regulation of coronary flow, antiarrhythmic effects, prevention of congestive heart failure, and decreased reinfarction. There are good arguments for the use of ACE inhibitors to achieve optimal postinfarct remodeling and protection. There are striking benefits of ACE inhibition in the treatment of early postinfarct heart failure (AIRE Study Investigators, 1993). Antianginal effects have not been proven and antiarrhythmic effects in humans still need to be established. Thus, the major sites of potential cardiovascular protection by ACE inhibitors at present are those situations in which there is abnormal wall stress on the myocardium or blood vessels, with the aim of lessening unwanted hypertrophic and mechanical changes. Multiple sites of action of ACE inhibitors are possible, acting both on the primary risk factors and on secondary postinfarct prevention. Thus, these agents have an important protective effect on the cardiovascular system, apart from their established use in hypertension and heart failure.

REFERENCES

Aberg G, Ferrer P. Effects of captopril on atherosclerosis in cynomolgus monkeys. *J Cardiovasc Pharmacol* 1990; 15 (Suppl 5): S65–S72.

Acute Infarction Ramipril Efficacy (AIRE) Study Investigators. Effect of ramipril on mortality and morbidity of survivors of acute myocardial infarction with clinical evidence of heart failure. *Lancet* 1993; 342: 821–828.

Asmar RG, Benetos A, Darne BM, et al. Converting enzyme inhibition: dissociation between antihypertensive and arterial effects. *J Human Hypertens* 1992; 6: 381–385.

Bairati I, Roy L, Meyer F. Double-blind, randomized, controlled trial of fish oil supplements in prevention of recurrence of stenosis after coronary angioplasty. *Circulation* 1992; 85: 950–956.

Bartels L, Remme WJ, van der Ent M, et al. The anti-ischemic effects of perindopril are more pronounced in patients with asymptomatic LV dysfunction than in those with normal LV function (abstr). *J Am Coll Cardiol* 1994; 21: 416A.

Bashir Y, Sneddon JF, Heald SC, et al. Changes in ventricular excitability during pharmacological unloading of the failing heart: contrasting effects of nitroprusside and captopril (abstr). *J Am Coll Cardiol* 1993; 21: 245A.

Cambien F, Poirier O, Lecerf L, et al. Deletion polymorphism in the gene for angiotensin-converting enzyme is a potent risk factor for myocardial infarction. *Nature* 1992; 359: 641–644.

CAPPP group. The Captopril Prevention Project: a prospective intervention trial of angiotensin converting enzyme inhibition in the treatment of hypertension. *J Hypertens* 1990; 8: 985–990.

Chinese CEI-AMI Trial Collaborative Group. Effects of captopril on the early mortality and complications in patients with AMI (pilot study) (abstr). Presented at Second International Symposium on ACE inhibition, London, UK, 17–21 February 1991.

Chobanian AV, Haudenschild CC, Nickerson C, Drago R. Antiatherogenic effect of captopril in the Watanabe heritable hyperlipidemic rabbit. *Hypertension* 1990; 15: 327–331.

Costa FV, Borghi C, Mussi A, Ambrosioni E. Hypolipidemic effects of long-term antihypertensive treatment with captopril. *Am J Med* 1988; 84 (Suppl 3A): 159–161.

De Mello WC, Crespo MJ, Altieri PI. Enalapril increases cardiac refractoriness. *J Cardiovasc Pharmacol* 1992; 20: 820–825.

Drexler H, Zeiher AM. Endothelial function in human coronary arteries in vivo. Focus on hypercholesterolemia. *Hypertension* 1991; 18 (Suppl II): II-90–II-99.

Dzau V, Braunwald E. Resolved and unresolved issues in the prevention and treatment of coronary artery disease: a workshop consensus statement. *Am Heart J* 1991; 221: 1244–1263.

Dzau V, Gibbons GH, Pratt RE. Molecular mechanisms of vascular renin-angiotensin system in myointimal hyperplasia. *Hypertension* 1991; 18 (Suppl II): II-100–II-105.

Enous R, Coetzee WA, Opie LH. Effects of the ACE inhibitor, perindoprilat, and of angiotensin-II on the transient inward current of guinea pig ventricular myocytes. *J Cardiovasc Pharmacol* 1992; 19: 17–23.

Farhy RD, Carretero OA, Ho K-L, Scicli AG. Role of kinins and nitric oxide in the effects of angiotensin-converting enzyme inhibitors on neointima formation. *Circ Res* 1993; 72: 1202–1210.

Fleckenstein A, Fleckenstein-Grun G, Frey M, Zorn J. Calcium antagonism and ACE inhibition. Two outstandingly effective means of interference with cardiovascular calcium overload, high blood pressure, and arteriosclerosis in spontaneously hypertensive rats. *Am J Hypertens* 1989; 2: 194–204.

Fletcher RD, Cintron GB, Johnson G, et al. Enalapril decreases prevalence of ventricular tachycardia in patients with chronic congestive heart failure. *Circulation* 1993; 87 (Suppl VI): VI-49–VI-55.

Ghirlanda G, Botta G, Bianchini G, et al. Influence of captopril on serum lipids in the long term treatment of hypertension associated with hyperlipidaemia (abstr). *Postgrad Med J* 1986; 62 (Suppl 1): 79.

GISSI-3 (Gruppo Italiano per lo Studio della Sopravvivenza Nell' Infarto Miocardico). GISSI-3: effects of lisinopril and trans-dermal glyceryl trinitrate singly and together on 6-week mortality and ventricular function after acute myocardial infarction. *Lancet* 1994; 343: 1115–1122.

ISIS-4 (Fourth International Study of Infarct Survival) — Ferguson JJ. Meeting highlights. *Circulation* 1994; 89: 545–547.

Jandrain B, Herbaut CR, V d Voorde KS. Long-term (1 year) acceptability of perindopril in Type II diabetic patients with hypertension. *Am J Med* 1992; 92 (Suppl 4B): 91S–94S.

James IM, Dickenson EJ, Burgoyne W, et al. Treatment of hypertension with captopril: preservation of regional blood flow and reduced platelet aggregation. *J Human Hypertens* 1988; 2: 21–25.

Janiak P, Pillon A, Prost J-F, Vilaine J-P. Role of angiotensin subtype 2 receptor in neointima formation after vascular injury. *Hypertension* 1992; 20: 737–745.

Kiowski W, Zuber M, Elsasser S, et al. Coronary vasodilatation and improved myocardial lactate metabolism after angiotensin-converting enzyme inhibition with cilazapril in patients with congestive heart failure. *Am Heart J* 1991; 122: 1382–1388.

Kloner RA, Przyklenk K. Cardioprotection with angiotensin-converting enzyme inhibitors: redefined for the 1990s. *Clin Cardiol* 1992; 15: 95–103.

Lacourciere Y, Gagne C. Influence of combination of captopril and hydrochlorothiazide on plasma lipids, lipoproteins and apolipoproteins in primary hypertension. *J Human Hypertens* 1993; 7: 149–152.

Lichtlen PR, Hugenholtz PG, Rafflenbeul W, et al on behalf of the INTACT group investigators. Retardation of coronary artery disease in humans by the calcium-channel blocker nifedipine: results of the INTACT Study (International Nifedipine Trial on Antiatherosclerotic Therapy). *Cardiovasc Drugs Ther* 1990; 4: 1047–1068.

Lubbe WF, Podzuweit T, Opie LH. Potential arrhythmogenic role of cyclic AMP and cytosolic calcium overload: implications for antiarrhythmic effects of beta-blockers and proarrhythmic effects of phosphodiesterase inhibitors. *J Am Coll Cardiol* 1992; 19: 1622–1633.

Malini PL, Strocchi E, Ambrosioni E, Magnani B. Long-term antihypertensive, metabolic and cellular effects of enalapril. *J Hypertens* 1984; 2 (Suppl 2): 101–105.

Masuo M, Toyo-oka T, Shin WS, Sugimoto T. Growth-dependent alterations of intracellular Ca^{2+}-handling mechanisms of vascular smooth muscle cells. PDGF negatively regulates functional expression of voltage-dependent, IP_3-mediated, and Ca^{2+}-induced Ca^{2+} release channels. *Circ Res* 1991; 69: 1327–1339.

(MERCATOR) Multicenter European Research Trial with Cilazapril after Angioplasty to Prevent Transluminal Coronary Obstruction and Restenosis Study Group. Does the new angiotensin-converting enzyme inhibitor cilazapril prevent restenosis after percutaneous transluminal coronary angioplasty? Results of the MERCATOR study: a multicenter, randomized, double-blind placebo-controlled trial. *Circulation* 1992; 86: 100–110.

Michel J-B, Dussaule J-C, Alhenc-Gelas F, et al. Can inhibition of the renin-angiotensin system have a cardioprotective effect? *J Cardiovasc Pharmacol* 1985; 7: S75–S79.

Muller CA, Opie LH, Peisach M, Pineda CA. Antiarrhythmic effects of the ACE inhibitor perindoprilat in a pig model of acute regional myocardial ischemia. *J Cardiovasc Pharmacol,* 1992; 19: 748–754.

Muller CA, Opie LH, Peisach M, Pineda CA. Chronic oral pretreatment with ACE inhibitor trandolapril decreases myocardial ACE activity and arrhythmias in a pig model of acute ischemia and reperfusion. *Eur Heart J* 1994, in press.

Okun R, Kraut J. Prazosin versus captopril as initial therapy. Effect on hypertension and lipid levels. *Am J Med* 1987; 82 (Suppl 1A): 58–63.

Opie LH, Clusin WT. Cellular mechanism for ischemic ventricular arrhythmias. *Ann Rev Med* 1990; 41: 231–238.

Pahor M, Gambassi G, Carbonin P. Antiarrhythmic effects of ACE inhibitors a matter of faith or reality? *Cardiovasc Res* 1994; 28: 173–182.

Pipilis A, Flather M, Collins R, et al. ISIS-4 pilot study: serial hemodynamic changes with oral captopril and oral isosorbide mononitrate in a randomized double-blind trial in acute myocardial infarction (abstr). *J Am Coll Cardiol* 1991; 17 (Suppl A): 115A.

Prince MJ, Stuart CA, Padia M, et al. Metabolic effects of hydrochlorothiazide and enalapril during treatment of the hypertensive diabetic patient. Enalapril for hypertensive diabetics. *Arch Intern Med* 1988; 148: 2363–2368.

Rakugi H, Jacob HJ, Krieger HJ, et al. Vascular injury induces angiotensinogen gene expression in the media and neointima. *Circulation* 1993; 87: 283–290.

Remme W. Neuroendocrine activation in ischemic cardiomyopathy without failure and in acute myocardial ischemia. *Cardiovasc Drugs Ther* 1989; 3: 987–994.

Ridker PM, Gaboury CL, Conlin PR, et al. Stimulation of plasminogen activator inhibitor in vivo by infusion of angiotensin-II. Evidence of a potential interaction between the renin-angiotensin system and fibrinolytic function. *Circulation* 1993; 87: 1969–1973.

Rolland PH, Charpiot P, Friggi A, et al. Effects of angiotensin-converting enzyme inhibition with perindopril on hemodynamics, arterial structure, and wall rheology in the hindquarters of atherosclerotic mini-pigs. *Am J Cardiol* 1993; 71: 22E–27E.

Rump AFE, Rosen R, Korth A, Klaus W. Deleterious effect of exogenous angiotensin-I on the extent of regional ischaemia and its inhibition by captopril. *Eur Heart J* 1993; 14: 106–112.

Sada T, Koike H, Ikeda M, et al. Cytosolic free calcium of aorta in hypertensive rats. Chronic inhibition of angiotensin converting enzyme. *Hypertension* 1990; 16: 245–251.

SAVE Study — Pfeffer MA, Braunwald E, Moye LA, et al. Effect of captopril on mortality and morbidity in patients with left ventricular dysfunction after myocardial infarction. Results of the Survival and Ventricular Enlargement Trial. *N Engl J Med* 1992; 327: 669–677.

Sbarouni E, Bradshaw A, Andreotti F, et al. Relationship between hemostatic abnormalities and neuroendocrine activity in heart failure. *Am Heart J* 1994; 127: 607–612.

Smalling RW, Redoubtable restenosis. *Circulation* 1992; 86: 325–327.

Sogaard P, Gotzsche C-O, Ravkilde J, Thygesen K. Effects of captopril on ischemia and dysfunction of the left ventricle after myocardial infarction. *Circulation* 1993; 87: 1093–1099.

SOLVD Investigators. Effect of enalapril on survival in patients with reduced left ventricular ejection fractions and congestive heart failure. *N Engl J Med* 1991; 325: 293–302.

SOLVD Investigators. Effect of enalapril on mortality and the development of heart failure in asymptomatic patients with reduced left ventricular fractions. *N Engl J Med* 1992; 327: 685–691.

Texter M, Lees RS, Pitt B, et al. The QUinapril Ischemic Event Trial (QUIET) design and methods: Evaluation of chronic ACE inhibitor therapy after coronary artery intervention. *Cardiovasc Drugs Ther* 1993; 7: 273–282.

TOMH Study. A randomized, placebo-controlled trial of a nutritional-hygienic regimen along with various drug monotherapies. *Arch Intern Med* 1991; 151: 1413–1423.

Waters D, Lesperance J, Francetich M, et al. A controlled clinical trial to assess the effect of a calcium channel blocker on the progression of coronary atherosclerosis. *Circulation* 1990; 82: 1940–1953.

Weber KT, Sun Y, Tyagi SC, Cleutjens JPM. Collagen network of the myocardium: function, structural remodeling and regulatory mechanisms. *J Mol Cell Cardiol* 1994; 26: 279–292.

Wiemer G, Scholkens BA, Becker RHA, Busse R. Ramiprilat enhances endothelial autacoid formation by inhibiting breakdown of endothelium-derived bradykinin. *Hypertension* 1991; 18: 558–563.

Winterton SJ, Sheridan DJ. Captopril affects cellular electrophysiology and is antiarrhythmic during myocardial ischaemia (abstr). *Eur Heart J* 1991; 11: 439.

Zanchetti A. Editorial Comment. ACE inhibitors and cardioprotection. *Cardiovasc Drugs Ther* 1989; 3: 855–857.

CHAPTER 12

ACE Inhibitors and Metabolic Cardiovascular Syndrome. Diabetic Nephropathy. Ageing.

The outstanding efficacy of ACE inhibitors in congestive heart failure and their prophylactic potential against postinfarct complications has now been extended to proof of protection against the renal complications of diabetes mellitus. Furthermore, if they could improve glucose tolerance or avoid atheroma in the early phases of this disease, then these agents could truly improve the outlook of diabetics or, in particular, of prediabetics.

INSULIN AND ATHEROMA

Insulin insensitivity and diabetes mellitus

Diabetes mellitus is a well established risk factor for ischemic heart disease and for acute myocardial infarction, as well as for stroke. Diabetes is also known to be associated with an increased incidence of an atherogenic blood lipid profile. Excess of circulating insulin is an early lesion in prediabetes (Fig. 12–1). Insulin is potentially atherogenic through at least two mechanisms. First, insulin excess and the lack of tissue metabolic effects of insulin, as found in non-insulin-dependent diabetes mellitus, is associated with hypertriglyceridemia, with an increased very low density lipoprotein, and with a corresponding decrease in the high density lipoprotein (Golay et al., 1987). One of the results is an increase in the highly atherogenic apolipoprotein E (DeFronzo, 1992). The mechanism for the fall in plasma high-density lipoprotein (HDL) levels may be due to an increase in the rate of breakdown of HDL and of associated apolipoprotein A-1 secondary to defects in carbohydrate metabolism (Golay et al., 1987). In nondiabetics, insulinemia is a condition often associated with hypertension, at least in white patients, and is positively correlated with triglyceride levels (Haffner et al., 1988).

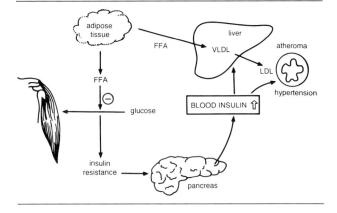

Figure 12–1. Proposed sequence of events leading to insulin resistance, based on inhibition of uptake of glucose by circulating free fatty acids (FFA). See also Martin et al. (1992). VLDL, very low density lipoproteins. Fig. © LH Opie.

In addition to effects on the blood lipid profile, insulin may directly be involved in atherogenesis acting as a growth factor (Stout et al., 1975) and as a stimulant of lipid synthesis in the arterial wall (Stout, 1968; Stout and Vallance-Owen, 1969; Opie, 1973). Insulin promotes proliferation of vascular smooth muscle cells, and stimulates synthesis of connective tissue (DeFronzo and Ferrannini, 1991), two processes that are integral components of the atherogenic process.

Although the links between insulin and atheroma have best been described in diabetic patients, they also exist in healthy persons in whom there is an association between hyperinsulinemia and coronary artery disease (Ducimetiere et al., 1980; Zavaroni et al., 1989). Thus excess circulating insulin may be the basic factor in the promotion of atheroma in diabetics, and resistance to its effects may explain the association of impaired glucose tolerance and coronary artery disease found in the large study on Whitehall civil servants in London (Fuller et al., 1980).

Insulin-resistance and metabolic cardiovascular syndrome

Recently the concept of insulin resistance in association with hypertension has received prominence (Fournier et al., 1986; Ferrannini et al., 1987; Bonora et al., 1987; DeFronzo and Ferrannini, 1991). *The hypothesis is that insulin resistance is clinically manifest as a pentad—obesity, non-insulin-dependent diabetes mellitus, hypertension, arteriosclerosis, and blood lipid disturbances* (Fig. 12–2). Alternatively, the name Syndrome X has been proposed (Reaven, 1988). This new name is not likely to appeal to cardiologists who already think of Syndrome X as a type of angina pectoris not associated with coronary artery disease. Better names are the *metabolic cardiovascular syndrome* (Arnesen, 1992) or the *insulin-resistance syndrome* (DeFronzo, 1992). The concept of insulin resistance is undoubtedly an important advance in conceptual thinking, because it explains the commonly found clinical association between obesity and hyperten-

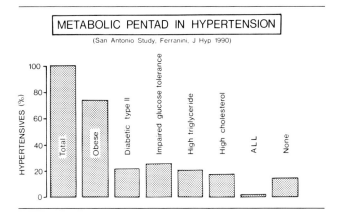

Figure 12–2. *The metabolic pentad thought to exist in hypertension is composed of obesity, type II diabetes, impaired glucose tolerance, high blood triglyceride levels, and high blood cholesterol levels. Of these, obesity is by far the most common. Data from Ferrannini et al. (1990) with permission of the author and the* Journal of Hypertension.

sion, at least in white patients. In other population groups, such as the Pima Indians and American blacks, there appears to be no relation between insulin resistance and hypertension (Saad et al., 1991). Therefore, important genetic considerations are also involved.

Mechanism of insulin resistance. The proposed explanations for the origin of insulin resistance are many and varied. One simple proposal is based on a modification of the *glucose-fatty acid cycle* of Randle et al. (1963). At about that time several workers, including our group (Shipp et al., 1961), showed that circulating free fatty acids could inhibit the uptake of glucose by muscle and therefore myocytes could become resistant to the normal effects of insulin in increasing the transport of glucose inwards. As a consequence, the pancreas would be called on to secrete more insulin. The result would be the combination of a high circulating insulin and resistance to its effects, as commonly found in prediabetes or obese diabetics (Martin et al., 1992). Obesity itself predisposes to higher than normal fasting levels of free fatty acids (next section). Exercise promotes uptake of glucose by muscle (Opie et al., 1971). Prolonged demand on the pancreas to continue to produce insulin may eventually lead to pancreatic exhaustion and late low insulin levels. Fatty acid suppression could be therapeutic (Kumar et al., 1994).

Obesity and blood free fatty acids (FFA). The mechanism whereby hyperglycemia is produced in Type II diabetes is thought to be by loss of the normal ability of insulin to suppress release of free fatty acids from adipose tissue (Reaven, 1988). Consequently, the abnormally high blood FFA levels are thought to stimulate formation of glucose in the liver (gluconeogenesis). Hence, the abnormalities of plasma FFA found in obesity come to be of interest. Fasting plasma FFA are higher in obese than in lean subjects (Opie and Walfish, 1963) which would be another metabolic link between obesity and Type II diabetes.

Postulated role of insulin resistance in production of hypertension. There is evidence linking insulin resistance to hypertension. First, in an Israeli study on 2475 randomly selected subjects, 83% of hypertensives (defined as a systolic blood pressure exceeding 145 mmHg or a diastolic blood pressure exceeding 93 mmHg) were either obese or had impaired glucose tolerance (Modan et al., 1985). In about half the subjects, the insulin values after the glucose load were measured. The mean increment in the plasma insulin, expressed as the sum of the values 60 minutes and 120 minutes after the glucose load, were as follows: 12 mU/L for hypertension alone, 47 mU/L for obesity alone, 52 mU/L for those with abnormal glucose tolerance alone, and 124 mU/L for the combination of all three. Similarly, in another large study conducted in San Antonio, hyperinsulinemia was positively correlated with blood pressure (Haffner et al., 1988).

Second, using an advance in technology, Ferrannini et al. (1987) directly measured insulin sensitivity with the euglycemic clamp technique—the amount of glucose that had to be infused to prevent the blood glucose from falling during a constant infusion of insulin (Fig. 12–3). The amount of glucose required equals the rate of disposal of glucose by the whole body, provided that there is no endogenous production of glucose. The latter was allowed for by measure-

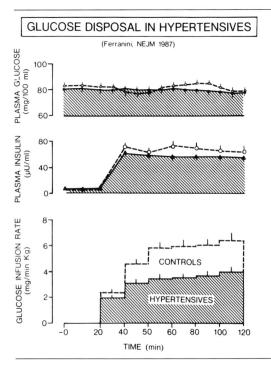

Figure 12–3. *In hypertensive patients infused with insulin, less glucose must concurrently be infused to keep the plasma glucose level the same (top panel). Therefore, there is decreased glucose disposal in the hypertensive subjects. For further details, see Ferrannini et al. (1987). Modified from original data with permission of authors and* New England Journal of Medicine.

ments of isotopic dilution, using infused tritiated glucose. In 13 young untreated subjects with moderately severe hypertension (mean blood pressure: 165/112 mmHg), insulin-induced glucose uptake was markedly impaired as shown by the much lower rate of glucose infusion required (see Fig. 12–3). The explanation is a reduced glucose uptake by skeletal muscle (Natali et al., 1991). Because glucose oxidation rates were unchanged, it follows that the defect in glucose disposal lies in the major nonoxidative fate of glucose, namely its conversion to glycogen (Natali et al., 1991). Interestingly, in heart muscle, glycogen is the major fate of insulin-stimulated glucose uptake, apart from oxidation (Chain et al., 1969). The latter authors proposed that insulin caused a specific stimulation of glycogen synthesis.

Are the high insulin levels in patients with hypertension the cause of or the consequence of the blood pressure elevation? This question can be answered by three studies. First, the fasting elevation of insulin found in patients with essential hypertension is not found in those with renovascular secondary hypertension (Marigliano et al., 1990). Second, insulin resistance can be evoked in rats by a high fructose diet and this procedure increases systolic blood pressure (Hwang et al., 1987). Third, when insulin sensitivity is restored to muscles by therapy with metformin in nondiabetic patients with hypertension, then fasting insulin levels fall and so does the blood pressure (DeFronzo, 1992).

The *mechanism* whereby insulin could be linked to hypertension remains obscure despite many postulates (DeFronzo and Ferrannini, 1991). One proposal is that insulin enhances adrenergic activity (Siani et al., 1990). When, however, insulin was chronically infused into dogs over 7 days, plasma catecholamine levels did not change (Hall et al., 1990). Alternatively, insulin may act on membrane pumps in vascular smooth muscle cells to increase cell sodium and calcium, thereby sensitizing the cells to vasoconstrictive stimuli (DeFronzo, 1992).

Whether insulin resistance by itself is sufficient to explain all the features of the clinical pentad seems unlikely. In contrast to the high incidence of insulin resistance in essential hypertension, the actual incidence of blood lipid disorders (dyslipidemia) is only about 12%, so that other factors, possibly genetic, may be involved in the association (Foster, 1989). "If insulin resistance is pathogenetic, it is more likely an accomplice than a sole killer." (Foster, 1989).

Reservations to the hypothesis linking insulin resistance to hypertension

First, the hypothesis linking insulin resistance to hypertension does not hold in black American subjects nor in Pima Indians, suggesting that the link is not directly between insulin and hypertension but rather may involve a genetic association (Saad et al., 1991). This lack of association is not likely to be limited to American blacks because in the South African Bantu the insulin response to an oral glucose load is only 50% of that found in whites (Rubenstein et al., 1969). Second, there are hypertensive patients in whom the relation between fasting serum insulin and glucose does not suggest hyperinsulinemia (Mbanya et al., 1988); and there are a number of other studies in which the association has not been found (Saad et al., 1991). Third, insulin also has vasodilator besides vasoconstrictor properties (Anderson and Mark, 1993). A new proposal is that insulin resistance is the result rather than the cause of the abnormalities of circulatory control found in skeletal muscle in hypertension. Nonetheless, the concept provides a useful framework for thought in linking non-insulin-dependent diabetes, obesity and hypertension as risk factors for atherosclerosis.

Insulin resistance and therapy for hypertension

The concept of insulin resistance has implications for the treatment of hypertension. First, nonpharmacological treatment can potentially improve insulin sensitivity. Thus, weight reduction and increased aerobic exercise should both act favorably to improve insulin resistance. Exercise increases glucose uptake by muscle and should, therefore, reduce insulin resistance (see Fig. 12–1). Exercise training is also antihypertensive (Kelemen et al., 1990). Second, because insulin resistance is not linked to hypertension in blacks, management of the insulin aspect does not warrant special consideration in their treatment. Third, certain antihypertensive drugs further impair insulin resistance.

In hypertensive whites treated with diuretics or diuretics and beta-blockers, plasma glucose and insulin were higher after a glucose load (Swislocki et al., 1989) and particularly after the combination (Fig. 12–4). These findings may explain why treatment involving these drugs is associated with an increased incidence of diabetes mellitus (Skarfors et al., 1989). Even a beta-blocker alone can impair glucose uptake and increase very low density lipoprotein as well as decreasing high density lipoprotein levels (HDL) in hypertensive patients (Pollare et al., 1989).

Other types of drugs, namely the ACE inhibitors, calcium antagonists and alpha-blockers, are likely to have neutral or beneficial effects on the insulin status (Lithell, 1991; Sheu et al., 1991; Shieh et al., 1992). Thus, changing from a beta-blocker to a ACE inhibitor may improve insulin resistance in a subset of hypertensive patients with marked insulin resistance (Berntorp et al., 1992).

ACE inhibition has been carefully compared with thiazide diuretic therapy for its effects on glucose and lipid metabolism in an important study by Pollare et al. (1989). In 50 patients with mild hypertension, captopril (mean daily dose 81 mg) was the antihypertensive equivalent of hydrochlorothiazide (mean daily dose 40 mg). Captopril improved glucose disposal, whereas the thiazide impaired it. Furthermore, the thiazide increased serum cholesterol and low density lipoprotein levels, as well as triglyceride levels. In contrast, captopril had none of these potentially deleterious effects. ACE inhibition also lessens the hypokalemic effects of insulin, thereby leading to improved glucose tolerance in nondiabetic hypertensive patients (Santoro et al.,

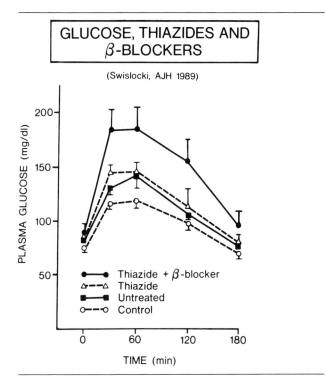

Figure 12–4. *In response to an oral glucose load, the plasma glucose rises very much higher in patients receiving thiazide and beta-blocker therapy than in controls. Note that untreated hypertensive subjects have values intermediate between the controls and those with impaired glucose tolerance. Thiazide-treated patients likewise have mild degrees of impairment of glucose tolerance. Reprinted by permission of Elsevier Science Publishing Co from Swislocki et al. (1989).*

1992). Hypothetically, the ACE inhibitor could be beneficial for those patients at risk of diabetes mellitus and/or coronary artery disease and the thiazide could be harmful, although this apparently attractive hypothesis still needs prospective confirmation.

DIABETES MELLITUS AND HYPERTENSION

Does ACE inhibition offer metabolic advantages over conventional therapy by thiazides and beta-blockers in hypertensive diabetic patients (Type I)? A review of the above evidence suggests that ACE inhibitors should. Yet, over a period of 36 months, captopril-treated patients fared no better than others as judged by fasting blood sugar, blood lipids, and glycosylated hemoglobin levels (Lacourciere et al., 1993). In a shorter study, over 9 months, equal control of blood pressure was achieved by verapamil or enalapril in the Swiss study on hypertensive diabetic patients, and there were no changes in a variety of metabolic parameters (Ferrier et al., 1992). In both of these studies, however, there was concomitant use of oral antidiabetics and of insulin, so that any specific metabolic benefit of the ACE inhibitors could have been overshadowed by such concomitant therapy. The real issue is whether ACE inhibitors prevent the appearance of overt diabetes in prediabetic hypertensive patients.

The specific question of the effects of ACE inhibitors on diabetic nephropathy will now be considered.

DIABETIC NEPHROPATHY

Diabetic nephropathy without hypertension

Logically, if the diabetic damage to the glomerular capillaries were sufficiently severe, then added hypertension would not be required to cause intraglomerular hypertension and hyperfiltration of albumin (Fig. 12–5). In this stage of diabetic renal disease, theoretical considerations suggest that relief of postglomerular arteriolar constriction and consequent relief of intraglomerular hypertension can be expected to follow ACE inhibitor therapy. Thus, Taguma et al. (1985) showed that captopril (37.5 mg daily) was able to improve heavy proteinuria in diabetics with renal failure, independently of any effect on the blood pressure.

Diabetic microalbuminuria

An important hypothesis is that ACE inhibition could specifically decrease the glomerular permeability to proteins by lessening the size of the selective pores (Morelli et al., 1990).

In early diabetic renal damage with microalbuminuria, therapy by the ACE inhibitor enalapril (20 mg daily for 6 months) reduced persistent protein loss when compared with placebo, presumably acting by a decrease of intraglomerular pressure; nonetheless, there was an associated decrease in the blood pressure level by about 10 mmHg, which could have reduced the intraglomerular pressure by

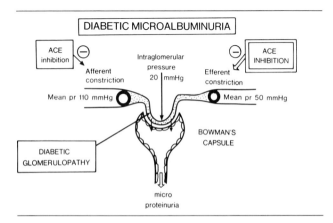

Figure 12–5. In diabetic microalbuminuria without hypertension, the problem is that of diabetic glomerular disease (glomerulopathy), so that the same intraglomerular pressure as normal causes loss of protein into the urine. Fig. © LH Opie.

reducing renal perfusion pressure (Marre et al., 1987). In an open study of the effect of captopril on blood pressure and albuminuria in normotensive insulin-dependent diabetic patients, Parving et al. (1989) showed that the albuminuria declined in the captopril treated group but rose in the controls. At the same time the mean blood pressure fell by 3 mmHg in the captopril group and rose by 6 mmHg in the control group, a total difference of 9 mmHg which is quite substantial in normotensive diabetic patients. Here again, the benefit of the ACE inhibitor on the microalbuminuria could not be dissociated from the effect on the blood pressure, as in another study using perindopril to decrease both blood pressure and microalbuminuria (Hermans et al., 1992).

In a further study from Parving's group (Mathiesen et al., 1991) on 21 normotensive diabetic patients followed for 4 years, captopril in an initial dose of 25 mg daily increased to 100 mg daily reduced microalbuminuria when compared with 23 controls, and only untreated patients developed overt clinical diabetic nephropathy. The latter was defined as persistent urinary albumin excretion exceeding 300 mg/ 24 hours. It is such patients that are more likely to suffer from a subsequent fall in the glomerular filtration rate with time (Feldt-Rasmussen et al., 1991). Although in the Mathiesen study (1991) it was claimed that the blood pressure was virtually unchanged, the 24 hour blood pressure profiles revealed clearly lower values for the captopril treated group than for the other group, so a primary hypotensive mechanism with reduced intraglomerular pressure still cannot be excluded.

Enalapril versus metoprolol. Arguing for a specific antiproteinuric effect of ACE inhibition in diabetic patients is the study of Bjorck et al. (1990) in which enalapril (mean daily dose 11 mg) plus furosemide (mean daily dose 96 mg) was compared with metoprolol (mean daily dose 117 mg) also plus furosemide (mean daily dose 58 mg). Although enalapril reduced the blood pressure better than metoprolol, the confounding effect of this greater fall in blood pressure could be corrected for by plotting blood pressure values against urinary albumin excretion. There are two reservations. First, the study was short in duration and, second, there was a higher dose of furosemide given to the patients receiving enalapril than to those receiving metoprolol. Thus, again, a specific antiproteinuric effect of the ACE inhibitor was not proven.

Enalapril versus hydrochlorothiazide. Also arguing for a specific antiproteinuric effect of ACE inhibition was the comparative study of enalapril versus hydrochlorothiazide in normotensive patients with insulin-dependent diabetes (Hallab et al., 1993). Enalapril 20 mg daily or hydrochlorothiazide 25 mg daily were given to 21 patients on a double-blind basis over 1 year, after a run-in period of 3 months. Enalapril decreased mean urinary protein excretion from 59 mg to 38 mg per 24 hours, whereas the diuretic did not. However, (1) the initial urine protein was twice as high in the diuretic group, and (2) there was a marginally greater fall in blood pressure in the enalapril group.

Postexercise proteinuria

Romanelli et al. (1989) exercised normotensive diabetic patients to produce microalbuminuria and studied the short-term effects of captopril (two 25 mg doses over 24 hours) in a double-blind trial. Captopril induced only small blood pressure changes which were not statistically significant, whereas there were large decreases in the amount of post-exercise albuminuria in captopril treated patients. That the effect could be specific to ACE inhibitors is shown by another study in which postexercise proteinuria was decreased by captopril but not by acebutolol, prazosin or indomethacin (Esnault et al., 1991).

Diabetic nephropathy with hypertension

Diabetic microangiopathy is the primary cause of glomerular damage, and, in addition, the effects of increased systemic blood pressure operate in those patients who have both diabetes and hypertension (Fig. 12–6). There is little doubt that antihypertensive treatment improves the prognosis in hypertensive patients with diabetic nephropathy (Parving et al., 1983) by lowering blood pressure and albuminuria, and decreasing the rate of fall of the glomerular filtration rate (Parving et al., 1988). An additional and important point to consider is that ACE inhibitor therapy or beta-blockade both improved microalbuminuria and hypertension in such patients, whereas a diuretic did not change the protein loss even though the blood pressure fell as

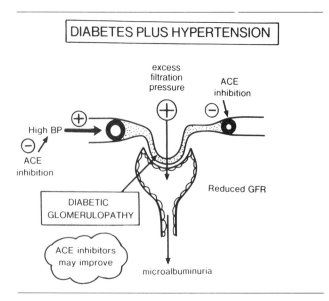

Figure 12–6. *When diabetes is combined with hypertension, then in addition to the diabetic glomerulopathy there is excess intraglomerular filtration pressure so that the microalbuminuria can become a marked proteinuria (nephrotic kidney of Kimmelstiel-Wilson). Fig. © LH Opie.*

much with the diuretic as with enalapril or atenolol (Stornello et al., 1991).

ACE inhibitors versus calcium antagonists for diabetic proteinuria

Captopril versus nifedipine. In an interesting study, first reported in a supplement (Insua et al., 1988) and later in full length (Mimran et al., 1988), it is suggested that captopril reduces urinary albumin excretion whereas nifedipine increases it, although these drugs were given to normotensive diabetic patients. The patients were insulin-dependent with incipient nephropathy, and 7 patients were given nifedipine, 8 were given captopril, and 7 were given placebo. The patients receiving placebo did not change urinary albumin excretion which, however, did rise in those receiving nifedipine and did fall in those receiving captopril. However, the blood pressure fell in the nifedipine-treated patients but not to the same extent as in the captopril-treated patients.

Captopril versus nicardipine. In Type II diabetics with overt proteinuria exceeding 500 mg per 24 hours, captopril 50 mg twice daily and nicardipine 20 mg three times daily gave equal reduction of blood pressure and of urinary protein (Stornello et al., 1989).

Enalapril versus nicardipine. In this small trial, Baba et al. (1989) studied 8 hypertensive non-insulin-requiring diabetic patients (Type II diabetes) with microalbuminuria in a cross-over trial comparing the ACE inhibitor enalapril (10–20 mg daily) with the calcium antagonist nicardipine (60–120 mg daily). Over a 4 week period of active treatment both drugs reduced microalbuminuria with similar hypotensive effects.

Enalapril versus nifedipine. In 102 diabetic patients (Type II) studied over one year, enalapril (40 mg per day, usually with a diuretic) reduced the blood pressure as much as nifedipine (60 mg per day). Enalapril reduced microalbuminuria whereas nifedipine did not (Chan et al., 1992). In contrast, enalapril but not nifedipine increased plasma creatinine (Chan et al., 1992).

Enalapril versus nitrendipine. An important preliminary communication shows that both of these agents, given over 15 months, to hypertensive diabetic patients (Type II) improved the glomerular filtration rate (Amuchastegui et al., 1993).

Enalapril versus verapamil. In the Swiss study, these agents were about equally antihypertensive, and indices of renal function did not change (Ferrier et al., 1992). Yet enalapril rather than verapamil reduced microalbuminuria, although not overt proteinuria.

Lisinopril versus diltiazem. In another small trial on non-insulin-dependent Type II diabetic patients, Bakris

(1990) compared the effects of the ACE inhibitor lisinopril with the calcium antagonist diltiazem in 8 patients with nephrotic range massive proteinuria (>3.5 g/24h). In this crossover study and at equally hypotensive doses, lisinopril (mean dose 60 mg twice daily) was the equivalent of diltiazem (mean dose 98 mg twice daily) in that the proteinuria fell equally in the two groups, whereas creatinine clearance did not change.

Perindopril versus nifedipine. In the Australian study from Melbourne, perindopril was as effective but no better than nifedipine tablets in reducing blood pressure and in preventing any increase in proteinuria over a period of 12 months (Melbourne Diabetic Nephropathy Study Group, 1991). Of the 43 patients who completed the trial, 30 were normotensive diabetics and 13 hypertensive, whereas 19 had Type I diabetes and 24 had Type II. The doses were 2 to 8 mg daily of perindopril and 20 to 80 mg daily of nifedipine tablets. In the hypertensive diabetic patients, both drugs decreased the mean blood pressure and the albuminuria, whereas in normotensive diabetic patients there was no significant reduction in the albuminuria with either drug. Albuminuria in the normotensive diabetic patients did not increase over one year, as might have been expected, suggesting that either drug was effectively preventing the occurrence of albuminuria. In these normotensive patients, perindopril did appear to reduce the magnitude of the microalbuminuria more than did nifedipine, but the numbers were too small to be statistically significant.

Assessment of results of comparative trials. At first sight there appears to be an apparent contradiction between the results of Bjorck et al. (1990) and those of the Melbourne Diabetic Nephropathy Study Group (1991) in that the former suggest a specific benefit of ACE inhibition in decreasing the albuminuria independently of the blood pressure, whereas the latter find no effect independent of blood pressure reduction. There are major differences between these trials in the duration of treatment, the severity and type of diabetes, and particularly in the extent of albuminuria in the two trials, making comparisons impossible. In the former trial, enalapril was compared with a beta-blocker and gave better blood pressure reduction than metoprolol. In contrast, perindopril was compared with a calcium antagonist and appeared to be equivalent. The latter trial was much longer in duration.

It is extremely difficult to evaluate the possible benefit of ACE inhibitors on diabetic albuminuria independently of any effect on blood pressure because in these trials different patient groups were studied for different times and the degree of renal failure varied greatly. The Melbourne study, the early study by Parving et al. (1983), and the abstract of Amuchastegui et al. (1993) all suggest that in diabetic patients it is blood pressure reduction and not the mode thereof that is crucial. The recent Italian study suggests that blood pressure reduction by ACE inhibition or beta-blockade is preferable to that achieved by a diuretic (Stornello et al., 1991). There is evidence favoring the use of most anti-hypertensives (including low-dose thiazides) in diabetics (National High Blood Pressure Education Program Working Party, 1994), with a marginal edge of preference for the ACE inhibitors (Perry and Beevers, 1989).

Combined ACE inhibitor and calcium antagonist therapy for diabetic hypertensive microalbuminuria. In two studies, verapamil has been combined with an ACE inhibitor (lisinopril or cilazapril) to give better reduction of microalbuminuria than with either agent alone, and the effect occurred independently of blood pressure changes (Fioretto et al., 1992; Bakris et al., 1992).

ACE inhibitors for diabetic nephropathy: new data

Besides the substantial theoretical advantages for the use of ACE inhibitors in diabetic nephropathy (Adler et al., 1993), there are now long-term studies showing that these agents delay progression to end-stage renal failure. As in the case of microalbuminuria of hypertension (Erley et al., 1993), the first aim must be to achieve meticulous control of the blood pressure (Stornello et al., 1991). In addition there is now solid evidence that the actual course of nephropathy can be changed in insulin-dependent diabetics.

Progression of microalbuminuria to overt disease. Captopril (50 mg twice daily) was given to 67 normotensive insulin-dependent diabetic patients (Type I) over 2 years. It decreased the rate of progression to overt proteinuria and

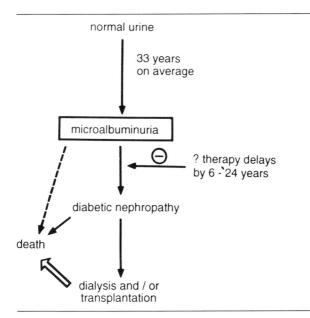

Figure 12–7. Model of progression of diabetic renal disease and possible benefits of antihypertensive treatment by an ACE inhibitor, according to Borch-Johnsen et al. (1993). For effect of ACE inhibition on hard end-points, see Lewis et al. (1993). Fig. © LH Opie.

prevented the glomerular filtration rate from falling (Laffel et al., 1993).

Remission of diabetic nephropathy with heavy proteinuria. Captopril given over 4.5 years to Type I patients with heavy proteinuria induced remission much more frequently than did placebo (Hebert et al., 1993).

Reduction of hard end-points. In this major trial on 409 patients over 3 years, the end-points were death, dialysis, or renal transplantation (Fig. 12–7) (Lewis et al., 1993). The patients were Type I diabetics with proteinuria and had an increased serum creatinine and retinopathy. Captopril (25 mg three times daily) decreased the risk of reaching each of the end-points by about half.

Comment. These three persuasive studies show that ACE inhibition can fundamentally change the course of Type I diabetic renal disease.

THE TICKING CLOCK HYPOTHESIS

To put observations on diabetic microalbuminuria into perspective, requires mention of the "ticking clock hypothesis." Based on an 8-year follow-up of 614 nondiabetic Mexican Americans in the San Antonio Heart Study, it appears that an atherogenic pattern of risk factors for coronary disease preceded the development of diabetes (Haffner et al., 1990). In such patients, the clock for atherosclerosis is hypothetically set in motion early in life by a constellation of genetic and environmental factors, including those regulating insulin secretion and sensitivity (Fig. 12–8). Conversely, the clock for microvascular complications, including ne-

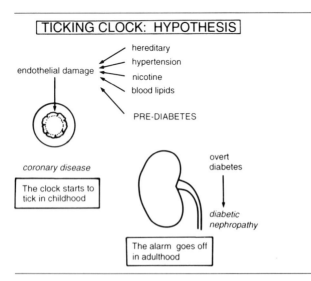

Figure 12–8. The ticking clock hypothesis whereby the clock regulating the development of coronary disease starts to tick long before the development of overt diabetes and nephropathy (Haffner et al., 1990; DeFronzo, 1992). Fig. © LH Opie.

phropathy, starts to tick much later in life with the onset of overt hyperglycemia (DeFronzo, 1992). Therefore, the real challenge is not how to control the hyperglycemia and ne-phropathy, but (1) to prevent the development of overt di-abetes in prediabetic patients, and (2) to promote a lifestyle counteracting the effects of insulin resistance. Prominent among the latter aims should be increased exercise, control of obesity, and a diet high in complex carbohydrates. Whether, in addition, ACE inhibition may play a preven-tative role is still a fascinating speculation.

AGEING

Last but not least in the list of metabolic challenges facing the ACE inhibitors is ageing. Theories of ageing are many (Martin et al., 1993) and include formation of free radicals. In highly select experimental conditions, ACE inhibitors re-duce the generation of free radicals (Sharma et al., 1993). Ageing is accompanied by increased fibrosis and other structural changes, especially in the cardiovascular system (Safar, 1990). ACE inhibitors could theoretically protect against such changes (see Chapters 4 and 11). But specu-lation is far from being fact. Of interest is a series of studies on various aspects of ageing in rats, the APRIL project (*A*geing and Perindo*pril*) in which the possible prophylactic benefit of ACE inhibition will be assessed. Preliminary re-ports suggest that ACE inhibition lessened the impact of age on endothelial and renal function (Harris, 1993). Such an approach is still very far from any clinical application.

Of greater immediate application is the prevention of systolic hypertension in the elderly.

Ageing and systolic hypertension

Loss of compliance of the major arteries is an excellent ex-planation for systolic hypertension. Thus a 35% decrease in compliance causes a 15% increase in systolic blood pressure and a 12% decrease in the diastolic blood pressure, while the mean pressure and cardiac output stay unchanged (Randall et al., 1984). When the loss of compliance goes up to 63%, then the systolic pressure rises by 18% and the di-astolic pressure falls by 24%, again with no changes in the overall mean blood pressure. In the latter situation, the car-diac output falls because the reduced compliance increases the afterload, compliance being one important component of the afterload, the other being the peripheral vascular resistance.

Thus an increasing loss of arterial compliance repre-sents an increasing load to the left ventricle and will in-crease the systolic blood pressure and decrease the diastolic blood pressure. The fact that the diastolic blood pressure is often normal or slightly high in elderly patients cannot be explained by a pure loss of arterial compliance (Randall et al., 1984). Rather, a further process such as that suggested in the hypothesis shown in Fig. 10–10 to increase periph-eral vascular resistance would adequately explain the rela-tive increase of diastolic blood pressure associated with sys-tolic hypertension.

Ageing and insulin resistance

As in younger patients, ACE inhibition improved insulin resistance in hypertensives (Paolisso et al., 1992). The drugs tested were captopril, enalapril, quinapril, ramipril, and lisinopril.

SUMMARY

Links between hypertension, insulin insensitivity, and diabetes mellitus are outlined. In early diabetic nephropathy, increasing evidence suggests that ACE inhibitors are beneficial against the microalbuminuria. Long-term outcome studies translating this observation into patient benefit are still awaited in Type II (non-insulin-dependent) diabetes. In insulin-dependent diabetic patients, ACE inhibition reduced hard end-points such as death, transplantation, or dialysis. A recent intriguing suggestion is that ACE inhibitors may be able to control some aspects of the ageing process.

REFERENCES

Adler SA, Nast C, Artishevsky A. Diabetic nephropathy: pathogenesis and treatment. *Ann Rev Med* 1993; 44: 303–315.

Amuchastegui CS, Casiraghi F, Mosconi P, et al. Long-term treatment with both nitrendipine (N) and enalapril (E) significantly increases glomerular filtration rate (GFR) in hypertensive microalbuminuric non-insulin dependent diabetics (NIDDs) with biopsy-proved diabetic glomerulopathy (abstr). *J Am Soc Nephrol* 1993; 4: 300.

Anderson EA, Mark AL. The vasodilator action of insulin. Implications for the insulin hypothesis of hypertension. *Hypertension* 1993; 21: 136–141.

Arnesen H. Introduction: the metabolic cardiovascular syndrome. *J Cardiovasc Pharmacol* 1992; 20 (Suppl 8): S1–S4.

Baba T, Murabayashi S, Takebe K. Comparison of the renal effects of angiotensin converting enzyme inhibitor and calcium antagonist in hypertensive Type 2 (non-insulin-dependent) diabetic patients with microalbuminuria: a randomised controlled trial. *Diabetologia* 1989; 32: 40–44.

Bakris GL. Effects of diltiazem or lisinopril on massive proteinuria associated with diabetes mellitus. *Ann Intern Med* 1990; 112: 707–708.

Bakris GL, Barnhill BW, Sadler R. Treatment of arterial hypertension in diabetic humans: importance of therapeutic selection. *Kidney Int* 1992; 41: 912–919.

Berntorp K, Lindgarde F, Mattiasson I. Long-term effects on insulin sensitivity and sodium transport in glucose-intolerant hypertensive subjects when beta-blockade is replaced by captopril treatment. *J Human Hypertens* 1992; 6: 291–298.

Bjorck S, Mulec H, Johnsen SA, et al. Contrasting effects of enalapril and metoprolol on proteinuria in diabetic nephropathy. *Br Med J* 1990; 300: 904–907.

Bonora E, Zavaroni I, Pezzarossa A, et al. Relationship between blood pressure and plasma insulin in non-obese and obese non-diabetic subjects. *Diabetologia* 1987; 30: 719–723.

Borch-Johnsen K, Wenzel H, Viberti GC, Mogensen CE. Is screening and intervention for microalbuminuria worthwhile in patients with insulin dependent diabetes? *Br Med J* 1993; 306: 1722–1723.

Chain EB, Mansford KRL, Opie LH. Effects of insulin on the pattern of glucose metabolism in the perfused working and Langendorff heart of normal and insulin-deficient rats. *Biochem J* 1969; 115: 537–546.

Chan JCN, Cockram CS, Nicholls MG, et al. Comparison of enalapril and nifedipine in treating non-insulin dependent diabetes associated with hypertension: one year analysis. *Br Med J* 1992; 305: 981–985.

DeFronzo RA. Insulin resistance, hyperinsulinemia, and coronary artery disease: a complex metabolic web. *J Cardiovasc Pharmacol* 1992; 20 (Suppl 11): S1–S16.

DeFronzo RA, Ferrannini E. Insulin resistance. A multifaceted syndrome responsible for NIDDM, obesity, hypertension, dislipidemia, and atherosclerotic cardiovascular disease. *Diabetes Care* 1991; 14: 173–194.

Ducimetiere P, Eschwege L, Papoz L, et al. Relationship of plasma insulin levels to the incidence of myocardial infarction and coronary artery disease mortality in a middle-aged population. *Diabetologia* 1980; 19: 205–210.

Erley CM, Haefele U, Heyne N, et al. Microalbuminuria in essential hypertension. Reduction by different antihypertensive drugs. *Hypertension* 1993; 21: 810–815.

Esnault VLM, Potironjosse M, Testa A, et al. Captopril but not acebutolol, prazosin or indomethacin decreases postexercise proteinuria. *Nephron* 1991; 58: 437–442.

Feldt-Rasmussen B, Mathiesen ER, Jensen T, et al. Effect of improved metabolic control on loss of kidney function in type I (insulin-dependent) diabetic patients: an update of the Steno studies. *Diabetologia* 1991; 34: 164–170.

Ferrannini E, Buzzigoli G, Bonadonna R, et al. Insulin resistance in essential hypertension. *N Engl J Med* 1987; 317: 350–357.

Ferrannini E, Haffner SM, Stern MP. Insulin sensitivity and hypertension. *J Hypertens* 1990; 8 (Suppl 7): S169–S173.

Ferrier C, Ferrari P, Weidmann P, et al. Swiss hypertension treatment programme with verapamil and/or enalapril in diabetic patients. *Drugs* 1992; 44 (Suppl 1): 74–84.

Fioretto P, Frigato F, Velussi M, et al. Effects of angiotensin-converting enzyme inhibitors and calcium antagonists on atrial natriuretic peptide release and action and on albumin excretion rate in hypertensive insulin-dependent diabetic patients. *Am J Hypertens* 1992; 5: 837–846.

Foster DW. Insulin resistance—a secret killer? *N Engl J Med* 1989; 320: 733–734.

Fournier AM, Gadia MT, Kubrusly DB, et al. Blood pressure, insulin, and glycemia in nondiabetic subjects. *Am J Med* 1986; 80: 861–864.

Fuller JH, Shipley MJ, Rose G, et al. Coronary-heart-disease risk and impaired glucose tolerance. *Lancet* 1980; 1: 1373–1376.

Golay A, Sech L, Shi M-Z, et al. High density lipoprotein (HDL) metabolism in non-insulin-dependent diabetes mellitus: measurement of HDL turnover using tritiated HDL. *J Clin Endocrinol Metab* 1987; 65: 512–518.

Haffner SM, Fong D, Hazuda HP, et al. Hyperinsulinemia, upper body adiposity, and cardiovascular risk factors in nondiabetics. *Metabolism* 1988; 37: 338–345.

Haffner SM, Stern MP, Hazuda HP, et al. Cardiovascular risk factors in confirmed prediabetic individuals. Does the clock for coronary artery disease start ticking before the onset of clinical diabetes? *JAMA* 1990; 263: 2893–2898.

Hall JE, Brands MW, Kivlighn SD, et al. Chronic hyperinsulinemia and blood pressure. Interaction with catecholamines? *Hypertension* 1990; 15: 519–527.

Hallab M, Gallois Y, Chatellier G, et al. Comparison of reduction in microalbuminuria by enalapril and hydrochlorothiazide in normotensive patients with insulin-dependent diabetes. *Br Med J* 1993; 306: 175–182.

Harris M. Do ACE inhibitors delay symptoms of aging? *Inpharma* 1993; 898: 5.

Hebert LA, Bain RP, Cattran D, et al. Remission (RM) of nephrotic-range proteinuria (NRP) in Type I diabetes: experience of the NIH multicenter controlled trial (T) of captopril (CAP) therapy in diabetic nephropathy (DN) (abstr). *J Am Soc Nephrol* 1993; 4: 303.

Hermans MP, Brichard SM, Colin I, et al. Long-term reduction of microalbuminuria after 3 years of angiotensin-converting enzyme inhibition by perindopril in hypertensive insulin-treated diabetic patients. *Am J Med* 1992; 92 (Suppl 4B): 102S–107S.

Hwang I-S, Ho H, Hoffman BB, Reaven GM. Fructose-induced insulin resistance and hypertension in rats. *Hypertension* 1987; 10: 512–516.

Insua A, Ribstein J, Mimran A. Comparative effect of captopril and nifedipine in normotensive patients with incipient diabetic nephropathy. *Postgrad Med J* 1988; 64 (Supple 3): 59–62.

Kelemen MH, Effron MB, Valenti SA, Stewart KJ. Exercise training combined with antihypertensive drug therapy. *JAMA* 1990; 263: 2766–2771.

Kumar S, Durrington PN, Bhatnagar IL. Suppression of non-esterified fatty acids to treat type A insulin resistance syndrome. *Lancet* 1994; 343: 1073–1074.

Lacourciere Y, Nadeau A, Poirier L, Tancrede G. Captopril or conventional therapy in hypertensive Type II diabetics. Three-year analysis. *Hypertension* 1993; 21: 786–794.

Laffel L, Gans DJ, McGill JB. Captopril decreases the rate of progression of renal disease in normotensive, insulin-dependent diabetes mellitus (IDDM) patients with microalbuminuria (abstr). *J am Soc Nephrol* 1993; 4: 304.

Lewis EJ, Hunsicker LG, Bain RP, Rohde RD for the Collaborative Study Group. The effect of angiotensin-converting enzyme inhibition on diabetic nephropathy. *N Engl J Med* 1993; 329: 1456–1462.

Lithell HO. Effect of antihypertensive drugs on insulin, glucose, and lipid metabolism. *Diabetes Care* 1991; 14: 203–209.

Marigliano A, Tedde R, Sechi LA, et al. Insulinemia and blood pressure. Relationships in patients with primary and secondary hypertension, and with or without glucose metabolism impairment. *Am J Hypertens* 1990; 3: 521–526.

Marre M, Leblanc H, Suarez L, et al. Converting enzyme inhibition and kidney function in normotensive diabetic patients with persistent microalbuminuria. *Br Med J* 1987; 294: 1448–1452.

Martin BC, Warram JH, Krolewski AS, et al. Role of glucose and insulin resistance in development of type 2 diabetes mellitus: results of a 25-year follow-up study. *Lancet* 1992; 340: 925–929.

Martin GR, Danner DB, Holbrook NJ. Aging—causes and defenses. *Ann Rev Med* 1993; 44: 419–429.

Mathiesen ER, Hommel E, Giese J, Parving H-H. Efficacy of captopril in postponing nephropathy in normotensive insulin dependent diabetic patients with microalbuminuria. *Br Med J* 1991; 303: 81–87.

Mbanya J-C, Thomas TH, Wilkinson R, et al. Hypertension and hyperinsulinemia: a relation in diabetes but not essential hypertension. *Lancet* 1988; 1: 733–734.

Melbourne Diabetic Nephropathy Study Group. Comparison between perindopril and nifedipine in hypertensive and normotensive diabetic patients with microalbuminuria. *Br Med J* 1991; 302: 210–216.

Mimran A, Insua A, Ribstein J, et al. Contrasting effects of captopril and nifedipine in normotensive patients with incipient diabetic nephropathy. *J Hypertens* 1988; 6: 919–923.

Modan M, Halkin H, Almog S, et al. Hyperinsulinemia. A link between hypertension obesity and glucose intolerance. *J Clin Invest* 1985; 75: 809–817.

Morelli E, Loon N, Meyer T, et al. Effects of converting-enzyme inhibition on barrier function in diabetic glomerulopathy. *Diabetes* 1990; 39: 76–82.

Natali A, Santoro D, Palombo C, et al. Impaired insulin action on skeletal muscle metabolism in essential hypertension. *Hypertension* 1991; 17: 170–178.

National High Blood Pressure Education Program Working Group. National high blood pressure education program working group report on hypertension in diabetes. *Hypertension* 1994; 23: 145–158.

Opie LH. Lipid metabolism of the heart and arteries in relation to ischaemic heart disease. *Lancet* 1973; 1: 192–195.

Opie LH, Walfish PG. Plasma free fatty acid concentrations in obesity. *N Engl J Med* 1963; 268: 757–760.

Opie LH, Owen P, Mansford KRL. Effects of increased heart work on glycolysis and on adenine nucleotides in the perfused heart of normal and diabetic rats. *Biochem J* 1971; 124: 475–490.

Paolisso G, Gambardella A, Verza M, et al. ACE inhibition improves insulin-sensitivity in aged insulin-resistant hypertensive patients. *J Human Hypertens* 1992; 6: 175–179.

Parving H-H, Andersen AR, Smidt UM, Svendsen PA. Early aggressive antihypertensive treatment reduces rate of decline in kidney function in diabetic nephropathy. *Lancet* 1983; 1: 1175–1178.

Parving H-H, Hommel E, Smidt UM. Protection of kidney function and decrease in albuminuria by captopril in insulin dependent diabetics with nephropathy. *Br Med J* 1988; 297: 1086–1091.

Parving H-H, Hommel E, Nielsen MD, Giese J. Effect of captopril on blood pressure and kidney function in normotensive insulin dependent diabetics with nephropathy. *Br Med J* 1989; 299: 533–536.

Perry IJ, Beevers DG. ACE inhibitors compared with thiazide diuretics as first-step antihypertensive therapy. *Cardiovasc Drugs Ther* 1989; 3: 815–819.

Pollare T, Lithell H, Berne C. A comparison of the effects of hydrochlorothiazide and captopril on glucose and lipid metabolism in patients with hypertension. *N Engl J Med* 1989; 321: 868–873.

Randall OS, Van den Bos GC, Westerhof N. Systemic compliance: does it play a role in the genesis of essential hypertension? *Cardiovasc Res* 1984; 18: 455–462.

Randle PJ, Garland PB, Hales CN, Newsholme EA. The glucose fatty acid cycle: its role in insulin sensitivity and the metabolic disturbances of diabetes mellitus. *Lancet* 1963; 1: 785–789.

Reaven GM. Banting Lecture 1988: role of insulin resistance in human disease. *Diabetes* 1988; 37: 1595–1607.

Romanelli G, Giustina A, Cimino A, et al. Short term effect of captopril on microalbuminuria induced by exercise in normotensive diabetics. *Br Med J* 1989; 298: 284–288.

Rubenstein AH, Seftel HC, Miller K, et al. Metabolic response to oral glucose in healthy South African White, Indian, and African subjects. *Br Med J* 1969; 1: 748–751.

Saad MF, Lillioja S, Nyomba BL, et al. Racial differences in the relation between blood pressure and insulin resistance. *N Engl J Med* 1991; 324: 733–739.

Safar M. Ageing and its effects on the cardiovascular system. *Drugs* 1990; 39 (Suppl 1): 1–8.

Santoro D, Natali A, Palombo C, et al. Effects of chronic angiotensin-converting enzyme inhibition on glucose tolerance and insulin sensitivity in essential hypertension. *Hypertension* 1992; 20: 181–191.

Sharma MK, Buettner GR, Kerber RE. Angiotensin-converting enzyme inhibitors reduce free radical generation during post-ischemic reperfusion of canine myocardium: a real-time study by electron spin resonance spectroscopy (abstr). *J Am Coll Cardiol* 1993; 410A: 949–42.

Sheu WHH, Swislocki ALM, Hoffman B, et al. Comparison of the effects of atenolol and nifedipine on glucose, insulin, and lipid metabolism in patients with hypertension. *Am J Hypertens* 1991; 4: 199–205.

Shieh SM, Sheu WHH, Fuh SMM, et al. Glucose insulin and lipid metabolism in doxazosin-treated patients with hypertension. *Am J Hypertens* 1992; 5: 827–831.

Shipp JC, Opie LH, Challoner D. Fatty acid and glucose metabolism in the perfused heart. *Nature* 1961; 189: 1018–1019.

Siani A, Strazzullo P, Giorgione N, et al. Insulin-induced increase in heart rate and its prevention by propranolol. *Eur J Clin Pharmacol* 1990; 38: 393–395.

Skarfors ET, Lithell HO, Selinus I, Aberg H. Do antihypertensive drugs precipitate diabetes in predisposed men? *Br Med J* 1989; 298: 1147–1152.

Stornello V, Valvo EV, Scapellato L. Hemodynamic, renal and humoral effects of the calcium entry blocker nicardipine and converting enzyme inhibitor captopril in hypertensive Type II diabetic patients with nephropathy. *J Cardiovasc Pharmacol* 1989; 14: 851–855.

Stornello M, Valvo EV, Scapellato L. Comparative effects of enalapril, atenolol and chlorthalidone on blood pressure and kidney function of diabetic patients affected by arterial hypertension and persistent proteinuria. *Nephron* 1991; 58: 52–57.

Stout RW. Insulin-stimulated lipogenesis in arterial tissue in relation to diabetes and atheroma. *Lancet* 1968; 2: 702–703.

Stout RW, Vallance-Owen J. Insulin and atheroma. *Lancet* 1969; 1: 1078–1079.

Stout RW, Bierman EL, Ross R. Effect of insulin on the proliferation of cultured primate arterial smooth muscle cells. *Circ Res* 1975; 36: 319–327.

Swislocki ALM, Hoffman BB, Reaven GM. Insulin resistance, glucose intolerance and hyperinsulinemia in patients with hypertension. *Am J Hypertens* 1989; 2: 419–423.

Taguma Y, Kitamoto Y, Futaki G, et al. Effect of captopril on heavy proteinuria in azotemic diabetes. *N Engl J Med* 1985; 313: 1617–1620.

Zavaroni I, Bonora E, Pagliara M, et al. Risk factors for coronary artery disease in healthy persons with hyperinsulinemia and normal glucose tolerance. *N Engl J Med* 1989; 320: 703–706.

APPENDIX 1 SUMMARY OF PHARMACOLOGIC PROPERTIES, CLINICAL INDICATIONS AND DOSES OF ACE INHIBITORS

Drug	Zinc ligand	Active drug	Elim T1/2 (hours)	Hypertension (usual daily dose)	CHF initial dose	CHF maintenance dose
Class I: captopril-like						
Captopril	SH	captopril	4–6 (total captopril)	25–50 mg 2x	6.25 mg	Up to 50 mg 3x
Class II: prodrugs						
Alacepril	carboxyl	captopril	8 (total captopril)	12.5–25 mg 2x	—	—
Benazepril	carboxyl	benazeprilat	21–22	5–80 mg 1-2 doses	2 mg	5–20 mg 1x
Cilazepril	carboxyl	cilazeprilat	8–24	2.5–5 mg 1x	—	—
Delapril	carboxyl	delaprilat	1.2–1.4	7.5–60 mg 1-2 doses	—	—
		5-OH-delaprilat				
Enalapril	carboxyl	enalaprilat	11	5–20 mg 1-2 doses	2.5 mg	Up to 10 mg 2x
Fosinopril	phosphoryl	fosinoprilat	12	10–40 mg 1x	—	—
Perindopril	carboxyl	perindoprilat	27–60	4–8 mg 1x	2 mg	2–8 mg 1x
Quinapril	carboxyl	quinaprilat	1.8	10–40 mg 1-2 doses	5 mg	5–40 mg 1-2 doses
Ramipril	carboxyl	ramiprilat	34–113	2.5–10 mg 1x	1.25 mg	2.5–5mg 1x
Spirapril	carboxyl	spiraprilat	<2	Not yet established	—	—
Trandolapril	carboxyl	trandolaprilat	16–24	0.5–2 mg 1x	—	—
Class III: water-soluble						
Lisinopril	carboxyl	lisinoprilat	7	10–40 mg 1x	2.5 mg	2.5–40 mg 1x

Elim T1/2, elimination (terminal) half-life; CHF, congestive heart failure

See Chapter 7 and Salvetti (1990)

APPENDIX 2 ACE INHIBITORS: SIDE-EFFECTS AND CONTRAINDICATIONS

1. Side-effects, Class

Cough—common

Hypotension—variable (renal artery stenosis; severe heart failure)

Deterioration of renal function (related to hypotension)

Angioedema (rare)

Renal failure (rare, bilateral renal artery stenosis)

Hyperkalemia (in renal failure, or with K-retaining diuretics)

Skin reactions

2. Side-effects first described for high-dose captopril

Neutropenia (cannot exclude Class effect)

Proteinuria

Loss of taste

Oral lesions

Scalded mouth syndrome (rare)

3. Contraindications

Renal—bilateral renal artery stenosis or equivalent lesions

Pre-existing hypotension

Severe aortic stenosis or obstructive cardiomyopathy

Pregnancy (NB: recent FDA warning)